What Experts Say About

EAT TO LIVE

"Finally, a diet book that looks at the science of eating in an accurate fashion. Most diet books have little basis in proven physiology. Dr. Fuhrman's book *Eat to Live* deals with why we gain weight, how to lose weight, and how to stay thin and healthy for life, and he backs it up with real scientific data. All the controversy ends after you read this book. It will be the final word in diet books and the one I recommend to my patients."

—Thomas Davenport, M.D., Massachusetts General Hospital

"Dr. Fuhrman's *Eat to Live* presents a compelling, scientific, practical approach to weight loss, health, and vitality that is a refreshing alternative to the plethora of popular but largely ineffective diets and weight-loss methods. For those who want to make dietary changes that will enable them to enjoy optimum health and appearance, this book is a must."

—James Craner, M.D., M.P.H., Occupational and Environmental Medicine, University of Nevada School of Medicine

"*Eat to Live* is a comprehensive, valuable, scientifically focused contribution empowering nutrition knowledge and a healthier life."

—Caldwell B. Esselstyn Jr., M.D., Preventive Cardiology Consultant, Cleveland Clinic, Cleveland, Ohio

"An awesome piece of work that fills the gap between the ivory tower–based nutrition research, which is difficult for the average person to interpret, and the unsubstantiated claims of New Age proponents of nutrition. For me this is a book that dropped out of heaven."

—Groesbeck P. Parham, M.D., Avon Scholar for
Cancer Control, University of Alabama
Comprehensive Cancer Center

"*Eat to Live* is a landmark publication, a gimmick-free guide to the food and exercise requirements for a robust life....Fuhrman deftly exposes the high protein and fad diets currently popular and includes case studies of the gratifying responses of his own patients to his simple food and exercise recommendations."

—William Harris, M.D., Hawaii
Permanente Medical Group

"Simply a great piece of work. Dr. Fuhrman has painstakingly taken the time to wade through the ever-burgeoning mountain of evidence which proves that the American diet and many physician-supported fad diets are not only unhealthy but are a contributing if not direct cause of our enormous public cardiovascular and cancer problem. His references are excellent and exhaustive. As individuals and as a nation we cannot ignore this book."

—Robert J. Warren, M.D.,
Fellow, American College of
Surgery and Orthopedic Surgery

"To write a great and informative book on the cutting edge of health care, one that can really help people, it would take a pioneer doctor. Such is the nature of *Eat to Live*, whose author, Dr. Fuhrman, is a hundred years ahead of his time. Fortunate is the reader who happens to come across this book. He or she walks under a lucky star."

—Roy A. Alterwein, M.D.,
Fort Lauderdale, Florida

"If you want or need to lose weight, this book will be of enormous practical value to you, showing you exactly what to do to become trim and healthy for the rest of your life. There are a lot of weight-loss books out there that aren't worth the paper they're printed on. This is a rare and priceless exception. It's a jewel. Get it. You'll be very glad you did."

—John Robbins, author of
The Food Revolution and
Diet for a New America

What Readers Say About

EAT TO LIVE

"It has truly turned back time; how wonderful to be 52 and feel 25. I feel younger every day!"
—Bobby Smith, 15 pounds in 1 month

"*Eat to Live* has helped me gain my life back and listen to my body!! Once you try it you will never go back!!" —Bobbi Freeman, 110 pounds in 2 years

"Start today and you will not believe how fast the weight will fall off!"
—Anthony Masiello, 160 pounds in 20 months

"I went from puffy and very sick to slim and energetic."
—Laurie McClain, 105 pounds in 11 months

"Thanks to *Eat to Live*, I lost 155 pounds, cured my asthma, and learned to love kale!"
—Cathy Stewart, 155 pounds in 4 years

"I lost weight and proved my cardiologist wrong. He said I could not lower my cholesterol/triglyceride levels without meds...my levels reduced by 62 percent...truly amazing results!"
—Mark Klein, 12 pounds in 6 weeks

"It's the fastest, easiest, best-feeling, way-to-live 'lifestyle' EVER! I went from size 10 to size 4 in 28 days." —Terri Newton, 60 pounds in 3 months

"*Eat to Live* is the education of a LIFETIME. It has been my health renaissance."

> —Freddie Palumbo, 60 pounds in 5 months

"I took the 6-Week Challenge, and now I am a believer! It works!"

> —Gerald Fanning, 20 pounds in 6 weeks

"ETL is not a fad diet. It's an education on diet. Here lies the secret of its success."

> —Rick Chavarria, 21 pounds in 6 weeks

"As an NCAA athlete, I struggled with weight holding back my times. I finally lost weight after years of trying!"   —Lauren Johnson, 20 pounds in 4 weeks

"In many cases, diseases that are labeled 'incurable' are NOT necessarily, especially when you *Eat to Live!* Try it—you have everything to gain and poor health to lose!!"   —Stacey Becker, recovered from lupus

"Lost 100 pounds and made my cystic acne disappear (like no medication ever could). *Eat to Live* changed my life."   —Andrew B., 100 pounds in 7 months

"I've transformed from an overweight, depressed, and unhealthy vegan into a fit, happy, and half-marathon-running vegan."

> —Ellen Murray, 135 pounds in 2 years

"Dubious? ETL launched a new life on so many levels; 70 pounds shed in 6 months, no regain 3 years later!"

> —Carla Gregston, 70 pounds in 6 months

"*Eat to Live* showed me how to recover from chronic back pain, two heart attacks, and type 2 diabetes. I had tried all the 'best' diet plans, but only got worse. *Eat to Live* works! No more heart problems; back pain almost gone; and diabetes eliminated!"

—Gearald Lautner, 63 pounds in 4 months

"I no longer take insulin. *Eat to Live* is the best thing that ever happened to me."

—Tina Brandenburg, 18 pounds in 3 months

"*CHOOSE to Live* should be the title of Dr. Fuhrman's book. My CHOICE to follow this program cured my hypothyroidism."

—Alba Jeanne MacConnell,
18 pounds in 11 months

"Bodybuilder finds lost abs under 40 pounds of fat! Stronger, healthier, fitter....Thank you, Dr. Fuhrman!"

—Joel Waldman, 40 pounds in 12 weeks

"Completely cured my diabetic problem; the VA said they had never seen anyone do what I did. Energy levels shot up and a feeling of well-being pervades."

—Jess Knepper, 96 pounds in 12 months

"*Eat to Live* has been a blessing: I no longer suffer from diverticulitis; my cholesterol went from 330 to 235 (and still dropping); and the added bonus: weight loss of 50 pounds." —Jean Nelson, 50 pounds in 3 months

"It showed me that depression isn't the mind crying out in pain, it's the body crying out for nutrition!"

—Jamie Baverstock, 17 pounds in 4 weeks

"I didn't know I was feeling bad until I started feeling great! I discovered that I can smell and taste better. I now have energy, I can jog up to 4 miles a day. Great eating standards to live by."

—Brad Kruse, 76 pounds in 8 months

"I lost 80 pounds, lowered my blood pressure, and became a group fitness instructor at my local YMCA."

—Marjorie Wimmersberger, 80 pounds in 2 years

"After over 20 years of dealing with a disabling illness and trying everything 'under the sun' to get better, I have found that following Dr. Fuhrman's nutritarian lifestyle is the ONLY way to get better!"

—Jean Mau, 15 pounds in 5 weeks

"Not only did I lose 15 pounds, but my hormones stabilized, allowing me to conceive my beautiful baby girl!"

—Christine Eason, 15 pounds in 3 months

"No faith; tried as experiment. Lost migraines, PMS, digestive troubles; slept better; quit Celexa. Five years later, weight still off!"

—Deborah Bennet, 55 pounds in 7 months

"I took control of my rheumatoid arthritis. *Eat to Live* gave me hope, control, and a healthy future. My doctor's response, 'Whatever you're doing, keep doing it.' I'm symptom free and medication free."

—Cheri Robbins, 45 pounds in 6 weeks

"*Eat to Live* has been the single most impacting publication in my 20 years as a professional coach to endurance athletes."

—James Herrera, 45 pounds in 6 months

"My addictions were transformed from cheese, meat, and medications to veggies, fruits, nuts, and seeds! You can do it too!"   —Mark Graves, 50 pounds in 1 year

"In 5 months I've lost so much more than 43 pounds! I've lost my self-disappointment, my sad reflection, my depression, medications, acne, migraines, and best of all…I lost my fat jeans. *Eat to Live* rocks!"

—Jessica Marie Barriere, 43 pounds in 5 months

"Absolutely, unequivocally the program all others should be judged by! You will find Dr. Fuhrman's program is the best obtainable!"

—Mike Springer, 40 pounds in 6 weeks

"I lost 40 pounds and feel better than I have in years. I'm a cancer survivor and also a Hep C survivor. With ETL…I'm on my way to total and complete recovery. I look younger and healthy."

—Rebecca Grant, 40 pounds in 2 months

"My cholesterol went down 100 points and I lost 37 pounds. I totally agree with Dr. Fuhrman that poor nutrition is a major public health crisis. I encourage all of my patients to read the book and start their journey to better health."

—Steve Hanor, M.D., 37 pounds in 3 months

"I tried every diet from the Zone to Blood Typing, and nothing worked long-term for me except *Eat to Live*. Friends tell me I look better now at 49 than I did when I was 17."

—Jay Kamhi, 35 pounds in 6 months

"No calorie counting? Count me in! I feel amazing and I've kept the weight off for almost 2 years by following these principles."

—Christopher Hansen, 30 pounds in 2 months

"Freedom to choose is so much better than calorie restrictions! My children have their mommy back!"

—Stephanie Harter, 27 pounds in 2 months

"Health occurs the way Nature requires, not the way Mankind desires."

—Gust Andrews, 23 pounds in 7 weeks

"Following Dr. Fuhrman's instructions, vitamin regimen, and diet, I have lost 24 pounds and cured myself of Hepatitis C."

—Mike Jourdan, 24 pounds in 6 months

ALSO BY JOEL FUHRMAN, M.D.

Eat for Health
Disease-Proof Your Child
Cholesterol Protection for Life
Fasting and Eating for Health

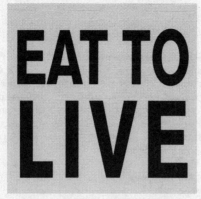

EAT TO LIVE

The Amazing Nutrient-Rich Program
for Fast and Sustained Weight Loss

Revised Edition

JOEL FUHRMAN, M.D.

Little, Brown and Company
New York Boston London

Little, Brown and Company
Hachette Book Group
237 Park Avenue, New York, NY 10017
www.hachettebookgroup.com

The publisher is not responsible for websites (or their content) that are not owned by the publisher.

The MyPyramid graphics are in the public domain and as such are not restricted by copyright. We ask, however, if you reproduce the MyPyramid graphics either electronically or in print, that you use them as originally designed; that they not be altered or modified; and that they be sourced to the USDA Center for Nutrition Policy and Promotion. If, however, you alter or modify their design, do not credit USDA or CNPP.

Printed in the United States of America

Originally published in hardcover by Little, Brown and Company, January 2003
Revised edition, January 2011
First mass market edition, May 2012

10 9 8 7 6 5 4 3 2 1

ATTENTION CORPORATIONS AND ORGANIZATIONS:
Most HACHETTE BOOK GROUP books are available at quantity discounts with bulk purchase for educational, business, or sales promotional use. For information, please call or write:

Special Markets Department, Hachette Book Group
237 Park Avenue, New York, NY 10017
Telephone: 1-800-222-6747 Fax: 1-800-477-5925

To my mother, Isabel,

for all her love and sacrifice

and

in memory of my father, Seymour,

for instilling in me an interest in superior nutrition

Contents

Foreword

Although the United States is the most powerful nation on earth, the one area in which this country does not excel is health. And the future is not bright. Almost a third of our young children are obese, and many do not exercise. No matter how much information becomes available about the dangers of a sedentary lifestyle and a diet heavily dependent on processed foods, we don't change our ways. Ideally, Americans should be able to translate financial well-being into habits that lead to longer and better lives, untroubled by expensive and chronic medical illnesses. Yet, in the United States, as well as western Europe, Russia, and many other affluent countries, the majority of adults are overweight and undernourished. While high-quality nutrition is readily available throughout the United States, the American public, rich and poor, is drawn to eating unhealthy food. Indeed, the list of top calorie sources for Americans includes many items I do not consider "real" foods, including milk, cola, margarine, white bread, sugar, and pasteurized processed American cheese.

Though smoking has received a lot of attention for the dangers it poses to public health, and cigarettes have been heavily lobbied against, obesity is a more important predictor of chronic ailments and quality of life than any other public scourge. In a recent survey of 9,500 Americans, 36 percent were overweight and 23 percent were obese, yet only 19 percent were daily smokers and 6 percent heavy drinkers. Several reasons for this epidemic of obesity in modern life have been offered. There is the pervasive role of advertising in Western society, the loss of family and social cohesiveness, the adoption of a sedentary lifestyle, and the lack of time to prepare fresh foods. In 1978, 18 percent of calories were eaten away from home; the figure is now 36 percent. In 1970, Americans ate 6 billion fast-food meals. By 2000, the figure was 110 billion.

Poor nutrition can also result in less productivity at work and school, hyperactivity among children and adolescents, and mood swings, all of which heighten feelings of stress, isolation, and insecurity. Even basic quality-of-life concerns such as constipation are affected, resulting in Americans spending $600 million annually on laxatives.

With time, the ravages of obesity predispose the typical American adult to depression, diabetes, and hypertension and increase the risks of death in all ages and in almost every ethnic and gender group. The U.S. Surgeon General has reported that 300,000 deaths annually are caused by or related to obesity. The incidence of diabetes alone has risen by a third since 1990, and treatment costs $100 billion a year.

The illnesses caused by obesity also lead to more lost workdays than any other single ailment and increase pharmaceutical and hospital expenditures to palliate untreatable degenerative conditions.

Government policy has had limited power to stem the tide of obesity, yet our nation's leaders have supported formal reports calling for a national effort to raise awareness of the dangers of being overweight. As a part of the Healthy People 2010 initiative, the federal government has proposed several steps to reduce chronic diseases associated with diet and weight through the promotion of better health and nutritional habits. It has set dietary guidelines and has encouraged physical exercise, but these efforts have not managed to change the minds, or strengthen the hearts, of most Americans. It is clear to the public that a minor change in one's eating habits will hardly transform one's life so readily. So the public turns to magic cures, pills, supplements, drinks, and diet plans that simply don't work or are unsafe. After a few failures, they give up hope.

Unlike for many diseases, the cure for obesity is known. Studies with thousands of participants have demonstrated that the combination of a dramatic change in eating habits and daily exercise results in weight loss, including a 60 percent reduction in the chance of developing chronic ailments, such as diabetes. Disseminating detailed information on these barriers is relatively easy, yet the plethora of diet books and remedies has created a complex and contradictory array of choices for those who are desperate to lose weight. With the publication of Dr. Joel Fuhrman's book, outlining a perfectly rational, straightforward, and sustainable diet, I believe we are witnessing a medical breakthrough. If you give this diet your complete commitment, there is no question in my mind that it will work for you.

In creating this plan, Dr. Fuhrman, a world expert in nutrition and obesity research, has gone beyond the dietary guidelines set up by the National Institutes of Health and the American Heart Association. Importantly, *Eat to Live* takes these nationally endorsed standards a quantum step further. Whereas conventional standards are designed for mass consumption and offer modest adjustments to our present eating habits, Dr. Fuhrman's recommendations are designed for those seeking breakthrough results. I have referred my patients to Dr. Fuhrman and have seen firsthand how his powerful methods excite and motivate people, and have witnessed wonderful results for both weight reduction and health restoration.

I am a cardiovascular surgeon infatuated with the challenge and promise of "high-tech" medicine and surgery. Nonetheless, I have become convinced that the most overlooked tool in our medical arsenal is harnessing the body's own ability to heal through nutritional excellence.

Dr. Fuhrman is doctor as teacher; he makes applying nutritional science to our own lives easy to learn, compelling, practical, and fun. His own common sense and his scientifically supported solutions to many diet-induced ailments will enable many readers to achieve unexpected degrees of wellness quickly and easily. He reminds us that not all fats or carbohydrates are good or bad and that animal proteins catalyze many detrimental side effects to our health. He pushes us to avoid processed foods and to seek the rich nutrients and phytochemicals available in fresh foods. Finally, he offers a meal plan that is tasty and easy to follow. However, make no mistake, the information you will find in this book will challenge you; the scientific evidence he cites will make it harder for you to ignore the long-term impact of the typical American diet. Indeed, it is a wake-up call for all of us to make significant changes in our lives. Now is the time to put this information into action to bring optimal health to all Americans. Go for it!

Mehmet C. Oz, M.D.
Director, Cardiovascular Institute
Columbia-Presbyterian Medical Center

EAT TO
LIVE

Introduction

Let me tell you about a typical day in my private practice. I'll see anywhere from two to five new patients like Rosalee. When Rosalee first walked through my door, she weighed 215 pounds and was on two medications (Glucophage and Glucotrol) to control her diabetes, as well as two more (Accupril and Maxide) to control her high blood pressure. She had tried every diet on the market and exercised but still couldn't manage to lose the weight she wanted to. She came to me desperate to regain a healthy weight but skeptical that my program could do anything more than what she experienced in the past—failure.

I asked her what in her wildest dreams she wanted her ideal weight to be and how long it should take her to attain that goal. She thought that her ideal weight should be 125 pounds and she would like to attain that within a year. I smiled and told her that I could design a diet for her to lose about five pounds the first month or twenty pounds the first month *and* reduce her medications. Not surprisingly, she picked the latter.

After hearing my explanation of the program I designed for her, Rosalee was psyched. Despite all that she had learned from reading about dieting, she never realized how all the mixed messages had led her down the wrong path. The plan I outlined for Rosalee made sense to her. She said, "If I can eat all that good-tasting food and still lose that much weight, I will definitely follow your instructions precisely." When Rosalee returned to my office the following month, she had lost twenty-two pounds and had been off the Glucotrol for four weeks and the Maxide for two weeks. Her blood pressure was normal and her glucose was under better control on less medication. It was now time to reduce her medication even further and move to the next phase of the diet.

Rosalee is typical of the thousands of patients I have helped in my practice, men and women who are no longer overweight and chronically ill. I get such a thrill from helping these patients regain optimal health and weight that I decided to write this book to place all the most important information for weight loss and health recovery in one clear document. I needed to do this. If you implement the information in the pages that follow, you too will see potentially lifesaving results.

I also see many young women who want to lose twenty to fifty pounds quickly in anticipation of an upcoming wedding or trip to the beach. This winter I saw a swimming coach who had to look great in her bathing suit come summer. These younger and healthier individuals are typically referred by their physicians or are informed enough to know that it can be dangerous to crash-diet. My plan is not only a healthful, scientifically designed diet calculated to supply optimal nutrition while losing weight quickly, it also meets the expectations of those desiring superb health and vitality while they find their ideal weight. My diet style can be combined with an exercise program for astonishing results, but it can also be used effectively by those too ill or too overweight to exercise sufficiently.

In spite of the more than $110 million consumers spend every day on diets and "reducing" programs (more than $40 billion per year), Americans are the most obese people in history. To be considered obese, more than one-third of a person's body must be made up of fat. A whopping 34 percent of all Americans are obese, and the problem is getting worse, not better.

Unfortunately, most weight-loss plans either don't work or offer only minor, usually temporary, benefits. There are plenty of "rules and counting" diets, diet drugs, high-protein programs, canned shakes, and other fads that might enable you to lose some weight for a period of time. The problem is that you can't stay on these programs forever. What's worse, many are dangerous.

For example, high-protein diets (and other diets rich in animal products and low in fruits and unrefined carbohydrates) are likely to significantly increase a person's risk of colon cancer. Scientific studies show a clear and strong relationship between cancers of the digestive tract, bladder, and prostate with low fruit consumption. What good is a diet that lowers your weight but also dramatically increases your chances of developing cancer? Because of such serious drawbacks, more and more desperate people are turning to drugs and surgical procedures for weight loss.

I have cared for more than ten thousand patients, most of whom first came to my office unhappy, sick, and overweight, having tried every dietary craze without success. After following my health-and-weight-loss formula, they shed the weight they always dreamed of losing, and they kept it off. For the first time in their lives, these patients had a diet plan that didn't require them to be hungry all the time.

Most patients who come to me say that they just can't lose weight, no matter what they do. They are not alone. It is almost universally accepted that obese patients cannot achieve an ideal weight or even an acceptable weight through traditional weight-loss programs. In one study of sixty overweight women who enrolled in a university diet-and-exercise program, none achieved her ideal weight.

My diet plan and recipes are designed for the hardest cases and those who have failed to lose the desired weight on other plans. Following the dietary advice offered in this book, you will achieve remarkable results, regardless of your previous experience. Weight loss averages fifteen pounds the first month and ten pounds each month thereafter. Some people lose as much as a pound a day. There is no hunger, and you can eat as much food as you desire (usually more food than you were eating before). It will work for everyone.

My patients experience other benefits as well. Many of them once suffered from chronic diseases that required multiple medications. A substantial number of my patients have been able to discontinue their medications as they recover from angina, high blood pressure, high cholesterol, diabetes, asthma, fatigue, allergies, and arthritis (to name just a few). More than 90 percent of my diabetic patients who are on insulin at the time of their first visit get off all insulin within the first month.

When I first saw Richard Gross, he had already had angioplasty and bypass surgery, and his doctors were recommending a second bypass operation because his chest pain had recurred and catheterization showed two out of the three bypassed vessels were severely blocked. Because he had suffered brain damage from the first bypass, Richard did not want to undergo another operation. Needless to say, he was very motivated to try my noninvasive approach. He followed my recommendations to the letter, and within two months on the plan his chest pains disappeared. His blood pressure normalized, his total cholesterol came down (without drugs) to 135, and he no longer required the six medications he had been taking for angina and hypertension. Now, seven years later, he is still free of any signs of vascular insufficiency.

I see numerous patients whose physicians have advised them to have angioplasty or bypass surgery but who have decided to try my aggressive nutritional management first. Those who follow the formula described in this book invariably find that their health improves and their chest pains gradually disappear. Of hundreds of cardiac patients treated in this manner, all but a few have done exceptionally well, with chest pain resolving in almost every case (only one went to repeat angioplasty because of a recurrence of chest symptoms), and I have had no patient die from cardiac arrest.

With the help of their doctors, most patients can slowly reduce—and eventually cease—their dependency on drugs. This program often enables my patients to avoid open-heart surgery and other invasive procedures. It often saves their lives.

However many details I provide of my patients' success, you are right to be skeptical. Thousands of patients with successful outcomes does not necessarily translate into your individual success. After all, you might point out, weren't these patients motivated by severe illness or the fear of death? Actually, many were relatively healthy people who came to me for routine medical care. They found a hidden benefit, and just decided to "eat to live" longer and healthier and lose the extra weight they did not need to carry, even if it was only ten to twenty pounds. When faced with the information in this book, they simply changed.

Dr. Fuhrman's Health Equation

These results sound fantastic, and they are. They are also true and predictable on my program. The key to this extraordinary diet is my simple formula: $H = N/C$.

Health = Nutrients/Calories

Your health is predicted by
your nutrient intake divided by your intake of calories.

$H = N/C$ is a concept I call the *nutrient density* of your diet. Food supplies us with both nutrients and calories (energy). All calories come from only three elements: carbohydrates, fats, and proteins. Nutrients are derived from noncaloric food factors—including vitamins, minerals, fibers, and phytochemicals. These noncaloric nutrients are vitally important for health. *Your key to permanent weight loss is to eat predominantly those foods that have a high proportion of nutrients (noncaloric food factors) to calories (carbohydrates, fats, and proteins). In physics a key formula is Einstein's $E = mc^2$. In nutrition the key formula is $H = N/C$.*

Every food can be evaluated using this formula. Once you begin to learn which foods make the grade—by having a high proportion of nutrients to calories—you are on your way to lifelong weight control and improved health.

Eating large quantities of high-nutrient foods is the secret to optimal health and permanent weight control. In fact, eating much larger portions of food is one of the beauties of the Eat to Live plan. You eat more, which effectively blunts your appetite, and you lose weight—permanently.

Eating to live does not require any deprivation. In fact, you do not have to give up any foods completely. However, as you consume larger and larger portions of health-supporting, high-nutrient foods, your appetite for low-nutrient foods decreases and you gradually lose your addiction to them. You will be able to make a complete commitment to this diet style for the rest of your life.

By following my menu plans with great-tasting recipes, you will significantly increase the percentage of high-nutrient foods in your diet and your excess weight will start dropping quickly and dramatically. This will motivate you even more to stick with it. This approach requires no denial or hunger. You can lose as much weight as you want even if diets have never worked for you in the past.

This book will allow everyone who stays on the program to become slimmer, healthier, and younger looking. You will embark on an adventure that will transform your entire life. Not only will you lose weight, you will sleep better, feel better physically and emotionally, and have more energy. You will also lower your chances of developing serious diseases in the future. You will learn why diets haven't worked for you in the past and why so many popular weight-loss plans simply do not meet the scientific criteria for effectiveness and safety.

My promise is threefold: substantial, healthy

weight reduction in a short period of time; prevention or reversal of many chronic and life-threatening medical conditions; and a new understanding of food and health that will continue to pay dividends for the rest of your life.

All the Information That You Need to Succeed

The main principle of this book is that for both optimal health and weight loss, you must consume a diet with a high nutrient-per-calorie ratio. Very few people, including physicians and dietitians, understand the concept of nutrient-per-calorie density. Understanding this key concept and learning to apply it to what you eat are the main focus of the book—but you must read the *entire* book. There are no shortcuts.

I have found that a comprehensive education in the subject is necessary for my patients to achieve the results they are looking for—but once they understand the concepts, they "own" them. They find it much easier to change. So make no mistake: the complete knowledge base of the book is essential if you want to achieve significant success, but I know that after you read this book you will say, "This makes sense." You will be a weight-loss and nutrition expert, and by the end you will have a strong foundation of knowledge that will serve you (and your newly slim self) for the rest of your life.

Why should you wait until you are faced with a life-threatening health crisis to want health excellence? Most people would choose to disease-proof their body and look great now. They just never thought they could do it so easily. Picture yourself in phenomenal health and in excellent physical condition at your ideal body weight. Not only will your waist be free of fat but your heart will be free of plaque.

Still, it is not easy to change: eating has emotional and social overtones. It is especially difficult to break an addiction. As you will learn, our American diet style is addictive, but not as addictive as smoking cigarettes. Stopping smoking is very hard, yet many still succeed. I have heard many excuses over the years, from smokers aiming to quit and sometimes even from failed dieters. Making any change is not easy. Obviously, most people know if they change their diet enough and exercise, they can lose weight—but they still can't do it.

After reading this book, you will have a better understanding of why changing has been so extremely difficult in the past and how to make it happen more easily. You will also discover dramatic results available to you that make the change exciting and well worthwhile. However, you still must first look deep within yourself and make a firm decision to do it.

I ask you to let me make my case, and try this plan for six weeks. After the first six weeks—the hardest on the plan—it becomes a lot easier. You may already have strong reasons to make a commitment to the Eat to Live plan, or you would not be reading this.

Even with patients determined to quit smoking, I insist that if they are faced with significant work-related stress, have an argument, get in a car accident, or experience any other calamity, they should not go back to smoking and use smoking as a stress reliever. I admonish them, "Call me, wake me in the middle of the night if you have to; I will help you, even prescribe medication if necessary, but just don't give yourself that option of self-medicating with cigarettes." It is not so different with your food addictions—accept no excuse to fall off the wagon in the first six weeks. You can break the addiction only if you give your body a fair chance. Do not say you will give it a try. Do not try; instead, make a commitment to do it right.

When you get married, does the religious figure or justice of the peace ask, "Do you swear to give this person a try?" When people tell me they will give it a try, I say don't bother, you have already decided to fail. It takes more than a try to quit addictions; it takes a commitment. A commitment is a promise that you stick with, no matter what.

Without that commitment, you are doomed to fail. Give yourself the chance to really succeed this time. If you commit to just six weeks on this program, you will change your life forever and turning back becomes much more difficult.

Make a clear choice between success and failure. It takes only three simple steps. One, buy the book; two, read the book; three, make the commitment.

The third step is the difficult choice, but that is all it is—another choice. Don't go there yet. First, read the entire book. Study this book; then it will become easier and logical to take the third step—making the commitment to follow the plan for at least six weeks. You must have the knowledge carefully and elaborately described in this book before that commitment is meaningful. It is like getting married. Don't commit to marriage unless you know your partner. It is an educated choice, a choice made from both emotion and knowledge. The same is true here.

Let me thank you for beginning the journey to wellness. I take it personally. I sincerely appreciate all people who take an interest in improving themselves and taking better care of their health. I am committed to your success. I realize that every great success is the result of a strong and sustained effort. I have no aspirations to change every person in America, or even a majority of people. But at least people should be given a choice. This book gives everyone who reads it that choice.

A lifetime of compromised health does not have to be your destiny, because this plan works and it works marvelously. If you weren't sure in the past that you could do it, let me repeat that taking that big step makes all the hard work worthwhile, because then you get the results you desire.

You have my respect and appreciation for making that choice to help yourself, your family, and even your country by earning back your health.

Put my ideas through this six-week test before evaluating your progress or deciding how healthy you feel. Do the grocery shopping. If you have lots of weight to lose, begin with my most powerful menu plans and instructions, without compromise, for the full six weeks. You will find the physiology of your body changing so significantly that you will never be the same. Your taste buds will become more sensitive, you will lose most of your cravings to overeat, you will feel so much better, and you will see such remarkable weight-loss results that it will be difficult ever to go back to your former way of eating. If you are on medication for diabetes or even for high blood pressure, make sure your physician is aware of your plan at the outset. He or she will need to monitor dosage to avoid overmedication. Read more about this in chapter seven.

Here is how the book works: Chapters one through four, considered together, are designed to be a comprehensive overview of human nutrition. The foundation of your success is based on the scientific information contained in these four chapters. In chapter one, you will see the problems with the standard American diet and learn how our food choices have the power to either cut short or add many years to our life. You may think you know all this, but let me surprise you with all that you don't know. Chapter two explains why obesity and chronic disease are the inevitable consequences of our poor food choices. I explain the link between low-nutrient foods and chronic disease/premature death as well as the connection between superior health/longevity and high-nutrient foods. In chapter three you will learn about those critical phytochemicals and the secret foods for both longevity and weight control. You will also learn why trying to control your weight by eating less food almost never works. The final chapter of this section of the book explains the problem with a diet rich in animal products and puts into perspective all the misleading advertising claims about foods that people have accepted as truth.

The next two chapters apply the concepts learned in the first four chapters by evaluating other diet plans and tackling many of the current controversies in human nutrition. Chapter five deepens your knowledge of the critical issues in order to understand the accurate information that is essential for maintaining your weight loss over the long term—your most important goal. Chapter six discusses food addiction and the differences between true hunger and toxic hunger.

Chapter seven illustrates the power of the Eat to Live plan to reverse illness and provides instruction on how to apply this plan to remedy your health problems and find your ideal weight. Applying the Eat to Live formula to reverse and prevent heart disease, autoimmune illnesses, and so much more opens your critical eye to a new way of looking at your well-being. Health care becomes self-care, with food your new weapon to prevent and defeat illnesses. This is a key chapter, not just for those with chronic medical problems but for all who want to live a longer, healthier life.

Chapters eight, nine, and ten put the advice into action and teach you how to make the healthy eating plan of this book taste great. Chapter eight explains the rules for swift and sustained weight loss and gives you the tools you need to adjust your diet to achieve the results you desire. It offers guidelines and a set program that allows you to plan your daily menus. Chapter nine contains cooking tips, menu plans, and recipes, including the more aggressive six-week plan designed for those who want to lose weight quickly, as well as vegetarian and nonvegetarian options. Frequently asked questions and answers are put forth in chapter ten, and I provide more practical information to aid you in your quest to regain your health.

It is my mission and my hope to give everyone the tools to achieve lifelong slimness and radiant health. Read on and learn how to put my health formula to work for you.

and a comprehensive plan that allows you to lose all daily requirements. Chapter nine outlines eating expectations, vitamins, and to help, including the more aggressive six-week plan. If we need to get there, you want to lose weight quicker, as well as nutrition and convenience, portion options. Frequently asked questions and pitfalls will naturally arise. Chapter ten provides more inspirational information to help you in your day-to-day journey. Here is the deal:

Let me arm you in advance, here to give you some of the tools to achieve the food addiction, and control health. Read this and learn how to get my health to health. I am here to work for you.

1

Digging Our Graves with Forks and Knives

THE EFFECTS OF THE AMERICAN DIET, PART I

Case Study:
Robert lost over sixty pounds and saved his life!

I was generally thin until about thirty-two years of age. I gained about thirty pounds seemingly over-night. At thirty-four, I began having labored breath-ing and was diagnosed with sarcoidosis, which caused significant scarring over a large area of my lungs. I began the standard treatment of a biopsy and steroids.

At age thirty-seven, I was fifty pounds over-weight. My life changed one afternoon at an all-you-can-eat buffet. The button on my last comfortable pair of pants snapped and the zipper broke. It was funny, embarrassing, and deadly serious all at the same time. That day, I decided I had to change and went to the bookstore to find some answers. I

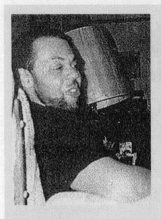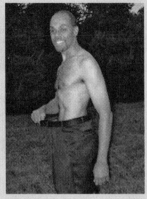

stumbled upon Dr. Fuhrman's book, and it made sense to me.

Six months later, I was sixty pounds lighter, but my wife brought to my attention a lump in my neck. The lump had been there for years, but without all my fat obscuring it, it was now readily visible. I had assumed that my gasping was a result of the sarcoidosis, but I had a massive thyroid cyst, which blocked my windpipe and cut off my air supply. The doctors decided that it needed to come out. A couple of days prior to surgery, I was given an MRI, which showed that I had no traces of the sarcoidosis. It had completely cleared up, just as Dr. Fuhrman had predicted.

During the surgery the cyst burst as soon as the surgeon attempted to cut it out with his scalpel, causing me to go into anaphylactic shock. Had the doctor not first drained the fluid with a needle, I might have died. Even more sobering is the fact that had I not adopted Dr. Fuhrman's advice, the cyst would have remained obscured and would have burst on its own. I would not have had the benefit of being on the operating table.

I am now forty-six years old, I run about twenty miles a week, and I have unbelievable stamina. My systolic blood pressure went from 140 to 108, and my current LDL cholesterol level is 40 (that is not a typo). I feel great. I look ten years younger than I did two years ago and take no medications. I have competed in several triathlons and am preparing for my first marathon.

Not long after my surgery, I sought out Dr. Fuhrman to thank him. You too can achieve your ideal weight, reverse disease, and, yes, even delay the aging process.

Americans have been among the first people worldwide to have the luxury of bombarding themselves with nutrient-deficient, high-calorie food, often called *empty-calorie or junk food.* By "empty-calorie," I mean food that is deficient in nutrients and fiber. More Americans than ever before are eating these high-calorie foods while remaining inactive—a dangerous combination.

The number one health problem in the United States is obesity, and if the current trend continues, by the year 2048 all adults in the United States will be overweight or obese.[1] The National Institutes of Health estimate that obesity is associated with a twofold increase in mortality, costing society more than $100 billion per year.[2] This is especially discouraging for dieters because after spending so much money attempting to lose weight, 95 percent of them gain all the weight back and then add on even more pounds within three years.[3] This incredibly high failure rate holds true for the vast majority of weight-loss schemes, programs, and diets.

Obesity and its sequelae pose a serious challenge to physicians. Both primary-care physicians and obesity-treatment specialists fail to make an impact on the long-term health of most of their patients. Studies show that initial weight loss is followed by weight regain.[4]

Those who genetically store fat more efficiently may have had a survival advantage thousands of years ago when food was scarce, or in a famine, but in today's modern food pantry they are the ones with the survival disadvantage. People whose parents are obese have a tenfold increased risk of being obese. On the other hand, obese families tend to have obese pets, which is obviously not genetic. So it is the combination of food choices, inactivity, and genetics that determines obesity.[5] More important, one can't change one's genes, so blaming them doesn't solve the problem. Rather than taking an honest look at what causes obesity, Americans are still looking for a miraculous cure—a magic diet or some other effortless gimmick.

Obesity is not just a cosmetic issue—extra weight leads to an earlier death, as many studies confirm.[6] Overweight individuals are more likely to die from all causes, including heart disease and cancer. Two-thirds of those with weight problems also have hypertension, diabetes, heart disease, or another obesity-related condition.[7] It is a major cause of early mortality in the United States.[8] Since dieting almost never works and the health risks of obesity are so life-threatening, more and more people are desperately turning to drugs and surgical procedures to lose weight.

Health Complications of Obesity

- Increased overall premature mortality
- Adult-onset diabetes
- Hypertension
- Degenerative arthritis
- Coronary artery disease
- Cancer

- Lipid disorders
- Obstructive sleep apnea
- Gallstones
- Fatty infiltration of liver
- Restrictive lung disease
- Gastrointestinal diseases

The results so many of my patients have achieved utilizing the Eat to Live guidelines over the past twenty years rival what can be achieved with surgical weight-reduction techniques, without the associated morbidity and mortality.[9]

Surgery for Weight Reduction and Its Risks

According to the National Institutes of Health (NIH), wound problems and complications from blood clots are common after-effects of gastric bypass and gastroplasty surgery. The NIH has also reported that those undergoing surgical treatment for obesity have had substantial nutritional and metabolic complications, gastritis, esophagitis, outlet stenosis, and abdominal hernias. More than 10 percent required another operation to fix problems resulting from the first surgery.[10]

GASTRIC BYPASS SURGERY COMPLICATIONS: 14-YEAR FOLLOW-UP[11]

Vitamin B$_{12}$ deficiency	239	39.9 percent
Readmit for various reasons	229	38.2 percent
Incisional hernia	143	23.9 percent
Depression	142	23.7 percent
Staple line failure	90	15.0 percent
Gastritis	79	13.2 percent
Cholecystitis	68	11.4 percent
Anastomotic problems	59	9.8 percent
Dehydration, malnutrition	35	5.8 percent
Dilated pouch	19	3.2 percent

Dangerous Dieting

In addition to undergoing extremely risky surgeries, Americans have been bombarded with a battery of gimmicky diets that promise to combat obesity. Almost all diets are ineffective. They don't work, because no matter how much weight you lose when you are on a diet, you put it right back on when you go off. Measuring portions and trying to eat fewer calories, typically called "dieting," almost never result in permanent weight loss and actually worsen the problem over time. Such "dieting" temporarily slows down your metabolic rate, so often more weight comes back than you lost. You wind up heavier than you were before you started dieting. This leads many to claim, "I've tried everything, and nothing works. It must be genetic. Who wouldn't give up?"

You may already know that the conventional "solution" to being overweight—low-calorie dieting—doesn't work. But you may not know why. It is for this simple yet much overlooked reason: for the vast majority of people, being overweight is not caused by how much they eat but by what they eat. The idea that people get heavy because they consume a high volume of food is a myth. Eating large amounts of the right food is your key to success and is what makes this plan workable for the rest of your life. What makes many people overweight is not that they eat so much more but that they get a higher percentage of their calories from fat and refined carbohydrates, or mostly low-nutrient foods. This low-nutrient diet establishes a favorable cellular environment for disease to flourish.

Regardless of your metabolism or genetics, you can achieve a normal weight once you start a high-nutrient diet style. Since the majority of all Americans are overweight, the problem is not primarily genetic. Though genes are an important ingredient, physical activity and food choices play a far more significant role. In studies on identical twins with the tendency to be overweight, scientists found that physical activity is the strongest environmental determinant of total body and central abdominal fat mass.[12] Even those with a strong family history of obesity effectively lose weight with increased physical activity and appropriate dietary modifications.

Most of the time, the reason people are overweight is too little physical activity, in conjunction with a high-calorie, low-nutrient diet. Eating a diet with plenty of low-fiber, calorie-dense foods, such as oil and refined carbohydrates, is the main culprit.

As long as you are eating fatty foods and refined carbohydrates, it is impossible to lose weight healthfully. In fact, this vicious combination of a sedentary lifestyle and eating typical "American" food (high-fat, low-fiber) is the primary reason we have such an incredibly overweight population.

Killing the Next Generation

This book may not appeal to individuals who are in denial about the dangers of their eating habits and those of their children. Many will do anything to continue their love affair with disease-causing foods and will sacrifice their health in the process. Many people prefer not to know about the dangers of their unhealthy diet because they think it will interfere with their eating pleasure. They are wrong. Healthy eating can result in even more pleasure.

If you have to give up something you get pleasure from, your subconscious may prefer to ignore solid evidence or defend illogically held views. Many ferociously defend their unhealthy eating practices. Others just claim, "I already eat a healthy diet," even though they do not.

There is a general resistance to change. It would be much easier if healthful eating practices and the scientific importance of nutritional excellence were instilled in us as children. Unfortunately, children are eating more poorly today than ever before.

Most Americans are not aware that the diet they feed their children guarantees a high cancer probability down the road.[13] They don't even contemplate that eating fast-food meals may be just as risky (or more so) as letting their children smoke cigarettes.[14]

> The 1992 Bogalusa Heart Study confirmed the existence of fatty plaques and streaks (the beginning of atherosclerosis) in most children and teenagers!

You wouldn't let your children sit around the table smoking cigars and drinking whiskey, because it is not socially acceptable, but it is fine to let them consume cola, fries cooked in trans fat, and a cheeseburger regularly. Many children eat doughnuts, cookies, cupcakes, and candy on a daily basis. It is difficult for parents to understand the insidious, slow destruction of their children's genetic potential and the foundation for serious illness that is being built by the consumption of these foods.[15]

It would be unrealistic to feel optimistic about the health and well-being of the next generation when there is an unprecedented increase in the average weight of children in this country and record levels of childhood obesity. Most ominous were the results reported by the 1992 Bogalusa Heart Study, which studied autopsies performed on children killed in accidental deaths. The study confirmed the existence of fatty plaques and streaks (the beginning of atherosclerosis) in most children and teenagers![16] These researchers concluded: "These results emphasize the need for preventive cardiology in early life." I guess "preventive cardiology" is a convoluted term that means eating healthfully.

Another autopsy study appearing in the *New England Journal of Medicine* found that more than 85 percent of adults between the ages of twenty-one and thirty-nine already have atherosclerotic changes in their coronary arteries.[17] Fatty streaks and fibrous plaques covered large areas of the coronary arteries. Everyone knows that junk foods are not healthy, but few understand their consequences—serious life-threatening illness. Clearly, the diets we consume as children have a powerful influence on our future health and eventual premature demise.[18]

There is considerable data to suggest that childhood diet has a greater impact on the later incidence of certain cancers than does a poor diet later in life.[19] It is estimated that as many as 25 percent of schoolchildren today are obese.[20] Early obesity sets the stage for adult obesity. An overweight child develops heart disease earlier in life. Mortality data suggests that being overweight during early adult life is more dangerous than a similar degree of heaviness later in adult life.[21]

Drugs Are Not the Solution

New drugs are continually introduced that attempt to lessen the effects of our nation's self-destructive eating behavior. Most often, our society treats disease after the degenerative illness has appeared, an illness that is the result of thirty to sixty years of nutritional self-abuse.

Drug companies and researchers attempt to develop and market medications to stem the obesity epidemic. This approach will always be doomed to fail. The body will always pay a price for consuming medicines, which usually have toxic effects. The "side" effects are not the only toxic effect of medications. Doctors learn in their introductory pharmacology course in medical school that all medications are toxic to varying degrees, whether side effects are experienced or not. Pharmacology professors stress never to forget that. You cannot escape the immutable biological laws of cause and effect through ingesting medicinal substances.

If we don't make significant changes in the foods we choose to consume, taking drugs prescribed by physicians will not improve our health or extend our lives. If we wish true health protection, we need to remove the cause. We must stop abusing ourselves with disease-causing foods.

Surprise! Lean People Live Longer

In the Nurses' Health Study, researchers examined the association between body mass index and overall mortality and mortality from specific causes in more than 100,000 women. After limiting the analysis to nonsmokers, it was very clear that the longest-lived women were the leanest.[22] The researchers concluded that the increasingly permissive U.S. weight guidelines are unjustified and potentially harmful.

Dr. I-Min Lee, of the Harvard School of Public Health, said her twenty-seven-year study of 19,297 men found there was no such thing as being too thin. (Obviously, it is possible to be too thin; however, it is uncommon and usually called anorexia, but that is not the subject of this book.) Among men who never smoked, the lowest mortality occurred in the lightest fifth.[23] Those who were in the thinnest 20 percent in the early 1960s were two and a half times less likely to have died of cardiovascular disease by 1988 than those in the heaviest fifth. Overall, the thinnest were two-thirds more likely to be alive in 1988 than the heaviest. Lee stated, "We observed a direct relationship between body weight and mortality. By that I mean that the thinnest fifth of men experienced the lowest mortality, and mortality increased progressively with heavier and heavier weight." The point is not to judge your ideal weight by traditional weight-loss tables, which are based on Americans' overweight averages. After carefully examining the twenty-five major studies available on the subject, I have found that the evidence indicates that optimal weight, as determined by who lives the longest, occurs at weights at least 10 percent below the average body-weight tables.[24] Most weight-guideline charts still place the public at risk by reinforcing an unhealthy overweight standard. By my calculations, it is not merely 70 percent of Americans who are overweight, it is more like 85 percent.[25]

The Longer Your Waistline, the Shorter Your Lifeline

As a good rule of thumb: for optimal health and longevity, a man should not have more than one-half inch of skin that he can pinch near his umbilicus (belly button) and a woman should not have more than one inch. Almost any fat on the body over this minimum is a health risk. If you have gained even as little as ten pounds since the age of eighteen or twenty, then you could be at significant increased risk for health problems such as heart disease, high blood pressure, and diabetes. The truth is that most people who think they are at the right weight still have too much fat on their body.

A commonly used formula for determining ideal body weight follows:

Women: Approximately ninety-five pounds for the first five feet of height and then four pounds for every inch thereafter.

| 5'4" | 95 + 16 = 111 |
| 5'6" | 95 + 24 = 119 |

Men: Approximately 105 pounds for the first five feet of height and then five pounds for every inch thereafter. Therefore, a 5'10" male should weigh approximately 155 pounds.

All formulas that approximate ideal weights are only rough guides, since we all have different body types and bone structure.

Body mass index (BMI) is used as a convenient indicator of overweight risk and is often used in medical investigations. BMI is calculated by dividing weight in kilograms by height in meters (squared). Another way to calculate BMI is to use this formula:

$$BMI = \frac{weight\ in\ pounds \times 703}{height\ in\ inches\ (squared)}$$

A BMI over 24 is considered overweight and greater than 30, obese. However, it is just as easy for most of us merely to use waist circumference.

I prefer waist circumference and abdominal fat measurements because BMI can be inaccurately high if the person is athletic and very muscular. Ideally, your BMI should be below 23, unless you lift weights and have considerable muscle mass. As an example, I am of average height and build (5'10" and 150 pounds) and my BMI is 21.5. My waist circumference is 30.5 inches. Waist circumference should be measured at the navel.

The traditional view is that men who have a waist circumference over forty inches and women with one over thirty-five inches are significantly overweight with a high risk of health problems and heart attacks. Evidence suggests that abdominal fat measurement is a better predictor of risk than overall weight or size.[26] Fat deposits around your waist are a greater health risk than extra fat in other places, such as the hips and thighs.

What if you feel you are too thin? If you have too much fat on your body but feel you are too thin, then you should exercise to build *muscle* to gain weight. I often have patients tell me they think they look too thin, or their friends or family members tell them they look too thin, even though they are still clearly overweight. Bear in mind that by their standards you may be too thin, or at least thinner than they are. The question to ask is, is their standard a healthy one? I doubt it. Either way: *Do not try to force yourself to overeat to gain weight!* Eat only as much food as your hunger drive demands, and no more. If you exercise, your appetite will increase in response. You should not try to put on weight merely by eating, because that will only add more fat to your frame, not muscle. Additional fat, regardless of whether you like the way you look when you are fatter or not, will shorten your life span.

Once you start eating healthfully, you may find you are getting thinner than expected. Most people lose weight until they reach their ideal weight and then they stop losing weight. Ideal weight is an individual thing, but it is harder to lose muscle than fat, so once the fat is off your body, your weight will stabilize. Stabilization at a thin, muscular weight occurs because your body gives you strong signals to eat, signals that I call "true hunger." *True hunger* maintains your muscle reserve, not your fat.

The Only Way to Significantly Increase Life Span

The evidence for increasing one's life span through dietary restriction is enormous and irrefutable. Reduced caloric intake is the only experimental technique to consistently extend maximum life span. This has been shown in *all* species tested, from insects and fish to rats and cats. There are so many hundreds of studies that only a small number are referenced below.

Scientists have long known that mice that eat fewer calories live longer. Research has demonstrated the same effect in primates (i.e., you). A study published in the *Proceedings of the National Academy of Sciences* found that restricting calories by 30 percent significantly increased life span in monkeys.[27] The experimental diet, while still providing *adequate* nourishment, slowed monkeys' metabolism and reduced their body temperatures, changes similar to those in the long-lived thin mice. Decreased levels of triglycerides and increased HDL (the good) cholesterol were also observed. Studies over the years, on many different species of animals, have confirmed that those animals that were fed less lived longest. In fact, allowing an animal to eat as much food as it desires can reduce its life span by as much as one-half.

High-nutrient, low-calorie eating results in dramatic increases in life span as well as prevention of chronic illnesses. From rodents to primates we see:

- Resistance to experimentally induced cancers
- Protection from spontaneous and genetically predisposed cancers
- A delay in the onset of late-life diseases
- Nonappearance of atherosclerosis and diabetes
- Lower cholesterol and triglycerides and increased HDL

- Improved insulin sensitivity
- Enhancement of the energy-conservation mechanism, including reduced body temperature
- Reduction in oxidative stress
- Reduction in parameters of cellular aging, including cellular congestion
- Enhancement of cellular repair mechanisms, including DNA repair enzymes
- Reduction in inflammatory response and immune cell proliferation
- Improved defenses against environmental stresses
- Suppression of the genetic alterations associated with aging
- Protection of genes associated with removal of oxygen radicals
- Inhibited production of metabolites that are potent cross-linking agents
- Slowed metabolic rate[28]

The link between thinness and longevity, and obesity and a shorter life span, is concrete. Another important consideration in other animal studies is that fat and protein restriction have an additional effect on lengthening life span.[29] Apparently, higher fat and higher protein intake promotes hormone production, speeds up reproductive readiness and other indicators of aging, and promotes the growth of certain tumors. For example, excess protein intake has been shown to raise insulin-like growth factor (IGF-1) levels,[30] which are linked to higher rates of prostate and breast cancer.[31]

In the wide field of longevity research there is only one finding that has held up over the years: eating less prolongs life, as long as nutrient intake is adequate.[32] All other longevity ideas are merely conjectural and unproven.[33] Such theories include taking hormones such as estrogen, DHEA, growth hormones, and melatonin, as well as nutritional supplements. So far, there is no solid evidence that supplying the body with any nutritional element over and above the level present in adequate amounts in a nutrient-dense diet will prolong life. This is in contrast to the overwhelming evidence regarding protein and caloric restriction.

This important and irrefutable finding is a crucial feature of the $H = N/C$ equation. We all must recognize that if we are to reach the limit of the human life span, we must not overeat on high-calorie food. Eating empty-calorie food makes it impossible to achieve optimal health and maximize our genetic potential.

To Avoid Overeating on High-Calorie Foods, Fill Up on Nutrient-Rich Ones

An important corollary to the principle of limiting high-calorie food is that the only way for a human being to safely achieve the benefits of caloric restriction while ensuring that the diet is nutritionally adequate is to avoid as much as possible those foods that are nutrient-poor.

Indeed, this is the crucial consideration in deciding what to eat. We need to eat foods with adequate

MORE NUTRIENTS AND FIBER WILL REDUCE
YOUR CALORIC DRIVE

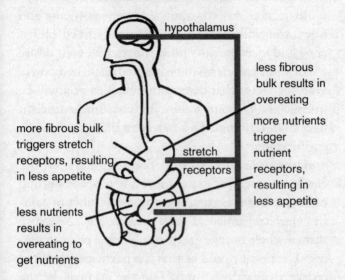

nutrients so we won't need to consume excess "empty" calories to reach our nutritional requirements. Eating foods that are rich in nutrients and fiber, and low in calories, "fills us up," so to speak, thus preventing us from overeating.

To grasp why this works, let us look at how the brain controls our dietary drive. A complicated system of chemoreceptors in the nerves lining the digestive tract carefully monitor the calorie and nutrient density of every mouthful and send such information to the hypothalamus in the brain, which controls dietary drive.

There are also stretch receptors in the stomach to signal satiety by detecting the *volume* of food eaten, not the *weight* of the food. If you are not filled up with nutrients and fiber, the brain will send out signals telling you to eat more food, or overeat.

In fact, if you consume sufficient nutrients and fiber, you will become *biochemically* filled (nutrients) and *mechanically* filled (fiber), and your desire to consume calories will be blunted or turned down. One key factor that determines whether you will be overweight is your failure to consume sufficient fiber and nutrients. This has been illustrated in scientific studies.[34]

How does this work in practice? Let's say we conduct a scientific experiment and observe a group of people by measuring the average number of calories they consumed at each dinner. Next, we give them a whole orange and a whole apple prior to dinner. The result would be that the participants would reduce their caloric intake, on the average, by the amount of calories in the fruit. Now, instead of giving them two fruits, give them the same amount of calories from fruit juice.

What will happen? They will eat the same amount of food as they did when they had nothing at the beginning of their meal. In other words, the juice did not reduce the calories consumed in the meal—instead, the juice became additional calories. This has been shown to occur with beer, soft drinks, and other sources of liquid calories.[35]

Liquid calories, without the fiber present in the whole food, have little effect in blunting our caloric drive. Studies show that fruit juice and other sweet beverages lead to obesity in children as well.[36]

If you are serious about losing weight, don't

drink your fruit—eat it. Too much fiber and too many nutrients are removed during juicing, and many of the remaining nutrients are lost through processing, heat, and storage time. If you are not overweight, drinking freshly prepared juice is acceptable as long as it does not serve as a substitute for eating those fresh fruits and vegetables. There is no substitute for natural whole foods.

There is a tendency for many of us to want to believe in magic. People want to believe that in spite of our indiscretions and excesses, we can still maintain optimal health by taking a pill, powder, or other potion. However, this is a false hope, a hope that has been silenced by too much scientific evidence. There is no magic. There is no miracle weight-loss pill. There is only the natural world of law and order, of cause and effect. If you want optimal health and longevity, you must engage the cause. And if you want to lose fat weight safely, you must eat a diet of predominantly unrefined foods that are nutrient- and fiber-rich.

What if I Have a Slow Metabolic Rate?

Your body weight may be affected slightly by genetics, but that effect is not strong. Furthermore, I am convinced that inheriting a slow metabolic rate with a tendency to gain weight is not a flaw or defect but rather a genetic gift that can be taken advantage of. How is this possible? A slower metabolism is associated with a longer life span in all species of animals. It can be speculated that if one lived sixty thousand or just a few hundred years ago, a slower metabolic rate might have increased our survival opportunity, since getting sufficient calories was difficult. For example, the majority of Pilgrims who arrived on our shores on the *Mayflower* died that first winter.[37] They could not make or find enough food to eat, so only those with the genetic gift of a slow metabolic rate survived.

As you can see, it is not always bad to have a slow metabolic rate. It can be good. Sure, it is bad in today's environment of relentless eating and when consuming a high-calorie, low-nutrient diet. Sure, it will increase your risk of diabetes and heart disease and cancer, given today's food-consumption patterns. However, if correct food choices are made to maintain a normal weight, the individual with a slower metabolism may age more slowly.

Our body is like a machine. If we constantly run the machinery at high speed, it will wear out faster. Since animals with slower metabolic rates live longer, eating more calories, which drives up our metabolic rate, will cause us only to age faster. Contrary to what you may have heard and read in the past, our goal should be the opposite: to eat less, only as much as we need to maintain a slim and muscular weight, and no more, so as to keep our metabolic rate relatively slow.

So stop worrying about your slower metabolic rate. A slower metabolic rate from dieting is not the primary cause of your weight problem. Keep these three important points in mind:

1. Resting metabolic rates do decline slightly during periods of lower caloric intake, but not enough to significantly inhibit weight loss.

2. Resting metabolic rates return to normal soon after caloric intake is no longer restricted. The lowered metabolic rate does not stay low permanently and make future dieting more difficult.

3. A sudden lowering of the metabolic rate from dieting does not explain the weight gain/loss cycles experienced by many overweight people. These fluctuations in weight are primarily from going on and getting off diets. It is especially difficult to stay with a reduced-calorie diet when it never truly satisfies the individual's biochemical need for nutrients, fiber, and phytochemicals.[38]

Those with a genetic tendency to be overweight may actually have the genetic potential to outlive the rest of us. The key to their successful longevity lies in their choosing a nutrient-rich, fiber-rich, lower-calorie diet, as well as getting adequate physical activity. By adjusting the nutrient-per-calorie density of your diet to your metabolic rate, you can use your slow metabolism to your advantage. When you can maintain a normal weight in spite of a slow metabolism, you will be able to achieve significant longevity.

An Unprecedented Opportunity in Human History

Science and the development of modern refrigeration and transportation methods have given us access to high-quality, nutrient-dense food. In today's modern society, we have available to us the largest variety of fresh and frozen natural foods in human history. Using the foods available to us today, we can devise diets and menus with better nutrient density and nutrient diversity than ever before possible.

This book gives you the information and the motivation you need to take advantage of this opportunity to improve your health and maximize your chances for a disease-free life.

You have a clear choice. You can live longer and healthier than ever before, or you can do what most modern populations do: eat to create disease and a premature death. Since you are reading this book, you have opted to live longer and healthier. "Eat to live" and you will achieve a happier and more pleasurable life.

Overfed, Yet Malnourished

THE EFFECTS OF THE AMERICAN DIET, PART II

Case Study:
Charlotte lost 130 pounds and reversed her heart disease and diabetes!

I had been heavy since childhood. It would be easy to blame my problems on heredity, since there is a history of obesity, heart disease, and diabetes on both sides of my family.

Through the years I tried many diets with only minimal and never lasting success. I reached a top weight of 263 pounds on a five-foot four-inch frame and had resigned myself to forever being a plus-size woman.

I was diagnosed with Type II diabetes (along with hypertension and high cholesterol) after suffering a stroke at age fifty-six. To control all these ills, I was prescribed medications that I was expected to take for life. About a year after the stroke, I was

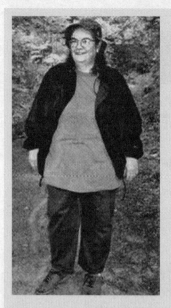 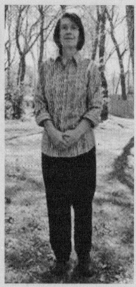

diagnosed with a serious form of tachycardia that required immediate medical attention. I ended up with two heart stents because of a 95 percent blockage and more prescriptions.

I avoided seeing doctors, because although they lectured me about my weight, the only solution they offered was a calorie-restricted version of the standard American diet on which I was always hungry and miserable. My husband, Clarence, searched the Internet for ways to help me become healthier and found Dr. Fuhrman and his book Eat to Live, *which claimed dramatic results through dietary changes.*

I quickly shed pounds, and my lab test results improved. Although my diabetes was controlled to the satisfaction of my doctors, Dr. Fuhrman said the first priority was to get rid of it completely through nutritional excellence. No physician I had seen had ever mentioned this as a possibility.

Now, about a year and a half later, I am no longer diabetic and have had no further heart problems. My fasting blood sugar averages 79 without treatment. Since July 29, 2003, my total cholesterol has dropped from 219 to 130, my triglycerides are down from 174 to 73, and my LDL cholesterol has gone from 149 to 70.

My current weight is around 130, slightly less than half my maximum. As hard as it is to imagine, the last time I was this weight, I was under age twelve. Less measurable, but important, benefits are that I no longer snore, have more energy, and have increased resistance to colds and flus that previously wore me down. There are many things I can do more easily now versus before when I was so overweight.

I owe all these positive changes to Dr. Fuhrman's Eat to Live program. I still have a hearty appetite, but my relationship to food is far less addictive. People may think I have lost weight through willpower, but that's not true. If I'd had any willpower, I would never have become so large in the first place. The Eat to Live program takes time and effort, but for me the results have been well worth it.

Now you know my formula for longevity (H = N/C) and that the key to this formula is the nutrient density of your diet. In other words, you must eat a diet rich in nutrients and fiber, with a very low percentage of foods that are not nutrient- and fiber-dense. It is the same formula that will enable your body to achieve slimness.

To help you learn how to apply this formula to your life, you first need to understand why you must follow it, exploring the relationships between diet, health, and disease. To do so, you need to take a look at the reality of how most people eat and what they gain or lose from such eating practices.

The Pros and Cons of Our "Natural Sweet Tooth"

Even though we have many unique human traits, we are genetically closely related to the great apes and other primates. Primates are the only animals on the face of the earth that can taste sweet and see color. We were designed by nature to see, grasp, eat, and enjoy the flavor of colorful, sweet fruits.

Fruit is an essential part of our diets. It is an indispensable requirement for us to maintain a high level of health. Fruit consumption has been shown in numerous studies to offer our strongest protection against certain cancers, especially oral and esophageal, lung, prostate, pancreatic, and colorectal cancer.[1] Thankfully, our natural sweet tooth directs us to those foods ideally "designed" for our

primate heritage—fruit. Fresh fruit offers us powerful health-giving benefits.

Researchers have discovered substances in fruit
that have unique effects on preventing aging and
deterioration of the brain.[2] Some fruits, especially
blueberries, are rich in anthocyanins and other
compounds having anti-aging effects.[3] Studies continue to provide evidence that more than any other
food, fruit is associated with lowered mortality
from all cancers combined.[4] Eating fruit is vital to
your health, well-being, and long life.

Regrettably, our human desire for sweets is typically satisfied by the consumption of products containing sugar, such as candy bars and ice cream—not
fresh fruit. The U.S. Department of Agriculture
(USDA) estimates that the typical American now
consumes an unbelievable thirty teaspoons of added
sugar a day.[5] That's right, in one day.

As we shall see, we need to satisfy our sweet
tooth with fresh, natural fruits and other plant substances that supply us not just with carbohydrates
for energy but also with the full complement of
indispensable substances that prevent illness.

Nutritional Lightweights: Pasta and White Bread

Unlike the fruits found in nature—which have a full
ensemble of nutrients—processed carbohydrates
(such as bread, pasta, and cake) are deficient in
fiber, phytonutrients, vitamins, and minerals, all of
which have been lost in processing.

Compared with whole wheat, typical pasta and bread are missing:

- 62 percent of the zinc
- 72 percent of the magnesium
- 95 percent of the vitamin E
- 50 percent of the folic acid
- 72 percent of the chromium
- 78 percent of the vitamin B_6
- 78 percent of the fiber

In a six-year study of 65,000 women, those with diets high in refined carbohydrates from white bread, white rice, and pasta had two and a half times the incidence of Type II diabetes, compared with those who ate high-fiber foods such as whole wheat bread and brown rice.[6] These findings were replicated in a study of 43,000 men.[7] Diabetes is no trivial problem; it is the seventh leading cause of death by disease in America, and its incidence is growing.[8]

Walter Willett, M.D., chairman of the Department of Nutrition at the Harvard School of Public Health and co-author of those two studies, finds the results so convincing that he'd like our government to change the Food Guide Pyramid, which recommends six to eleven servings of any kind of carbohydrate. He says, "They should move refined grains, like white bread, up to the sweets category because metabolically they're basically the same."

These starchy (white-flour) foods, removed from nature's packaging, are no longer real food. The fiber and the majority of minerals have been removed, so such foods are absorbed too rapidly, resulting in a sharp glucose surge into the blood-stream. The pancreas is then forced to pump out insulin faster to keep up. Excess body fat also causes us to require more insulin from the pancreas. Over time, it is the excessive demand for insulin placed on the pancreas from both refined foods and increased body fat that leads to diabetes. Refined carbohydrates, white flour, sweets, and even fruit juices, because they enter the bloodstream so quickly, can also raise triglycerides, increasing the risk of heart attack in susceptible individuals.

Every time you eat such processed foods, you exclude from your diet not only the essential nutri-ents that we are aware of but hundreds of other undiscovered phytonutrients that are crucial for normal human function. When the nutrient-rich outer cover is removed from whole wheat to make it into white flour, the most nutritious part of the food is lost. The outer portion of the wheat kernel con-tains trace minerals, phytoestrogens, lignans, phytic acid, indoles, phenolic compounds, and other phy-tochemicals, as well as almost all the vitamin E in the food. True whole grain foods, which are associ-ated with longer life, are vastly different from the processed foods that make up the bulk of calories in the modern American diet (MAD).[9]

Medical investigations clearly show the dangers of consuming the quantity of processed foods that we do. And because these refined grains lack the fiber and nutrient density to satisfy our appetite, they also cause obesity, diabetes, heart disease, and significantly increased cancer risk.[10]

One nine-year study involving 34,492 women between the ages of fifty-five and sixty-nine showed a two-thirds increase in the risk of death from heart disease in those eating refined grains.[11] Summarizing fifteen epidemiological studies, researchers concluded that diets containing refined grains and refined sweets were consistently linked to stomach and colon cancer, and at least fifteen breast cancer studies connect low-fiber diets with increased risks.[12] Eating a diet that contains a significant quantity of sugar and refined flour does not just cause weight gain, it also leads to an earlier death.

Refined Foods Are Linked To:

- Oral cavity cancer
- Stomach cancer
- Colorectal cancer
- Intestinal cancer
- Breast cancer
- Thyroid cancer
- Respiratory tract cancer
- Diabetes
- Gallbladder disease
- Heart disease[13]

If you want to lose weight, the most important foods to avoid are processed foods: condiments, candy, snacks, and baked goods; fat-free has nothing to do with it. Almost all weight-loss authorities agree on this—you must cut out the refined carbohydrates, including bagels, pasta, and bread. As far as the human body is concerned, low-fiber carbohydrates such as pasta are almost as damaging as white sugar. Pasta is not health food—it is hurt food.

Now I can imagine what many of you are thinking: "But, Dr. Fuhrman! I love pasta. Do I have to give it up?" I enjoy eating pasta, too. Pasta can sometimes be used in small quantities in a recipe that includes lots of green vegetables, onions, mushrooms, and tomatoes. Whole grain pastas and bean pastas, found in health-food stores, are better choices than those made from white flour. The point to remember is that all refined grains must be placed in that limited category—foods that should constitute only a small percentage of our total caloric intake.

What about bagels? Is the "whole wheat" bagel you just bought at the bagel store really made from whole grain? No; in most cases, it is primarily white flour. It is hard to tell sometimes. Ninety-nine percent of pastas, breads, cookies, pretzels, and other grain products are made from white flour. Sometimes a little whole wheat or caramel color is added and the product is called whole wheat to make you think it is the real thing. It isn't. Most brown bread is merely white bread with a fake tan. Wheat grown on American soil is not a nutrient-dense food to begin with, but then the food manufacturers remove the most valuable part of the food and add bleach, preservatives, salt, sugar, and food coloring to make breads, breakfast cereals, and other convenience foods. Yet many Americans consider such food healthy merely because it is low in fat.

Soil Depletion of Nutrients Is Not the Problem—Our Food Choices Are

Contrary to many of the horror stories you hear, our soil is not depleted of nutrients. California, Washington, Oregon, Texas, Florida, and other states still have rich, fertile land that produces most of our fruits, vegetables, beans, nuts, and seeds. America provides some of the most nutrient-rich produce in the world.

Our government publishes nutritional analyses of foods. It takes food from a variety of supermarkets across the country, analyzes it, and publishes the results. Contrary to claims of many health-food and supplement enthusiasts, the produce grown in this country is nutrient-rich and high in trace minerals, especially beans, nuts, seeds, fruits, and vegetables.[14] American-produced grains, however, do not have the mineral density of vegetables. Grains and animal-feed crops grown in the southeastern states are the most deficient, but even in those states only a small percentage of crops are shown to be deficient in minerals.[15]

Thankfully, by eating a diet with a wide variety of natural plant foods, from a variety of soils, the threat of nutritional deficiency merely as a result of soil inadequacy is eliminated. Americans are not nutrient-deficient because of our depleted soil, as some nutritional-supplement proponents claim. Americans are nutrient-deficient because they do not eat a sufficient quantity of fresh produce. Over 90 percent of the calories consumed by Americans come from refined foods or animal products. With such a small percentage of our diet consisting of unrefined plant foods, how could we not become nutrient-deficient?

Since more than 40 percent of the calories in the American diet are derived from sugar or refined grains, both of which are nutrient-depleted, Americans are severely malnourished. Refined sugars cause us to be malnourished in direct proportion to how much we consume them. They are partially to blame for the high cancer and heart attack rates we see in America.

It is not merely dental cavities that should concern us about sugar. If we allow ourselves and our children to utilize sugar, white flour products, and oil to supply the majority of calories, as most American families do, we shall be condemning ourselves to a lifetime of sickness, medical problems, and a premature death.

Refined sugars include table sugar (sucrose), milk sugar (lactose), honey, brown sugar, high-fructose corn syrup, molasses, corn sweeteners, and fruit juice concentrates. Even the bottled and boxed fruit juices that many children drink are a poor food; with no significant nutrient density, they lead to obesity and disease.[16] Processed apple juice, which is not far from sugar water in its nutrient score, accounts for almost 50 percent of all fruit servings consumed by preschoolers.[17] For example, apple juice contains none of the vitamin C originally present in the whole apple. Oranges make the most nutritious juice, but even orange juice can't compare

with the original orange. In citrus fruits, most of the
anti-cancer compounds are present in the membranes and pulp, which are removed in processing
juice. Those cardboard containers of orange juice
contain less than 10 percent of the vitamin C present in an orange and even less of the fiber and phytochemicals. Juice is not fruit, and prepackaged
juices do not contain even one-tenth of the nutrients
present in fresh fruit.

Processed carbohydrates, lacking in fiber, fail to slow
sugar absorption, causing wide swings in glucose levels.

Empty calories are empty calories. Cookies,
jams, and other processed foods (even those from
the health-food store) sweetened with "fruit juice"
sound healthier but are just as bad as white-sugar
products. When fruit juice is concentrated and used
as a sweetener, the healthy nutritional components
are stripped away—what's left is plain sugar. To your
body, there is not much difference between refined
sugar, fruit juice sweeteners, honey, fruit juice concentrate, and any other concentrated sweetener.
Our sweet tooth has been put there by nature to
have us enjoy and consume real fruit, not some imi-
tation. Fresh-squeezed orange juice and other fresh
fruit and vegetable juices are relatively healthy foods
that contain the majority of the original vitamins
and minerals. But sweet fruit juices and even carrot
juice should still be used only moderately, as they
still contain a high concentration of sugar calories
and no fiber. They are not an ideal food for those

desiring to lose weight. I often use these juices as part of salad dressings and other dishes rather than alone as a drink. Fresh fruits and even dried fruits do contain an assortment of protective nutrients and phytochemicals, so stick with the real thing.

Lester Traband's Yearly Checkup

My patient Les Traband came in for his yearly checkup. He was not overweight and had been following a vegetarian diet for years. I did a dietary review of what he ate regularly. He was eating "healthy" flaxseed waffles for breakfast, lots of pasta, whole wheat bread, and vegan (no animal products) prepared frozen meals on a regular basis.

I spent about thirty minutes pointing out that he was certainly not following my dietary recommendations for excellent health and presented him with some menu suggestions and an outline of my nutritional prescription for superior health, which he agreed to follow.

Twelve weeks later, he had lost about eight pounds and I rechecked his lipid profile, because I didn't like the results we received from the blood test taken the day of his checkup.

The results speak for themselves:

	2/1/2001	5/2/2001
Cholesterol	230	174
Triglycerides	226	57
HDL	55	78
LDL	130	84
Cholesterol/HDL ratio	4.18	2.23

Enrichment with Nutrients Is a House Made of Straw

White or "enriched" rice is just as bad as white bread and pasta. It is nutritionally bankrupt. You might as well just eat the Uncle Ben's cardboard box it comes in. Refining the rice removes the same important factors: fiber, minerals, phytochemicals, and vitamin E. So, when you eat grains, eat whole grains.

Refining foods removes so much nutrition that our government requires that a few synthetic vitamins and minerals be added back. Such foods are labeled as enriched or fortified. Whenever you see those words on a package, it means important nutrients are missing. Refining foods lowers the amount of hundreds of known nutrients, yet usually only five to ten are added back by fortification.

As we change food through processing and refining, we rob the food of certain health-supporting substances and often create unhealthy compounds, thus making it a more unfit food for human consumption. As a general rule of thumb: the closer we eat foods to their natural state, the healthier the food.

Not All Whole Wheat Products Are Equal

"Whole grain" foods are not always nutrient-dense, healthy foods. Many whole grain cold cereals are so processed that they do not have a significant fiber per serving ratio and have lost most of their nutritional value.

Eating fragmented and unbalanced foods causes many problems, especially for those trying to lose weight.

Whole wheat that is finely ground is absorbed into the bloodstream fairly rapidly and should not be considered as wholesome as more coarsely ground and grittier whole grains. The rapid rise of glucose triggers fat storage hormones. Because the more coarsely ground grains are absorbed more slowly, they curtail our appetite better.

Whole grain hot cereals are less processed than cold cereals and come up with better nutritional scores. They can be soaked in water overnight so you do not have to cook them in the morning.

Unlike eating whole grain foods, ingesting processed foods can subtract nutrients and actually create nutritional deficiencies, as the body utilizes nutrients to digest and assimilate food. If the mineral demands of digestion and assimilation are greater than the nutrients supplied by the food, we may end up with a deficit—a drain on our nutrient reserve funds.

For most of their lives, the diets of many American adults and children are severely deficient in plant-derived nutrients. I have drawn nutrient levels on thousands of patients and have become shocked at the dismal levels in supposedly "healthy" people. Our bodies are not immune to immutable biological laws that govern cellular function. Given enough time, disease will develop. Even borderline deficiencies can result in various subtle defects in human health, leading to anxiety, autoimmune disorders, cancer, and poor eyesight, to name a few.[18]

Fat and Refined Carbohydrates: Married to Your Waist

The body converts food fat into body fat quickly and easily: 100 calories of ingested fat can be converted to 97 calories of body fat by burning a measly 3 calories. Fat is an appetite stimulant: the more you eat, the more you want. If a food could be scientifically engineered to create an obese society, it would have fat, such as butter, mixed with sugar and flour.

The combination of fat and refined carbohydrates has an extremely powerful effect on driving the signals that promote fat accumulation on the body. Refined foods cause a swift and excessive rise in blood sugar, which in turn triggers insulin surges to drive the sugar out of the blood and into our cells. Unfortunately, insulin also promotes the storage of fat on the body and encourages your fat cells to swell.

As more fat is packed away on the body, it interferes with insulin uptake into our muscle tissues. Our pancreas then senses that the glucose level in the bloodstream is still too high and pumps out even more insulin. A little extra fat around our midsection results in so much interference with insulin's effectiveness that two to five times as much insulin may be secreted in an overweight person than in a thin person.

The higher level of insulin in turn promotes more efficient conversion of our caloric intake into body fat, and this vicious cycle continues. People get heavier and heavier as time goes on.

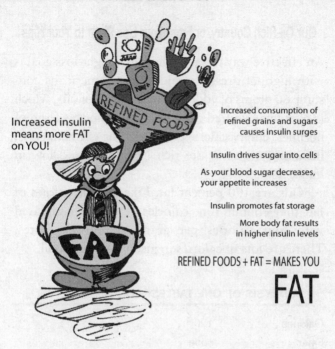

Increased insulin means more FAT on YOU!

Increased consumption of refined grains and sugars causes insulin surges

Insulin drives sugar into cells

As your blood sugar decreases, your appetite increases

Insulin promotes fat storage

More body fat results in higher insulin levels

REFINED FOODS + FAT = MAKES YOU

FAT

Eating refined carbohydrates—as opposed to complex carbohydrates in their natural state—causes the body's "set point" for body weight to increase. Your "set point" is the weight the body tries to maintain through the brain's control of hormonal messengers. When you eat refined fats (oils) or refined carbohydrates such as white flour and sugar, the fat-storing hormones are produced in excess, raising the set point. To further compound the problem, because so much of the vitamin and mineral content of these foods has been lost during processing, you naturally crave more food to make up for the missing nutrients.

Our Oil-Rich Country, or From Your Lips Right to Your Hips

An effective way to sabotage your weight-loss goal is with high-fat dressings and sauces. Americans consume 60 grams of added fat in the form of oils, which is over five hundred calories a day from this form of no-fiber, empty calories.[19] Refined or extracted oils, including olive oil, are rich in calories and low in nutrients.

Oils are 100 percent fat. Like all other types of fat, they contain nine calories per gram, compared with four calories per gram for carbohydrates. There are lots of calories in just a little bit of oil.

ANALYSIS OF ONE TABLESPOON OF OLIVE OIL

Calories	120
Fiber	none
Protein	none
Fat	13.5 gm
Saturated fat	1.8 gm
Minerals	none (trace, less than .01 mg of every mineral)
Vitamins	none (trace of vitamin E, less than 1 IU)

Fat, such as olive oil, can be stored on your body within minutes, without costing the body any caloric price; it is just packed away (unchanged) on your hips and waist. If we biopsied your waist fat and looked at it under an electron microscope, we could actually see where the fat came from. It is stored there as pig fat, dairy fat, and olive oil fat—just as it was in the original food. It goes from your lips right to your hips. Actually, more fat from your last meal is deposited around your waist than on your hips, for both men and women.[20] Analyzing these body-fat deposits is an accurate way for research scientists to discern food intake over time.[21] Having research subjects remember what they ate (dietary recall analysis) is not as accurate as a tissue biopsy, which reports exactly what was really eaten.

Foods cooked in oil or coated with oil soak up more oil than you think. A low-calorie "healthy" food easily becomes fattening. Most Americans eat negligible amounts of salad vegetables, but when they do eat a small salad, they consume about three leaves of iceberg lettuce in a small bowl and then proceed to pour three or four tablespoons of oily dressing on top. Since oil is about 120 calories per tablespoon, they consume some 400 (empty) calories from dressing and about 18 from lettuce. They might as well forget the lettuce and just drink the dressing straight from the bottle. One key to your success is to make healthful salad dressings from my recipes in chapter nine or use other low-calorie and low-salt options.

The message Americans are hearing today from the media and health professionals is that you don't need to go on a low-fat diet, you merely need to replace the bad fats (saturated fats mostly from animal products and trans fats in processed foods) with olive oil. Americans are still confused and receive conflicting and incorrect messages. Olive oil and other salad and cooking oils are not health foods and are certainly not diet foods.

There is considerable evidence to suggest that consuming monounsaturated fats such as olive oil is less destructive to your health than the dangerous saturated and trans fats. But a lower-fat diet could be more dangerous than one with a higher level of fat if the lower-fat diet has more saturated and trans fats. Also, reducing fat and adding more low-nutrient carbohydrates such as bread, white flour, pasta, white rice, and white potatoes is not a significant improvement in nutritional quality. Low-fat does not mean nutritious and healthful.

In the 1950s people living in the Mediterranean, especially on the island of Crete, were lean and virtually free of heart disease. Yet over 40 percent of their caloric intake came from fat, primarily olive oil. If we look at the diet they consumed back then, we note that the Cretans ate mostly fruits, vegetables, beans, and some fish. Saturated fat was less than 6 percent of their total fat intake. True, they ate lots of olive oil, but the rest of their diet was exceptionally healthy. They also worked hard in the fields, walking about nine miles a day, often pushing a plow or working other manual farm equipment. Americans didn't take home the message to eat loads of vegetables, beans, and fruits and do loads of exercise; they just accepted that olive oil is a health food.

Today the people of Crete are fat, just like us. They're still eating a lot of olive oil, but their consumption of fruits, vegetables, and beans is down.

Meat, cheese, and fish are their new staples, and their physical activity level has plummeted. Today heart disease has skyrocketed and more than half the population of both adults and children in Crete is overweight.[22]

Even two of the most enthusiastic proponents of the Mediterranean diet, epidemiologist Martijn Katan of Wageningen Agricultural University in the Netherlands and Walter Willett of the Harvard School of Public Health, concede that the Mediterranean diet is viable only for people who are close to their ideal weight.[23] That excludes the majority of Americans. How can a diet revolving around a fattening, nutrient-deficient food like oil be healthy?

Ounce for ounce, olive oil is one of the most fattening, calorically dense foods on the planet; it packs even more calories per pound than butter (butter: 3,200 calories; olive oil: 4,020).

The bottom line is that oil will add fat to our already plump waistlines, heightening the risk of disease, including diabetes and heart attacks. Olive oil contains 14 percent saturated fat, so you increase the amount of artery-clogging saturated fat as you consume more of it. I believe consuming more fattening olive oil in your diet will raise your LDL (bad) cholesterol, not lower it. Weight gain raises your cholesterol; unprocessed foods such as nuts, seeds, and vegetables, utilized as a source of fat and calories instead of oil, contain phytosterols and other natural substances that lower cholesterol.[24] Also, keep in mind that in Italy, where they consume all that supposedly healthy olive oil, people have twice the chance of getting breast cancer as in Japan, where they have a significantly lower intake of oil.[25]

The Mediterranean diet looked better than ours because of the increased consumption of vegetation, not because of the oil. People who use olive oil generally put it on vegetables such as salads and tomatoes, so its use is correlated with higher consumption of produce. Their diets were better in spite of the oil consumption, not because of it.

If you are thin and exercise a lot, one tablespoon of olive oil a day is no big deal, but the best choice for most overweight Americans is no oil at all.

The Popularity of the Mediterranean Diet

I have only a few bones to pick with those advocating the Mediterranean diet style. First, they claim that cooking food in olive oil increases phytochemical absorption and that eating vegetables without a high-fat topping is not as nutritious since the phytochemicals are not absorbed. When vegetables are cooked, or eaten with fat, some nutrients are more efficiently absorbed and other heat-sensitive nutrients are lost or rendered less absorbable. Many studies show that raw fruits and vegetables offer the highest blood levels of cancer-protective nutrients and the most protection against cancer of any other foods, including cooked vegetation.[26] Any advice not recognizing that raw vegetables and fresh fruits are the two most powerful anti-cancer categories of foods is off the mark. Plus, when you use raw seeds and nuts instead of oil, you receive dramatic health benefits without all the empty colories because of the high micronutrient content.

Paul Talalay, M.D., of the Brassica Chemoprotection Laboratory at the Johns Hopkins School of Medicine is involved with researching the effects of cooking on phytochemicals. He reports "widely different effects on the compounds in vegetables that protect against cancer."[27] These compounds are both activated and destroyed by various cooking methods.

I recognize that raw, uncooked vegetables and fruits offer the most powerful protection against disease, and I encourage my patients to eat huge salads and at least four fresh fruits per day. Diets with little raw foods are not ideal. As the amount of raw fruits and vegetables are increased in a person's diet, weight loss and blood pressure are lowered effortlessly.[28]

Additionally, raw foods contain enzymes, some of which can survive the digestive process in the stomach and pass into the small intestines. These heat-sensitive elements may offer significant nutritional advantages to protect against disease, according to investigators from the Department of Biochemistry at Wright State University School of Medicine.[29] These researchers concluded that "most foods undergo a decrease in nutritive value in addition to the well-known loss of vitamins when cooked and/or processed." Most vitamins are heat-sensitive, for example 20 to 60 percent of vitamin C is lost, depending on the cooking method.[30] Thirty to 40 percent of minerals are lost in cooking vegetables as well.[31] Consuming a significant quantity of raw foods is essential for superior health.

For the best results, your diet should contain a huge amount of raw foods, a large amount of the less calorically dense cooked vegetation, and a lesser amount of the more calorically rich cooked starchy vegetables and grains. Cooking your food in oil will make your diet less effective and you will not lose weight as easily. You may not even lose any weight at all.

Keep in mind, weight loss slows down over time. Most people starting almost any diet after eating haphazardly lose some weight initially. It is easy to drop a few pounds by merely counting calories, but many overweight individuals with a strong genetic tendency to obesity and slow metabolism who need to lose lots of weight may lose very little or none at all. Some may lose an initial five to fifteen pounds, but then when further weight loss becomes even more difficult, they give up.

Another problem with the Mediterranean diet is the preponderance of pasta and Italian bread, which not only causes difficulty with weight control but is also an important factor in increasing colon cancer risk in populations with this eating style.[32]

For the very overweight individual, the Mediterranean diet, like other conventional weight-loss programs, is neither restrictive enough nor filling enough to achieve the results desired. Because olive oil adds so many extra calories to their diet, the dieters still have to carefully count calories and eat tiny portions. All those calories supplied by olive oil, almost one-third of the total caloric intake, make the diet significantly lower in nutrients and fiber.

You can always lose weight by exercising more, and I am all for it. However, many very overweight patients are too ill and too heavy to exercise much. As a former athlete, and today as a physician, I am an exercise nut and a fanatic about recommending exercise to my patients, but many people cannot comply with a substantial exercise program until they are in better health or lose some more weight first. They need a diet that will drop weight effectively, *even if they can't do lots of exercise.*

I have tested my recommendation on more than two thousand patients. The average patient loses the most weight in the first four to six weeks, with the average being about twenty pounds. The weight loss continues nicely—those following this program continue to lose about ten pounds the second month and about a pound and a half per week thereafter. The weight loss continues at this comparatively quick rate until they reach their ideal weight.

The bottom line about healthy fats is that raw nuts, seeds, and avocados contain healthy fats. However, you should consume a limited amount of these foods, especially if you wish to lose weight. Also remember that oil, including olive oil, does not contain the nutrients and phytonutrients that were in the original olive. The oil has little nutrients (except a little vitamin E) and a negligible amount of phytochemical compounds. If you eat the quantities of oil permitted on the typical Mediterranean diet, where all the vegetables are cooked in oil, you will have difficulty taking off the weight you need to lose.

You can add a little bit of olive oil to your diet if you are thin and exercise a lot. However, using a small amount of raw seeds and nuts in salad dressings and dips is a better, more healthful option. Plus, the more oil you add, the more you are lowering the nutrient-per-calorie density of your diet—and that is not your objective, as it does not promote health.

The "Magic" of Fiber—A Critical Nutrient

When we think of fiber, we usually think of bran or Metamucil, something that we take to prevent constipation and that tastes like cardboard. Change that thinking. Fiber is a vital nutrient, essential to human health. Unfortunately, the American diet is dangerously deficient in fiber, a deficiency that leads to many health problems (for example, hemorrhoids, constipation, varicose veins, and diabetes) and is a major cause of cancer. As you can see, if you get fiber naturally in your diet from great-tasting food, you get much more than just constipation relief.

When you eat mostly natural plant foods, such as fruits, vegetables, and beans, you get large amounts of various types of fiber. These foods are rich in complex carbohydrates and both insoluble and water-soluble fibers. The fibers slow down glucose absorption and control the rate of digestion. Plant fibers have complex physiological effects in

HOW YOUR BODY BENEFITS
FROM THE FIBER FOUND IN PLANT FOODS

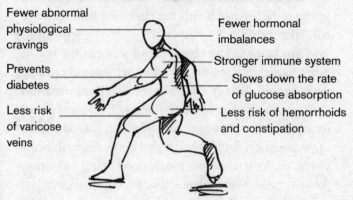

Fewer abnormal physiological cravings

Prevents diabetes

Less risk of varicose veins

Fewer hormonal imbalances

Stronger immune system

Slows down the rate of glucose absorption

Less risk of hemorrhoids and constipation

the digestive tract that offer a variety of benefits, such as lowering cholesterol.[33]

Because of fiber, and because precious food components haven't been lost through processing, natural plant foods fill you up and do not cause abnormal physiological cravings or hormonal imbalances.

Confusion in the Marketplace over the Role of Fiber

Some people are so confused that they do not know what to believe anymore. For example, two studies about fiber received sensational coverage by the media after appearing in the *New England Journal of Medicine*.[34] Newspapers proclaimed the bold headlines HIGH-FIBER DIET DOES NOT PROTECT AGAINST COLON CANCER. No wonder our population is so confused by conflicting messages about nutrition. Some people have actually given up trying to eat healthfully because one day they hear one claim and the next week they hear the opposite. There's a lesson to be learned here: Don't get your health advice from the media.

I am bringing up this issue so you realize not to jump to conclusions on the basis of one study or one news report. You can see how research information is often (mis)reported in the news. I have reviewed more than two thousand nutritional research papers in preparation for this book and many more in prior years, and there is not much conflicting evidence. As in a trial, the evidence has become overwhelming and irrefutable—high-fiber foods offer significant protection against both cancer (including colon cancer) and heart disease. I didn't say *fiber;* I said high-fiber *foods*. We can't just add a high-fiber candy bar or sprinkle a little Metamucil on our doughnut and french fries and expect to reap the benefits of eating high-fiber foods, yet this is practically what the first study did.

The studies mentioned above did not show that a diet high in fresh fruits, vegetables, beans, whole grains, and raw nuts and seeds does not protect against colon cancer. It has already been adequately demonstrated in hundreds of observational studies that such a diet does offer such protection from cancer at multiple sites, including the colon.

The first study merely added a fiber supplement to the diet. I wouldn't expect adding a 13.5-gram fiber supplement to the disease-causing American diet to do anything. It is surprising that this study was actually conducted. Obviously, adding supplemental fiber does not capture the essence of a diet rich in these protective plant foods.

The second study compared controls against a group of people who were counseled on improving their diet. The participants continued to follow their usual (disease-causing) diet and made only a moderate dietary change—a slight reduction in fat intake, with a modest increase in fruits and vegetables for four years. The number of colorectal adenomas four years later was similar. Colorectal adenomas are not colon cancer; they are benign polyps. Only a very small percentage of these polyps ever advance to become colon cancer, and the clinical significance of small benign adenomas is not clear. In any case, it is a huge leap to claim that a diet high in fruits and vegetables does not protect against cancer. This study did not even attempt to address colon cancer, just benign polyps that rarely progress to cancer.

In both studies, even the groups supposedly consuming a high-fiber intake were on a low-fiber diet by my standards. The group consuming the most fiber only ate 25 grams of fiber a day. A high-fiber intake is a marker of many anti-cancer properties of natural foods, especially phytochemicals. The diet plan I recommend is not based on any one study, but on more than two thousand studies and the results I've seen with thousands of my own patients. Following this plan, you will consume between 50 and 100 grams of fiber (from real food, not supplements) per day.

In an editorial, published in the same issue of the *New England Journal of Medicine,* Tim Byers,

M.D., M.P.H., basically agreed, stating, "Observational studies around the world continue to find that the risk of colorectal cancer is lower among populations with high intakes of fruits and vegetables and that the risk changes on adoption of a different diet."[35] He further explained that the three- or four-year period assessed by these trials is too brief and cannot assess the effects of long-term dietary patterns that have already been shown to protect against colorectal cancer.

The reality is that healthy, nutritious foods are also very rich in fiber and that those foods associated with disease risk are generally fiber-deficient. Meat and dairy products do not contain any fiber, and foods made from refined grains (such as white bread, white rice, and pasta) have had their fiber removed. Clearly, we must substantially reduce our consumption of these fiber-deficient foods if we expect to lose weight and live a long, healthy life.

Fiber intake from food is a good marker of disease risk. The amount of fiber consumed may better predict weight gain, insulin levels, and other cardiovascular risk factors than does the amount of total fat consumed, according to studies reported in the *Journal of the American Medical Association*.[36] Again, data show that removing the fiber from food is extremely dangerous.

People who consume the most high-fiber foods are the healthiest, as determined by better waist measurements, lower insulin levels, and other markers of disease risk. Indeed, this is one of the key themes of this book—for anyone to consider his or her diet healthy, it must be predominantly composed of high-fiber, natural foods.

It is not the fiber extracted from the plant package that has miraculous health properties. It is the entire plant package considered as a whole, containing nature's anti-cancer nutrients as well as being rich in fiber.

3

Phytochemicals: Nature's "Magic" Pills

Case Study:
Julia lost over one hundred pounds and has turned her life around!

After three heart attacks within three months and five angioplasties in a three-year period, I knew my health was in a critical state. I almost died after the last angioplasty and had internal bleeding that was difficult to stop. The torture of all my medical problems made me think I would be better off if I had died. I weighed 225 pounds, suffered from unstable angina, and could not walk one block. I was on ten medications and considered myself a cardiac cripple at the age of sixty.

Luckily, I learned about Dr. Fuhrman and read his books. I felt as if it was my last chance to try to get back any quality of life. I was determined. Within three months of following his plan, my chest pain

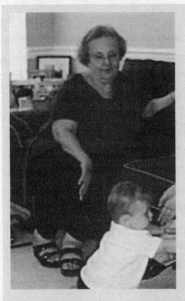
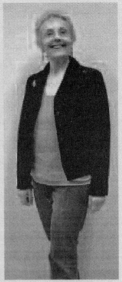

was gone and I went from not being able to walk one block to being able to walk two miles with no problems. Within seven months, I weighed 135 pounds. I had lost ninety pounds without even trying to lose weight. I just wanted to be healthier and live again. I continued with the plan and kept losing weight.

I had always considered myself a vegetarian but never liked vegetables! So at first, the whole vegetable thing was difficult for me. In the beginning I ate a lot of the same things over and over again because I liked them the best. It probably took me a month to get over the toxic cravings. Then I began to enjoy the natural flavors of food, and I liked everything. Kale, which I had never tried before, became my favorite vegetable. I never felt hungry.

I enjoy every day of my life now. I exercise. I garden. I cook. I do everything that I couldn't do for more than ten years of my life. I look and feel healthy. It's wonderful. I'm having a love affair with a plant-based diet.

When I think back to how sick I was, it is frightening. In addition to my cardiac ailments, I suffered from daily migraines and had bleeding ulcers from all the medications that I was on. Today I weigh 120 pounds, walk three miles a day, go to yoga classes, and enjoy life immensely. I know I would not be alive if it was not for Dr. Fuhrman's program. I am so grateful.

You have to just do it. Keep your eyes on the prize. I always said that to myself every day— "Think of what lies ahead."

There are clear reasons why heart attacks and cancer prevail as our number one and number two killers. Let's examine them.

The American Diet: Designed for Disease

Americans currently consume about 25.5 percent of their calories from fiberless animal foods and another 62 percent from highly processed refined carbohydrates and extracted oils.[1] Almost half of all vegetables consumed are potatoes, and half of the potatoes consumed are in the form of fries or chips.

Furthermore, potatoes are one of the least nutritious vegetables.

The same studies that show the anti-cancer effects of green leafy vegetables and fruits and beans suggest that potato-heavy diets are not healthy and show a positive association with colon cancer.[2]

U.S. FOOD CONSUMPTION BY CALORIES[3]

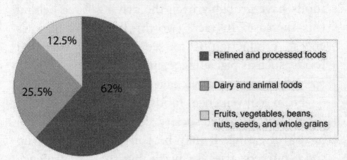

12.5%

25.5%   62%

■ Refined and processed foods

▨ Dairy and animal foods

□ Fruits, vegetables, beans, nuts, seeds, and whole grains

100 CALORIES OF	BAKED POTATO	BAKED SWEET POTATO	FROZEN SPINACH
Protein	2.1 g	1.7 g	12.2 g
Fiber	1.6 g	3.0 g	17.36 g
Calcium	5.4 mg	28 mg	462 mg
Iron	.38 mg	.45 mg	8.5 mg
Magnesium	27 mg	20 mg	242 mg
Zinc	.31 mg	.29 mg	1.8 mg
Selenium	.32 mcg	.7 mcg	5.8 mcg
Vitamin C	13.8 mg	24 mg	100 mg
Vitamin E	.43 mg	.28 mg	4.0 mg
Vitamin A	near zero	21,822 IU	32,324 IU
Volume	1 cup	½ cup	3 cups

Possibly this association exists because of the way potatoes are consumed—fried or with butter or other dangerous fats. Excluding potatoes, Americans consume a mere 5 percent of their calories from fruits, vegetables, and legumes.

Cheese consumption increased 180 percent between 1970 and 2003, and cheese is the primary source of saturated fat in our diet.[4] Convenience foods have probably been the driving force behind this increase. In fact, two-thirds of our nation's cheese production is for commercially prepared foods, such as pizza, tacos, nachos, fast-food meals, spreads, sauces, and packaged snacks.

From convenience foods to fast-food restaurants, our fast-paced society has divorced itself from healthful eating. It may be convenient to pick up soda, burgers, fries, or pizza, but that convenience is not without its price; the result is that we are sicker than ever, and our medical costs are skyrocketing out of control.

I insist that our low consumption of unrefined plant foods is largely responsible for our dismal mortality statistics.[5] Most of us perish prematurely as a result of our dietary folly.

Populations with low death rates from the major

THE MAJOR KILLERS OF AMERICANS

	PERCENT OF ALL DEATHS[6]
Heart attacks, diabetes, and strokes	40
All cancers	22

MAJOR FOODS: U.S. PER CAPITA FOOD SUPPLY, 2008[7]

	PERCENTAGE BY CALORIES
Meats	14.7
Eggs	1.4
Dairy	11.9
Fruits and vegetables	**5.4**
White potatoes	2.5
Refined oils	21.1
Sweeteners	17.2
Wheat flour (over 95% white)	16.3
Other processed foods	9.6

UNREFINED PLANT FOOD CONSUMPTION VS. THE KILLER DISEASES[8]

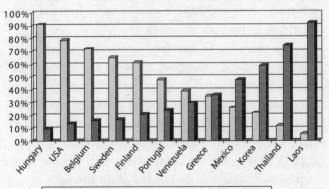

☐ Percentage of deaths from heart disease and cancer
■ Percentage of calories from unrefined plant foods

killer diseases—populations that almost never have overweight members—consume more than 75 percent of their calories from unrefined plant substances. This is at least ten times more than what the average American consumes.

So why is this the case? Why do we see so much heart disease and cancer in wealthier societies? Is it animal products that are so deadly? Are refined carbohydrates solely to blame? Or is it just that plant foods are so miraculously wonderful at protecting us against disease? Or is it all three?

Obviously, the economically poorer regions of the world have significant public health problems: poor sanitation; poverty and malnutrition; high infant-mortality rates; high rates of infectious disease, including AIDS, parasitic diseases, and even tuberculosis. However, in spite of all these things that cause an early death, if we look at the cause-of-death statistics from the World Health Organization (WHO) for people between the ages of fifty-five and seventy-five, we find very few cancer deaths and heart attack deaths in those poor societies.

The diseases of poverty are mostly infectious diseases and are found in areas of the world with compromised nutrition. Heart attacks and the most common cancers (breast, colon, prostate) are found in rich societies where nutritional extravagance is the rule. Nowhere in the world today can we find a society that combines economic wealth with a high intake and variety of unrefined plant foods.

Can you imagine the health potential of a society that would be able to enjoy excellent sanitation, emergency medical care, refrigeration, clean water, flush toilets, and availability of fresh produce year-round and yet avoid nutritional ignorance and nutritional extravagance? We have this opportunity today, an unprecedented opportunity in human history, the opportunity to live a long and healthy life without the fear of disease. This opportunity can be yours.

Nutritional Powerhouses: Plant Foods

Natural plant foods, though usually carbohydrate-rich, also contain protein and fats. On average, 25 percent of the calories in vegetables are from protein. Romaine lettuce, for example, is rich in both protein and essential fatty acids, giving us those healthy fats our bodies require. For more information about essential fats and the protein content of vegetables and various other foods, see chapter five.

Many large-scale epidemiological studies have shown conclusively that certain plant foods play a role in protecting the body against diseases that affect—and kill—at least 500,000 Americans each year. There is no longer any question about the importance of fruits and vegetables in our diet. The greater the quantity and assortment of fruits and vegetables consumed, the lower the incidence of heart attacks, strokes, and cancer.[9] There is still some controversy about which foods cause which cancers and whether certain types of fat are the culprits with certain cancers, but there's one thing we know for sure: raw vegetables and fresh fruits have powerful anti-cancer agents. Studies have repeatedly shown the correlation between consumption of these foods and a lower incidence of various cancers, including those of the breast, colon, rectum, lung, stomach, prostate, and pancreas.[10] This means that your risk of cancer decreases with an increased intake of fruits and vegetables, and the earlier in life you start eating large amounts of these foods, the more protection you get.

Humans are genetically adapted to expect a high intake of natural and unprocessed plant-derived substances. Cancer is a disease of maladaptation. It results primarily from a body's lacking critical substances found in different types of vegetation, many of which are still undiscovered, that are metabolically necessary for normal protective function. Natural foods unadulterated by man are highly complex—so complex that the exact structure and the majority of compounds they contain are not precisely known. A tomato, for example, contains more than ten thousand different phytochemicals.

It may never be possible to extract the precise symphony of nutrients found in vegetation and place it in a pill. Isolated nutrients extracted from food may never offer the same level of disease-protective effects of whole natural foods, as nature "designed" them. Fruits and vegetables contain a variety of nutrients, which work in subtle synergies, and many of these nutrients cannot be isolated or extracted. Phytochemicals from a variety of plant foods work together to become much more potent at detoxifying carcinogens and protecting against cancer than when taken individually as isolated compounds.

Authorities Join the Unrefined-Plant-Food Bandwagon

After years of examining the accumulating evidence, eight top health organizations joined forces and agreed to encourage Americans to eat more unrefined plant food and less food from animal sources, as revealed in the dietary guidelines published in the *Journal of the American Heart Association*. These authorities are the Nutrition Committee of the American Heart Association, the American Cancer Society, the American Academy of Pediatrics, the Council on Cardiovascular Disease in the Young, the Council on Epidemiology and Prevention, the American Dietetic Association, the Division of Nutrition Research of the National Institutes of Health, and the American Society for Clinical Nutrition.

Their unified guidelines are a giant step in the right direction. Their aim is to offer protection against the major chronic diseases in America, including heart disease and cancer. "The emphasis is on eating a variety of foods, mostly fruits and vegetables, with very little simple sugar or high-fat foods, especially animal foods," said Abby Bloch, Ph.D., R.D., chair of the American Cancer Society at the time. Based on a culmination of years of research, these health experts' conclusion was that too much animal-source food is one of the leading causes of heart disease, cancer, strokes, diabetes, obesity, etc.—all the major chronic diseases that cost 1.4 million Americans their lives each year (more than two-thirds of all deaths in the United States).

The Phytochemical Revolution

We are on the verge of a revolution. Substances newly discovered in broccoli and cabbage sprouts sweep toxins out of cells. Substances found in nuts and beans prevent damage to our cells' DNA. Other compounds in beets, peppers, and tomatoes fight cancerous changes in cells. Oranges and apples protect our blood vessels from damage that could lead to heart disease. Nature's chemoprotective army is alert and ready to remove our enemies and shield us from harm.

Hardly a day goes by when some new study doesn't proclaim the health-giving properties of fruits, vegetables, and beans. Unprocessed plant foods contain thousands of compounds, most of which have not yet been discovered, that are essential for maintaining health and maximizing genetic potential. Welcome to the phytochemical revolution.

Phytochemicals, or plant-derived chemicals, occur naturally in plants (*phyto* means "plant"). These nutrients, which scientists are just starting to discover and name, have tremendously beneficial effects on human physiology. The effects of our not consuming sufficient amounts of them are even more astounding—premature death from cancer and atherosclerosis.

Eating a wide variety of raw and conservatively cooked plant foods (such as steamed vegetables) is the only way we can ensure that we get a sufficient amount of these essential health-supporting elements. Taking vitamin and mineral supplements or adding some vitamins to processed foods will not prevent the diseases associated with eating a diet containing a low percentage of calories from whole natural foods.

Scientists cannot formulate into pills nutrients that have not yet been discovered! If the pills did contain sufficient amounts of all the phytonutrients and other essential substances, we would have to swallow a soup bowl full of pills and powders. To date, researchers have discovered more than ten thousand phytochemicals. No supplement can contain a sufficient amount. Thankfully, you can get all these nutrients *today* by eating a wide variety of plant-based foods.

Please bear in mind that I am not against nutritional supplements. In fact, I recommend various supplements to many of my patients with various health problems, and a high-quality multivitamin/multimineral to almost everyone.

I do *not* recommend that most people consume supplements containing vitamin A, isolated beta-carotene, or folic acid, as there are risks associated with excess consumption of these nutrients. The point to be emphasized is that supplements alone cannot offer optimal protection against disease and that you cannot make an unhealthy diet into a healthy one by consuming supplements.

You Cannot Buy Your Health in a Bottle—You Must Earn It!

When your nutrient intake is out of balance, health problems may result. For example, beta-carotene has been touted as a powerful antioxidant and anti-cancer vitamin. However, in recent years we have discovered that beta-carotene is only one of about five hundred carotenoids. Scientists are finding that taking beta-carotene supplements is not without risk, and supplements are certainly a poor substitute for the real thing—the assortment of various carotenoid compounds found in plants.

The reason researchers believed beta-carotene had such a powerful anti-cancer effect was that populations with high levels of beta-carotene in their bloodstream had exceedingly low rates of cancer. More recently we found out that these people were protected against cancer because of *hundreds* of carotenoids and phytochemicals in the fruits and vegetables they were consuming. It wasn't that beta-carotene was responsible for the low incidence of cancer; it merely served as a flag for those populations with a high fruit and vegetable intake. Unfortunately, many scientists confused the flag for the ship.

Recently, large-scale studies have shown that taking beta-carotene (or vitamin A) in supplemental form may not be such a great idea.[11]

In Finnish trials, taking beta-carotene supplements failed to prevent lung cancer and actually increased its incidence.[12] This study was halted when the researchers discovered that the death rate from lung cancer was 28 percent higher among participants who had taken the high amounts of beta-carotene and vitamin A. Furthermore, the death rate from heart disease was 17 percent higher for those who had taken the supplements than for those just given a placebo.[13]

Another study showed a similar correlation between beta-carotene supplementation and increased occurrence of prostate cancer. At this point, as a result of these European studies, as well as similar studies conducted here in the United States, articles in the *Journal of the National Cancer Institute,* the *Lancet,* and the *New England Journal of Medicine* all advise us to avoid taking beta-carotene supplements.[14] A meta-analysis of the studies on this subject in 2007 recognized a 16 percent increased mortality in people who took vitamin A supplements and a 7 percent increased mortality in people who took beta-carotene supplements.[15]

We can learn a lesson from this research. A high intake of isolated beta-carotene may impair the absorption of other carotenoids. Taking beta-carotene or vitamin A may hinder carotenoid anti-cancer activity from zeaxanthin, alpha-carotene, lycopene, lutein, and many other crucial plant-derived carotenoids. When my patients ask what multivitamin they should use, I tell them I'd prefer they take a high-quality multi that does not contain vitamin A or plain beta-carotene. (See recommended products at my website, DrFuhrman.com.)

A high intake of just one nutrient when nature has combined it with many others may make things worse, not better. We humans, especially physicians, are notorious for interfering with nature, thinking we know better. Sometimes we do—all too often we don't. Only later, when it may be too late, do we realize that in fact we have made things worse.

While it still may take decades longer to understand how whole foods promote health, we must accept the fact that the foods found in nature are ideally suited to the biological needs of the species. "The most compelling evidence of the last decade has indicated the importance of protective factors, largely unidentified, in fruits and vegetables," said Walter C. Willett, M.D., Ph.D., chairman of the Department of Nutrition at Harvard's School of Public Health and a speaker at the American Association for Cancer Research.[16]

In other words, a diet in which fruits, vegetables, and other natural plant foods supply the vast majority of calories affords us powerful protection against disease. Phytochemicals in their natural state are potent cancer inhibitors. For example, a study published in the *Journal of the National Cancer Institute* reported that men who ate three or more servings of cruciferous vegetables a week had a 41 percent reduced risk of prostate cancer compared with men who ate less than one serving a week.[17] Cruciferous vegetables, such as broccoli and cabbage, are high in isothiocyanates, which activate enzymes present in all cells that detoxify carcinogens. Eating a variety of other vegetation lowered risk even further. Green vegetables, onions, and leeks also contain organosulfur phytonutrients that inhibit abnormal cellular changes that eventually lead to cancer. A wide variety of wholesome plant-based foods is the only real anti-cancer strategy.

SOME ANTI-CANCER SUBSTANCES
IN NATURAL PLANT FOODS

Allium compounds	Flavonoids	Phenolic acids
Allyl sulfides	Glucosinolates	Phytosterols
Anthocyanins	Indoles	Polyacetylenes
Caffeic acid	Isoflavones	Polyphenols
Catechins	Isothiocyanates	Protease inhibitors
Coumarins	Lignans	Saponins
Dithiolthiones	Liminoids	Sulforaphane
Ellagic acid	Pectins	Sterols
Ferulic acid	Perillyl alcohol	Terpenes

The list above is only a small sample of beneficial compounds, and more are being discovered daily. Cancer-prevention studies attempting to dissect the precise ingredients or combination of ingredients in fruits and vegetables are ongoing; but these studies, like the many others before them, are likely to be a huge waste of resources. There are simply too many protective factors that work synergistically to expect significant benefit from taking a few isolated substances. These beneficial compounds have overlapping and complementary mechanisms of action. They inhibit cellular aging, induce detoxification enzymes, bind carcinogens in the digestive tract, and fuel cellular repair mechanisms.[18]

Cancer Is Much More Preventable Than Treatable

The process of carcinogenesis entails an accumulation of mutations or damage to our DNA (the

FIVE WAYS PHYTOCHEMICALS PREVENT CANCER

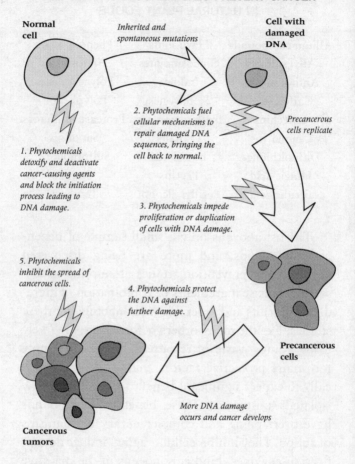

Normal cell

Inherited and spontaneous mutations

Cell with damaged DNA

Precancerous cells replicate

2. Phytochemicals fuel cellular mechanisms to repair damaged DNA sequences, bringing the cell back to normal.

1. Phytochemicals detoxify and deactivate cancer-causing agents and block the initiation process leading to DNA damage.

3. Phytochemicals impede proliferation or duplication of cells with DNA damage.

5. Phytochemicals inhibit the spread of cancerous cells.

4. Phytochemicals protect the DNA against further damage.

Precancerous cells

More DNA damage occurs and cancer develops

Cancerous tumors

cellular blueprint) over the course of twenty to forty years. You must start protecting yourself today, not after you find out you have cancer. Cancer is much more preventable than treatable. Instead, many try to dig a well after their house is on fire.

The process of cellular disintegration is extremely

prolonged, and we know that many pre-neoplastic lesions (abnormal, but not yet cancer) disappear spontaneously.[19] Studies on both humans and animals have shown that plant-derived nutrients are able to prevent the occurrence of, and even reverse, DNA damage that may later result in cancer.[20] Fortunately, we have the potential to suppress the progression of cancer in its early stages by how we choose to eat. The ability to remove and fix these partially damaged cells is proportional to their exposure to phytochemicals.

When we consume a sufficient variety and quantity of phytochemical substances to maximally arm our immune defenses against cancer, we afford ourselves the ability to repair DNA damage, detoxify cancer-causing agents, and resist disease in general. These same substances also activate other immune-enhancing mechanisms that improve our defenses against viruses and bacteria, making our body disease-resistant in general.

Green Plant Foods vs. Animal Foods

So now you know that it is not merely excess fat that causes disease. It is not merely eating empty-calorie food that causes disease. And it is not merely the high consumption of animal foods such as dairy, meat, chicken, and fish that leads to premature death in America. These factors are important, but what is most crucial is what we are missing in our diets by not eating enough produce. Let's take a look at some more of the reasons why plant foods are so protective and essential for human health.

To illustrate the powerful nutrient density of green vegetables, let us compare the nutrient density of steak with the nutrient density of broccoli and other greens.

Now, which food has more protein—broccoli or steak? You were wrong if you thought steak.

Steak has only 6.4 grams of protein per 100 calories and broccoli has 11.1 grams, almost twice as much.[21]

Keep in mind that most of the calories in meat come from fat; green vegetables are mostly protein. (All calories must come from fat, carbohydrate, or protein.)

Popeye Was Right—Greens Pack a Powerful Punch

The biggest animals—elephants, gorillas, rhinoceroses, hippopotamuses, and giraffes—all eat predominantly green vegetation. How did they get the protein to get so big? Obviously, greens pack a powerful protein punch. In fact, all protein on the planet was formed from the effect of sunlight on green plants. The cow didn't eat another cow to form the protein in its muscles, which we call steak. The protein wasn't formed out of thin air—the cow ate grass. Not that protein is such a big deal or some special nutrient to be held in high esteem. I am making this point because most people think animal products are necessary for a diet to include adequate protein. I am merely illustrating how easy it is to consume more than enough protein while at the

NUTRIENTS PRESENT IN 100-CALORIE PORTIONS OF SELECTED FOODS[22]

	BROCCOLI	STEAK	ROMAINE LETTUCE	KALE
Protein	11 g	6 g	7 g	7 g
Calcium	118 mg	2 mg	194 mg	257 mg
Iron	2.2 mg	.8 mg	5.7 mg	3.2 mg
Magnesium	46 mg	6 mg	82 mg	64 mg
Potassium	507 mg	74 mg	1,453 mg	814 mg
Fiber	11 g	0	12 g	7.1 g
Phytochemicals	very high	0	very high	very high
Antioxidants	very high	0	very high	very high
Folate	200 mcg	2 mcg	800 mcg	46 mcg
Riboflavin	.29 mg	.06 mg	.40 mg	.25 mg
Niacin	1.6 mg	1.1 mg	1.8 mg	1.8 mg
Zinc	1.0 mg	1.2 mg	1.4 mg	.9 mg
Vitamin C	143 mg	0	141 mg	146 mg
Vitamin A	3,609 IU	0 IU	51,232 IU	48,641 IU
Beta-carotene	2,131 mcg	0	30,739 mcg	29,186 mcg
Vitamin E	4.7 mg	.07 mg	.76 mg	3.0 mg
Cholesterol	0	22 mg	0	0
Saturated fat	0	3.1g	0	0
Weight	357 g	29 g	588 g	357 g
	(12.6 oz)	(1.0 oz)	(20.7 oz)	(12.6 oz)

same time avoiding risky, cancer-promoting effects of too many animal products. Consuming more plant protein is also the key to achieving safe and successful weight loss.

Now, which has more vitamin E or vitamin C—broccoli or steak? I'm sure you are aware that steak has no vitamin C or vitamin E. It is also almost totally lacking in fiber, folate, vitamin A, beta-carotene, lutein, lycopene, vitamin K, flavonoids, and thousands of other protective phytochemicals. Meat does have certain vitamins and minerals, but even when we consider the nutrients that meat does contain, broccoli has lots more of them. For many important nutrients, broccoli has more than ten times as much as steak. The only exception is vitamin B_{12}, which is not found in plant fare.

When you consider the fiber, phytochemicals, and other essential nutrients, green vegetables win the award for being the most nutrient-dense of all foods. We will give greens a score of 100 and judge all other foods against this criterion.

The Secret of Extreme Longevity

Interestingly, there is one food that scientific research has shown has a strong positive association with increased longevity in humans. So which food do you think that is?

The answer is raw, leafy greens, normally referred to as salad.[23] Leafy greens such as romaine lettuce, kale, collards, Swiss chard, and spinach are the most nutrient-dense of all foods.

Most vegetables contain more nutrients per calorie than any other food and are rich in all necessary amino acids. For example, romaine lettuce, which gets 18 percent of its calories from fat and almost 50 percent of its calories from protein, is a rich powerhouse with hundreds of cancer-fighting phytonutrients that protect us from a variety of threatening illnesses. Being healthy and owning a disease-resistant body is not luck; it is earned.

In a review of 206 human-population studies, raw vegetable consumption showed the strongest protective effect against cancer of any beneficial food.[24] However, fewer than one in a hundred Americans consumes enough calories from vegetation to ensure this defense.

I tell my patients to put a big sign on their refrigerator that says THE SALAD IS THE MAIN DISH.

The word *salad* here means any *vegetable* eaten raw or uncooked, e.g., a bowl of cold pasta in olive oil with a token vegetable is *not* a salad. I encourage my patients to eat two *huge* salads a day, with the goal of consuming an entire head of romaine or other green lettuce daily. I suggest that you go and make the sign and tape it to your fridge now—and then come back. If you plan on doing it later, you may forget. If you learn but one practical habit from this book, let it be this one.

Green Salad Is Less Than 100 Calories per Pound

Did you notice that 100 calories of broccoli is about twelve ounces of food, and 100 calories of ground sirloin is just one ounce of food? With green vegetables you can get filled up, even stuffed, yet you will not be consuming excess calories. Animal products, on the other hand, are calorie-dense and relatively low in nutrients, especially the crucial anti-cancer nutrients.

What would happen if you attempted to eat like

a mountain gorilla, which eats about 80 percent of its diet from green leaves and about 15 percent from fruit? Assuming you are a female, who needs about 1,600 calories a day, if you attempted to get 1,200 of those calories from greens, you would need to eat over fifteen pounds of greens. That is quite a big salad! Since your stomach can only hold about one liter of food (or a little over a quart), you would have a problem fitting it all in.

You would surely get lots of protein from this gorilla diet. In fact, with just five pounds of greens you would exceed the recommended daily allowance (RDA) for protein and would get loads of other important nutrients. The problem with this gorilla diet is that you would develop a *calorie deficiency.* You would become too thin. Believe it or not, I do not expect you to eat exactly like a gorilla. However, the message to take home is that the more of these healthy green vegetables (both raw and cooked) you eat, the healthier you will be and the thinner you will become.

Now let's contrast this silly and extreme gorilla example with another silly and extreme way of eating, the American diet.

If you attempt to follow the perverted diet that most Americans eat, or even if you follow the precise recommendations of the USDA's pyramid— eight to eleven servings of bread, cereal, rice, and pasta (consumed as 98 percent refined grains by Americans) with four to six servings of dairy, meat, poultry, or fish—you would be eating a diet rich in calories but extremely low in nutrients, antioxidants, phytochemicals, and vitamins. You would be overfed and malnourished, the precise nutritional profile that causes heart disease and cancer.

Weighing Food and Trying to Eat Smaller Portions Is Futile

Earlier I compared 100 calories of greens with 100 calories of meat. I did not contrast them by weight or by portion size, as is more customary.

I compared equal caloric portions because it is meaningless to compare foods by weight or portion size. Let me provide an example to explain why this is the case. Take one teaspoon of melted butter, which gets 100 percent of its calories from fat. If I take that teaspoon of butter and mix it in a glass of hot water, I can now say that it is 98 percent fat-free by weight. One hundred percent of its calories are still from fat. It doesn't matter how much water or weight is added, does it?

In fact, if a food's weight were important, it would be easy to lose weight; we would just have to drink more water. The water would trigger the weight receptors in the digestive tract and our appetite would diminish. Unfortunately, this is not the way our body's appestat—the brain center in the hypothalamus that controls food intake—is controlled. As explained in chapter one, bulk, calories, and nutrient fulfillment, not the weight of the food, turn off our appestat. Since the foods Americans consume are so calorie-rich, we have all been trying to diet by eating small portions of low-nutrient foods. We not only have to suffer hunger but also wind up with perverted cravings because we are nutrient-deficient to boot.

We must consume a certain level of calories daily to feel satisfied. So now I ask you to completely rethink what you consider a typical portion size. To achieve superior health and a permanently thin physique, you should eat large portions of green foods. When considering any green plant food, remember to make the portion size huge by conventional standards. Eating large portions of these super-healthy foods is the key to your success.

The Nutrient-Weight "Conflabulation"

Nutrient-weight ratios hide how nutrient-deficient processed food is and make animal-source food look not so fatty. Could this be why the food industry and the USDA chose this method? Could it be a conspiracy to have consumers not realize what they are really eating?

For example, a Burger King bacon double cheeseburger is clearly not a low-fat food. If we calculate its percentage of fat by weight and include the ketchup and the bun, we can accurately state that it is only 18 percent fat (over 80 percent fat-free). However, as a percentage of calories it is 54 percent fat, and the hamburger patty alone is 68 percent fat. McDonald's McLean Deluxe burger was advertised in the early 1990s as 91 percent fat-free using the same numbers trick, when in fact 49 percent of its calories came from fat.

Likewise, so-called low-fat 2 percent milk is not really 2 percent fat. Thirty-five percent of its calories come from fat. They can call it 98 percent fat-free (by weight) only because of its water content. Low-fat milk is not a low-fat product at all, and neither are low-fat cheeses and other low-fat animal foods when you recalculate their fat on a per calorie percentage basis. This is just a sad trick played on Americans. Incidentally, 49 percent of the calories in whole milk come from fat.

The U.S. Department of Meat, Milk, and Cheese

Using weight instead of calories in nutrient-analysis tables has evolved into a ploy to hide how nutritionally unsound many foods are. The role of the USDA was originally to promote the products of the animal agriculture industry.[25] Over fifty years ago, the USDA began promoting the so-called four basic food groups, with meat and dairy products in the number one and two spots on the list. Financed by the meat and dairy industry and backed by nutritional scientists on the payroll of the meat and dairy industry, this promotion ignored science.[26]

This program could be more accurately labeled "the four food myths." It was taught in every classroom in America, with posters advocating a diet loaded with animal protein, fat, and cholesterol. The results of this fraudulent program were dramatic—in more ways than one. Americans began eating more and more animal foods. The campaign sparked the beginning of the fastest-growing cancer

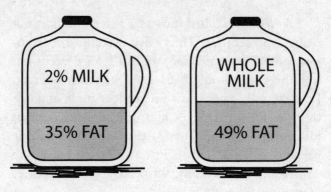

2% MILK

35% FAT

WHOLE MILK

49% FAT

epidemic in history, and heart attack rates soared to previously unheard-of levels.

For years and years the USDA resisted lowering cholesterol and dietary fat recommendations in spite of the irrefutable evidence that Americans were committing suicide with food. Heavy political pressure, lobbyists, and money blocked the path to change.[27]

Promoting nutrient analysis of foods by weight instead of by calorie became a great way to keep excess calories, cholesterol, and saturated fat in the diet—a terrific strategy to create a nation with an epidemic of obesity, heart disease, and cancer. A foreign enemy out to destroy America could not have devised a more effective and insidious plot. How ironic that this was the program designed by our own government, promoted with our own tax dollars, and justified on the ground that it served the public interest.

With all the scientific data available today, including massive investigational studies on human health and diet, you would think that people would know which foods are best to eat and why—but most people are still confused about diet and nutrition. Why?

Part of the problem is that most of us are slow to make changes, especially when they involve personal habits and family traditions. Most people do not embrace change. They are more comfortable with familiarity and cling to long-held but incorrect information. In spite of a vast increase in nutritional information, much of it is contradictory and has led to only more confusion.

Our government spends over $20 billion on price supports that benefit the dairy, beef, and veal industries.[28] This money is given to farmers to artificially reduce the cost of crops used to feed cows, thereby helping to reduce the prices we pay for dairy foods, fowl, and meat. Fruits and vegetables grown primarily for human consumption are specifically excluded from USDA price supports.

Out of one pocket, we pay billions of our tax dollars to support the production of expensive, disease-causing foods. Out of the other pocket, we pay medical bills that are too high because our overweight population consumes too much of these rich, disease-causing foods. Our tax dollars are actually used to make our society sicker and keep our health insurance costs high.

The Food Pyramids That Will Turn You into a Mummy

The USDA Food Pyramid (Figure 1) was in place until 2005, when it was replaced with MyPyramid

USDA FOOD GUIDE PYRAMID

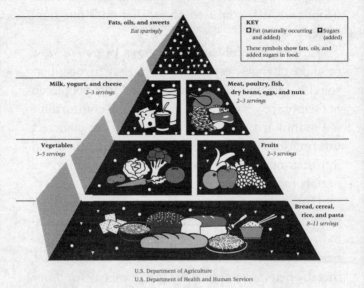

U.S. Department of Agriculture
U.S. Department of Health and Human Services

Figure 1

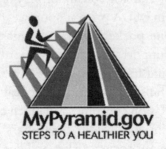

Figure 2

(Figure 2). MyPyramid includes twelve intake levels, from 1,000 calories per day to 3,200 per day, and is designed to help consumers find the right caloric balance.

The MyPyramid recommendations for a 2,000-calorie diet are:

Grains, 6 ounces daily
Vegetables, 5 servings or 2½ cups daily
Fruits, 4 servings or 2 cups daily
Oil, 6 teaspoons daily
Milk, 3 cups daily
Meat and beans, 5½ ounces daily

Since early childhood we have been bombarded with incorrect nutritional dietary advice, and unfortunately the scandal continues today. Even after decades of scientific research refuting its recommendations, the latest USDA recommendation—MyPyramid—is only a slight improvement. While the recommended servings of vegetables and fruits have been increased and exercise is recommended, it still reinforces the deadly dietary errors that people have become accustomed to making.

The food pyramid endorses a level of animal-food consumption that causes the diseases that kill us: heart attacks and cancer.

Foods also are grouped in ways that don't make sense. Meat and beans are in the same food group because they are considered protein-rich foods. Nuts and seeds are not even shown. However, while nuts, seeds, and beans have been shown to reduce cholesterol levels and heart disease risk, meat is linked to increased risk.

MyPyramid would lead people to believe that milk should be consumed on a daily basis. Including milk as its own very prominent group implies that it is an essential part of a healthy diet, which is anything but the truth, especially with the strong association of milk with prostate cancer.[29] The pyramid offers little help for those really wanting to reduce their health risks.

This is an exercise in political correctness, not nutritional science. Could it be possible that the USDA continues to be unduly influenced by political pressure exerted by food industry groups? A pyramid based on science and science alone would have to place vegetables at the foundation!

After many years of our population being advised to increase its consumption of produce, half of all Americans still don't eat three vegetable servings a day. That total even includes those heart attack–causing foods that are fried in trans fats—french fries and potato chips. On any given day, no fruit whatsoever passes the lips of half of all Americans.

In 2010 the National Cancer Institute budgeted about four million dollars to promote the virtues of fruits and vegetables. Compare that with McDonald's $1.2 billion spent on U.S. marketing. The major cause of all diseases afflicting Americans today is a produce-deficient diet.

Based on an exhaustive look at research data from around the world over the past fifteen years, my recommendation is that your diet should contain over 90 percent of calories from unrefined plant foods. This high percentage of nutrient-dense plant foods in the diet allows us to predict freedom from cancer, heart attacks, diabetes, and excess body weight. Fruits, vegetables, and beans must be the base of your food pyramid; otherwise, you will be in a heap of trouble down the road.

The diseases that afflict, and eventually kill, almost all Americans can be avoided. You can live a high-quality, disease-free life and remain physically active and healthy. You can die peacefully and uneventfully at an old age, as nature intended.

To achieve the results in preventing and reversing disease, and attaining a permanent healthy body weight, we must be concerned with the *nutritional quality* of our diet.

The picture is becoming crystal clear—the key to what will make you thin will also make you healthy. Once you learn to "eat to live," thinness and health will walk hand in hand, happily ever after.

4

The Dark Side of Animal Protein

Case Study:
ReBecca lost over 320 pounds and found sound nutrition and restored energy!

I saw Dr. Fuhrman on TV in 2003 and became really fired up about his eating program. I told my friend, who was so thrilled that I was showing concern for my health that she bought me a copy of Eat to Live. I read the book from cover to cover! To this day, I still carry it with me. It is my second bible. I really LIVE by the book: passages are underlined, notes are in the margins, etc. Yes, I experienced headaches and cravings the first five to seven days, but because I could eat without weighing food or counting calories, I felt it was an even exchange.

After a few weeks, I truly felt energized! My poor body was getting some sound nutrition. I did not get weighed before I began the program, but I

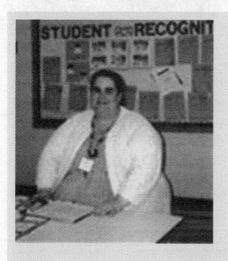 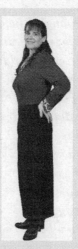

estimate that I weighed about 482 pounds. During the first eight weeks, I lost 72½ pounds. From that moment on, I never looked back!

Week after week, I continued to lose weight. Eight and a half months later, I had lost a total of 133 pounds. By the following year, I had lost another 100 pounds, and another 50 pounds by the next year. As I approach my ideal weight, the weight is coming off more slowly. I now belong to a gym and have incorporated walking and weight training into my weekly routine.

Today I embrace my new high-nutrient eating lifestyle. I don't eat cheese, bread of any type, rice, or pasta. I eat to live. People are confused when they see how I eat, questioning how I can eat so much and still lose weight or how I am satisfied eating a plant-based diet. My own family doctor is amazed at my transformation. Yes, my life has changed! Before I committed to losing weight, the bigger I became, the more invisible I became. I went from a world of being all alone with a good friend or two (who saw the real me hiding under all that weight) to this world of so many people. I am still adjusting to this, too, as it can be overwhelming. Previously, I shopped late at night to avoid people making comments during "normal" shopping hours. I bought clothes from big women's magazines. The clothes had no style and were just big, baggy dresses. I avoided restaurants. I could not fit in a booth, and having a chair pulled to the end of the table was so embarrassing. I could never use a public bathroom because I could not fit in the stall.

I owe my life to the Eat to Live lifestyle. Dr. Fuhrman saved me from literally eating myself to death. How grateful and blessed I am. Whatever lies ahead, I am ready for it!

One day we hear that a high-fat diet causes cancer, and the next day a study shows that those on low-fat diets do not have lower cancer rates. The public is so confused and fed up that they just eat anything, and the number of overweight people continues to grow.

How much do you know about nutrition? True or false?

1. We need milk to get enough calcium to protect us against osteoporosis.

2. A diet high in protein is healthy.

3. The best source of protein is animal foods such as meat, chicken, eggs, fish, and dairy.

4. Plant foods do not have complete protein.

5. To get adequate protein from a plant-based diet, you should combine certain foods to make sure you receive a complete complement of the necessary amino acids at each meal.

6. We can protect ourselves against cancer by switching to low-fat animal foods such as chicken, fish, and skim milk and by omitting red meat.

Answers provided below.

The China Project

Fortunately, evidence from a massive series of scientific investigations has shed some light on the confusion. The China-Cornell-Oxford Project (also known as the China Project) is the most comprehensive study on the connection between diet and disease in medical history. The *New York Times* called this investigation the "Grand Prix of all epidemiological studies" and "the most comprehensive large study ever undertaken of the relationship between diet and the risk of developing disease."[1]

Spearheaded by T. Colin Campbell, Ph.D., of Cornell University, this study has made discoveries that have turned the nutritional community upside down. To the surprise of many, the China Project has revealed many so-called nutritional facts as demonstrably false. For example, the answer to all the nutrition quiz questions above is false.

China was an ideal testing ground for this comprehensive project because the people in one area of China ate a certain diet and the people just a few hundred miles away may have eaten a completely different diet. Unlike in the West, where we all eat very similarly, rural China was a "living laboratory" for studying the complex relationship between diet and disease.[2]

The China Project was valid because it studied populations with a *full range of dietary possibilities,* from a completely plant-food diet to diets that included a significant amount of animal foods. Adding small quantities of a variable is how scientists can best detect the risk or value of a dietary practice. It's the same principle as comparing nonsmokers with those who smoke half a pack a day to best observe the dangers of smoking. Comparing a fifty-cigarette-per-day habit with a sixty-cigarette-per-day habit may not reveal much more additional damage from those last ten cigarettes.

In China, people lived their entire lives in the towns they were born in and rarely migrated, so the dietary effects that researchers looked at were present for the subjects' entire lives. Furthermore, as a result of significant regional differences in the way people ate, there were dramatic differences in the prevalence of disease from region to region. Cardiovascular disease rates varied twentyfold from one place to another, and certain cancer rates varied by several hundredfold. In America, there is little difference in the way we eat; therefore, we do not see a hundredfold difference in cancer rates between one town and another.

Fascinating findings were made in this study. The data showed huge differences in disease rates based on the amount of plant foods eaten and the availability of animal products. Researchers found that as the amount of animal foods increased in the diet, even in relatively small increments, so did the emergence of the cancers that are common in the West. Most cancers occurred in direct proportion to the quantity of animal foods consumed.

In other words, as animal-food consumption approached zero, cancer rates fell. Areas of the country with an extremely low consumption of animal foods were virtually free of heart attacks and cancer. An analysis of the mortality data from 65 counties and 130 villages showed a significant association with animal protein intake (even at relatively low levels) and heart attacks, with a strong protective effect from the consumption of green vegetables.[3]

All animal products are low (or completely lacking) in the nutrients that protect us against cancer and heart attacks—fiber, antioxidants, phytochemicals, folate, vitamin E, and plant proteins. They are rich in substances that scientific investigations have shown to be associated with cancer and heart disease incidence: saturated fat, cholesterol, and arachidonic acid.[4] Diets rich in animal protein are also associated with high blood levels of the hormone IGF-1, which is a known risk factor for several types of cancer.[5]

The China Project showed a strong correlation between cancer and the amount of animal protein, not just animal fat, consumed.[6] Consumption of lean meats and poultry still showed a strong correlation with higher cancer incidence. These findings indicate that even low-fat animal foods such as skinless white-meat chicken are implicated in certain cancers.

Heart Health—It's Not Just Fat and Cholesterol

There was also a relationship between animal protein and heart disease. For example, plasma apolipoprotein B is positively associated with animal-protein intake and inversely associated (lowered) with vegetable-protein intake (e.g., legumes and greens). Apolipoprotein B levels correlate strongly with coronary heart disease.[7] Unknown to many is that animal protein has a significant effect on raising cholesterol levels as well, while plant protein lowers it.[8]

Scientific studies provide evidence that animal protein's effect on blood cholesterol may be significant. This is one of the reasons those switching to a low-fat diet do not experience the cholesterol lowering they expect unless they also remove the low-fat animal products as well. Surprising to most people is that yes, even low-fat dairy and skinless white-meat chicken raise cholesterol. I see this regularly in my practice. Many individuals do not see the dramatic drop in cholesterol levels unless they go all the way by cutting all animal protein from their diet.

Red meat is not the only problem. The consumption of chicken and fish is also linked to colon cancer. A large study examined the eating habits of 32,000 adults for six years and then watched the incidence of cancer for these subjects over the next six years. Those who avoided red meat but ate white meat regularly had a more than 300 percent increase over those who ate no white meat in colon cancer incidence.[9] The same study showed that eating beans, peas, or lentils at least twice a week was associated with a 50 percent lower risk than never eating these foods.

CHOLESTEROL CONTENT IN	BEEF, TOP SIRLOIN	CHICKEN BREAST, NO SKIN[10]
100 grams	90 mg	85 mg
100 calories	33 mg	51 mg

Chicken has about the same amount of cholesterol as beef, and the production of those potent cancer-causing compounds called heterocyclic amines (HCAs) is even more concentrated in grilled chicken than in beef.[11] Another study from New Zealand that investigated heterocyclic amines in meat, fish, and chicken found the greatest contributor of HCAs to cancer risk was chicken.[12] Likewise, studies indicate that chicken is almost as dangerous as red meat for the heart. Regarding cholesterol, there is no advantage to eating lean white instead of lean red meat.[13]

The best bet for overall health is to significantly limit or eliminate all types of meat—red and white. Dr. Campbell further explains his view that animal protein (in addition to animal fats) is implicated in disease causation:

> I really believe that dietary protein—both the kind and the amount—is more significant, as far as cholesterol levels are concerned, than is saturated fat. Certainly it is more significant than dietary cholesterol. We do know that animal protein has a quick and major impact on enzymes involved in the metabolism of cholesterol. Whether it is the immune system, various enzyme systems, the uptake of carcinogens into the cells, or hormonal activities, animal protein generally only causes mischief.[14]

It may be impossible to extricate which component of animal food causes the most mischief. However, it is clear that while Americans struggle in vain to even marginally reduce the amount of fat in their diet, they still consume high levels of animal products and very little unrefined produce.

Cholesterol levels can be decreased by reducing both saturated fat and animal protein while eating more plant protein.

Remember, those countries and areas of China with extremely low rates of Western diseases did not achieve them merely because their diets were low in fat. It was because their diets were rich in unrefined plant products—they were not eating fat-free cheesecake and potato chips.

Never forget that coronary artery disease and its

end result—heart attacks, the number one killer of all American men and women—are almost 100 percent avoidable. Poring over nation-by-nation mortality data collected by the World Health Organization, I found that most of the poorer countries, which invariably consume small amounts of animal products, have less than 5 percent of the adult population dying of heart attacks.[15] The China Project confirmed that there were virtually no heart attacks in populations that consume a lifelong near-vegetarian diet and almost no heart attacks in populations consuming a diet that is rich in natural plant foods and receives less than 10 percent of its calories from animal foods.

My observation of the worldwide data is supported by studies of American vegetarians and non-vegetarians.[16] These studies show that the major risk factors associated with heart disease—smoking, physical inactivity, eating processed food, and animal-product consumption—are avoidable. Every heart attack death is even more of a tragedy because it likely could have been prevented.

Understanding the Conflicting and Confusing Cancer Studies

The China Project data also helps explain findings from the Nurses' Health Study in Boston, which showed that American women who reduced their fat intake surprisingly did not have a decreased risk of breast cancer.[17] First of all, those on the lower-fat diet consumed 29 percent of their calories from fat.

This is still a high-fat diet (by my standards) and even higher than the group with the highest fat intake in China. It's like cutting back on smoking from three packs a day to two and expecting to get a significant decrease in lung cancer risk. By the way, the lowest-fat group in China, whose diet was almost entirely composed of plants, was getting 6 percent of their calories from fat, and the high-fat group in China consumed about 24 percent of their calories from fat.

Second, these women who reported eating less fat in the Nurses' Health Study actually consumed just as much as or more calories from animal protein than those on the higher-fat diet, and the amount of unrefined plant produce did not increase. The low-fat group in China was not eating anywhere near the quantity of processed foods that we do in America. Their cancer rates were so low not solely because the diet was low in fat and animal protein but also because, unlike Americans, they actually ate lots of vegetables.

Generally speaking, the reason the evidence from the China Project is so compelling is that results from population studies in the West are not very accurate. They generally study adults who have made some moderate dietary change later in life, and all subjects are past the age when dietary influence has the most effect. Certain cancers, such as breast and prostate cancer, are strongly influenced by how we eat earlier in life, especially right before and after puberty.

After studying multiple diseases, not just one

type of cancer, the researchers involved in the China Project concluded: "There appears to be no threshold of plant-food enrichment or minimization of animal product intake beyond which further disease prevention does not occur. These findings suggest that even moderate intakes of foods of animal origin are associated with significant increases in plasma cholesterol concentration, which are associated, in turn, with significant increases in chronic degenerative disease mortality rates."[18] In other words, populations with very low cholesterol levels have not only low heart disease rates but low cancer rates as well.

The insight provided by the research is simple: As long as Americans continue to practice nutritional indifference, they will suffer the consequences. Don't expect any significant protection from marginal changes.

Cancer Is a Fruit- and Vegetable-Deficiency Disease

Fruits and vegetables are the two foods with the best correlation with longevity in humans. Not whole wheat bread, not bran, not even a vegetarian diet shows as powerful a correlation as a high level of fresh fruit and raw green salad consumption.[19] The National Cancer Institute recently reported on 337 different studies that all showed the same basic information:[20]

1. Vegetables and fruits protect against all types of cancers if consumed in large enough quantities. Hundreds of scientific studies document

this. The most prevalent cancers in our country are mostly plant-food-deficiency diseases.

2. Raw vegetables have the most powerful anti-cancer properties of all foods.

3. Studies on the cancer-reducing effects of vitamin pills containing various nutrients (such as folate, vitamin C, and vitamin E) give mixed reviews; sometimes they show a slight benefit, but most show no benefit. Occasionally studies show that taking isolated nutrients is harmful, as was discussed in chapter three regarding beta-carotene.

4. Beans in general, not just soy, have additional anti-cancer benefits against reproductive cancers, such as breast and prostate cancer.[21]

Most Americans would prefer to take a pill so they could continue eating what they are accustomed to. Can you imagine a pill made by a pharmaceutical company that could reduce cancer rates by 80 percent or more? Wouldn't that be the most financially successful pharmaceutical product of all time? You would be crazy not to take this life-extending gift.

The anti-cancer and disease-protective qualities of food demonstrate the crux of the failure of modern medicine. After billions and billions of dollars allocated and donated to cancer research, we have nothing to show for it. We are losing the war on cancer because we are on an incessant search for the impossible-to-find cure, when in fact removing the causes is the only way to win.

You can close this book and put it away right

now as long as you can incorporate this crucial dietary change into your life: consume high levels of fruits, green vegetables, and beans. This is the key to both weight loss and better health. Exactly how much veggies and beans you need to eat and how to incorporate them into your diet and make them taste great are covered in chapter eight.

A Vegetarian Diet Is No Guarantee of Good Health

People who omit meat, fowl, and dairy but fill up on bread, pasta, pretzels, bagels, rice cakes, and crackers may be on a low-fat diet, but because their diet is also low in vitamins, minerals, phytochemicals, important essential fatty acids, and fiber, it is conspicuously inadequate and should not be expected to protect against cancer. Additionally, because these refined grains are low in fiber, they do not make you feel full until after you have taken in too many calories from them. In other words, both their nutrient-to-calorie and nutrient-to-fiber ratios are extremely low.

Let me repeat this again to be clear: Following a strict vegetarian diet is not as important as eating a diet rich in fruits and vegetables. A vegetarian whose diet is mainly refined grains, cold breakfast cereals, processed health-food-store products, vegetarian fast foods, white rice, and pasta will be worse off than a person who eats a little chicken or eggs, for example, but consumes a large amount of fruits, vegetables, and beans.

Studies have confirmed this. Multiple studies have shown that vegetarians live quite a bit longer than nonvegetarians do.[22] But when we take a close look at the data, it appears that those who weren't as strict had longevity statistics that were equally impressive as long as they consumed a high volume of a variety of unrefined plant foods.

Remember, long-term vegans (strict vegetarians who consume no dairy or other foods of animal origin) almost never get heart attacks. If you have heart disease or a strong family history of heart disease, you should consider avoiding all animal-based products. To quote a respected authority, William Castelli, M.D., director of the famed Framingham Heart Study in Massachusetts:

> We tend to scoff at vegetarians, but they're doing much better than we are. Vegans have cholesterol levels so low, they almost never get heart attacks. Their average blood cholesterol is about 125 and we've never seen anyone in the Framingham study have a heart attack with a level below 150.

The research shows that those who avoid meat and dairy have lower rates of heart disease, cancer, high blood pressure, diabetes, and obesity.[23] The data is conclusive: vegetarians live longer in America, probably a lot longer.

How Much Longer Do Vegetarians Live?

This is a difficult question to answer accurately, as there are few studies on lifelong vegetarians in countries with electricity, refrigeration, good sanitation, and adequate nutrition. American studies conducted in 1984 on Seventh-Day Adventists, a religious group that provides dietary and lifestyle advice to its members, sheds some light on this issue. Adventist leadership discourages the consumption of meat, fowl, and eggs; pork is prohibited. Because eating animal products is only discouraged and not necessarily prohibited, there is a large range in animal-product consumption. Some Adventists never eat meat and eggs, whereas others consume them daily. When we take a careful look at the Seventh-Day Adventist data, those who lived the longest were those following the vegetarian diet the longest, and when we look at the subset who had followed a vegetarian diet for at least half their life, it appears they lived about thirteen years longer than their average, nonsmoking Californian counterparts.[24] Most of the participants in this study were converted to the religion, not born into it. There was no data on those following such a diet since childhood. However, the data from this carefully constructed study was compelling; and what is of considerable interest to me is the association of green salad consumption and longer life.[25] Leafy greens, the most nutrient-rich foods on the planet, were the best predictor of extreme longevity.

Some nutritional experts would argue that a strict vegetarian who follows a diet rich in natural vegetation, not refined grains, has the longest longevity potential, as indicated by evaluating the China Project data together with hundreds of the smaller food-consumption studies—but, of course, this is still educated speculation. Let's not argue whether it is all right to eat a little bit of animal foods or not, and thereby miss the point that cannot be contradicted or disagreed with:

> Whether you eat a vegetarian diet or include a small amount of animal foods, for optimal health you must receive the majority of your calories from unrefined plant foods. It is the large quantity of unrefined plant foods that grants the greatest protection against developing serious disease.

The Breast and Prostate Cancer Mystery Unraveled

So much has been written about the causes of breast cancer (there are entire books devoted to the subject), yet women are still confused. This section should not be skipped over by men. Men have mothers, daughters, sisters, and wives they must help protect, and the same factors that cause breast cancer cause prostate cancer. Men with a family history of breast cancer have an increased risk of prostate cancer, and women with a family history of prostate cancer have an increased risk of breast cancer.[26] So there is a strong link between these two hormonally sensitive cancers.

American women are now twice as likely to develop breast cancer as they were a century ago, and most of this increase has occurred in the past fifty years. In spite of all the fear and publicity, American women are still in the dark about what they can do to protect themselves, and researchers looking for a simple cause have met with frustration. The reason is that breast cancer, like most cancers, is multicausal. Considering a number of contributing factors simultaneously is essential to understand the rapid climb in the incidence of breast cancer in recent decades. We know much today about the causes of breast cancer, and the good news is that genetics plays a minor role and the disease does not strike at random. The war against breast cancer can be won.

Understanding the Factors Involved in the Development of Cancer

Carcinogenesis, the process that leads to cancer, is believed to occur in a series of steps. It is a multistage process that begins with precancerous cellular damage that gradually proceeds to more malignant changes. The first step is the development of cellular abnormalities, which eventually leads to cancer. This usually occurs during adolescence, and soon after puberty.[27] Remember that unhealthy childhood nutritional practices cause excessive sex hormone production and early pathologic changes in the breast tissue that set the stage for cancer many years later.

We know that puberty at an earlier age is a significant marker of increased risk, and we know that there is overwhelming evidence that ovarian hormones play a crucial role, at all stages, in the development of breast cancer.[28] It is common knowledge among physicians that the earlier a woman matures, as measured by the age of her first menstrual period, the higher her risk for breast cancer.[29] Both early menarche (the onset of menstruation) and greater body weight are markers of increased risk of breast cancer.[30]

Women are not the only sex affected; the same increased risk as a result of early maturation is seen with both prostate cancer and testicular cancer.[31] If we grow and mature more rapidly, we increase our cancer risk and age faster. We see the same thing in lab animals; if we feed them so they grow faster, they die younger.[32]

Ominously, the onset of menstruation has been occurring at a younger and younger age in Western societies during the past century.[33] The average age in the United States is now about twelve years. According to the World Health Organization, the average age at which puberty began in 1840 was seventeen.[34]

During the time period that the age of menarche has decreased from seventeen to about twelve in western Europe and the United States, there has been a concomitant change in Western eating habits. There has been an increased consumption of fat, refined carbohydrates, cheese, and meat and a huge decrease in the consumption of complex carbohydrates such as starchy plants. Modern studies of girls on vegetarian diets characterized by more complex carbohydrates and no meat show a later age of menarche and, as one would expect, a significant reduction of acne as well.[35] A greater consumption of animal foods leads to a higher level of hormones related to early reproductive function and growth.[36] These hormonal abnormalities persist into adulthood.[37] Uterine fibroids also develop from a diet deficient in fruits and vegetables and heavy in meat. As the consumption of meat increases and vegetation decreases, one's risk of fibroids increases proportionately.[38] In other words, the stage is set by our poor dietary habits early in life. Breast and prostate cancer are strongly affected by our dietary practices when we are young.

First European and then American studies have indicated that the protein richness of one's diet is a more sensitive marker of early menarche than

AGE OF PUBERTY OVER TIME

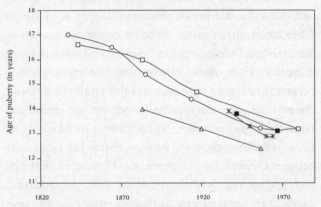

Source: Tanner, J. M. 1973. Trend toward earlier menarche in London, Oslo, Copenhagen, the Netherlands and Hungary. *Nature* 243: 75–76.

increased body weight.[39] This conclusion is consistent with the data relating earlier menarche with increased animal protein use in South African girls.[40] Then in the 1990s, when the data from the massive China-Cornell-Oxford Project was dissected, we again saw the high correlation between breast cancer incidence and the consumption of animal products.[41]

In China, animal-food consumption correlated well with early menarche and increasing levels of sex hormones. Serum testosterone levels had the best correlation with breast cancer, even better than estrogen. Of note is that increasing levels of testosterone significantly increases the risk of both breast cancer and prostate cancer. Testosterone rises as well with increasing levels of obesity, and being overweight is another consistent risk factor.[42]

What makes the data from the China Project so intriguing is that breast cancer incidence is so low in China compared with Western countries and that animal-food consumption is so much lower than in America. Even those consuming the most animal products in China consume less than half the amount Americans do. As animal-food intake increased from about once a week in the lowest third to about four times a week in the highest third, breast cancer rates increased by 70 percent. Of note is that the only difference among the diets was the addition of meat in varying amounts. Consumption of fresh vegetables in all groups was about the same, offering little chance of confounding variables. There was a strong increase in the occurrence of breast cancer mortality with increasing animal-product consumption.

In this country, we consume an enormous amount of cheese. Our record-high increase in cheese consumption is alarming: a 182 percent increase in the past thirty years.[43] Cheese has more saturated fat and more hormone-containing and promoting substances than any other food, and the incidence of our hormonally sensitive cancers has skyrocketed.

In spite of studies that do not show an impressive association with small differences in fat consumption later in life, large changes early in life have huge repercussions.[44] When we consider the diet consumed throughout our life, meat and dairy continue to be implicated as a strong causal factor in breast cancer.[45] There is almost no breast cancer at all in populations that consume less than 10 percent of their calories from animal products.[46] After reviewing many studies on this issue for the *Journal of the National Cancer Institute,* a group of prominent scientists concluded that the studies that failed to show the relationship between animal-product consumption and breast cancer suffered from methodological problems.[47]

Unraveling the Protein Myth

We have been indoctrinated since early childhood to believe that animal protein is a nutrient to be held in high esteem. We have been brought up with the idea that foods are good for us if they help us grow bigger and faster. Nothing could be further from the truth.

The public as well as the media are confused about this issue. They continue to associate the term *better nutrition* with earlier maturity and larger stature resulting from our greater consumption of animal protein and animal fats. These unfavorable trends are repeatedly reported as positive events. Earlier writers and nutritionists have mistakenly equated rapid growth with health. I believe an increased rate of growth is not a good thing. The slower a child grows, the slower he or she is aging. Slower growth, taking longer to reach maturity, is predictive of a longer life in animal studies.[48] We are finding the same thing in humans: an unnaturally rapid growth and premature puberty are risk factors for cancers and other diseases later in life. Evidence continues to mount that these same factors leading to early maturity and excessive growth in childhood increase the occurrence of cancer in general, not just breast and prostate cancer.[49] Excluding malnutrition or serious disease, the slower we grow and mature, the longer we live.

The other side of the story is that it is not just the fat in animal foods that causes cancer and heart disease. Animal protein is also getting a bad rap by legitimate nutritional researchers and scientists in studies. Scientists have discovered a link between animal protein and cancer in both laboratory and human epidemiological studies, and reducing one's consumption of animal protein slows the aging process.[50]

Animal-product consumption in general is proportionally associated with multiple types of cancer. A massive international study that amassed data from fifty-nine different countries showed that men who ate the most meat, poultry, and dairy products were the most likely to die from prostate cancer, while those who ate the most unrefined plant foods and nuts were the least likely to succumb to this disease.[51]

Another study from Germany found colon cancer and rectal cancer decreased by about 50 percent in adult vegetarians. However, a significantly greater reduction of cancer and all-cause mortality (about a 75 percent reduction) was related to being on a vegetarian diet for more than twenty years.[52] The degree of protection correlated well with number of years on a vegetarian diet. Other studies on vegetarian diet in different countries show almost the same thing.[53] The causes start accumulating early.

There is considerable evidence that exposure to certain outlawed chemicals, especially PCBs and DDT, may promote further pathologic changes. Women who have breast cancer have a higher concentration of these chemicals in their breast tissue than do women who do not have cancer.[54] This has also been noted in Long Island, New York, where there is a particularly high rate of breast cancer. Researchers hypothesize that the increased exposure to these chemicals, still in our environment, is the result of eating coastal fish. Added to all of this is the exposure to trans fats and cancer-causing compounds that are released when meat, fish, or fowl is grilled, fried, or barbecued.[55] Clearly, cancer causation is a complicated, multifactorial issue.

Cancers Associated with Increased Consumption of Animal Products[56]

Bladder cancer	Lung cancer
Brain cancer	Lymphoma
Breast cancer	Oropharyngeal cancer
Colon cancer	Ovarian cancer
Endometrial cancer	Pancreatic cancer
Intestinal cancer	Prostate cancer
Kidney cancer	Skin cancer
Leukemia	Stomach cancer

Exercise Powerfully Reduces Cancer Risk

Researchers at the University of Tromsø in Norway report that women who exercise regularly reduce their risk of developing breast cancer substantially. Their study involved more than 25,000 women ages twenty to fifty-four at the time of their entry into the study. The researchers found that younger, premenopausal women (under forty-five years old) who exercised regularly had 62 percent less risk than sedentary women. The risk reduction was highest for lean women who exercised more than four hours per week; these women had a 72 percent reduction in risk.

Diet and exercise have a much more important role to play in cancer prevention than mammograms and other detection methods. Keep in mind that mammograms merely detect, not prevent, cancer; they show disease only after the cancerous cells have been proliferating for many years.[57] By that time the majority of cancers have already spread from their local site and surgically removing the tumor is not curative. Only a minority of women who have their breast cancers detected by a mammogram have their survival increased because of the earlier detection.[58] The majority would have done just as well to find it later. I am not aiming to discourage women ages fifty to sixty-five from having mammograms; rather, my message is that this alone is insufficient. Mammograms, which do nothing to prevent breast cancer, are heavily publicized, while women hear nothing else about what they can do to prevent and protect themselves against breast cancer in the first place.

Do not underestimate the effect of a superior diet on gradually removing and repairing damage caused by years of self-abuse. Do not be discouraged just because you cannot bring your risk down to zero because of your mistakes in the past. The same thing could be said for cigarette smokers. Should they not quit smoking, merely because their risk of lung cancer can't be brought down to zero when they quit? Actually, lung cancer rates are considerably lower (about one-fifth) in countries that have a high vegetable consumption, even though they may smoke like crazy.[59] Raw fruits and vegetables offer powerful protection; leafy greens are the most protective.[60]

My main point is that our population has been ignoring those interventions that can most effectively save lives. We search for more answers because the ones we have found are not to our liking. Our most powerful artillery on the war against breast cancer, and cancer in general, is to follow the overall advice presented in this book and begin at as young an age as possible.

Increasing the Survival of Cancer Patients

It would be difficult for anyone to disagree that superior nutrition has a protective effect against cancer. The question that remains is this: Can optimal nutrition or nutritional intervention be an effective therapeutic approach for patients who already have cancer? Can the diet you eat make a difference if you have cancer? Scientific data indicates that the answer is yes.

Researchers looking for answers to these questions studied women with cancer and found that saturated fat in the diet promoted a more rapid spread of the cancer.[61] Other researchers found similar results. For a woman who already has cancer, her risk of dying increased 40 percent for every 1,000 grams of fat consumed monthly.[62] Studies also indicate that high fruit and vegetable intake improved survival, and fat on the body increases the risk of a premature death.[63]

Similar findings are found in the scientific literature regarding prostate cancer and diet, indicating that diet has a powerful effect on survival for those with prostate cancer.[64] For humans, *too much processed food and too many animal products are toxic.*

ANIMAL PROTEIN	PLANT PROTEIN
Raises cholesterol	Lowers cholesterol
Cancer promoter	Cancer protector
Promotes bone loss	Promotes bone strength
Promotes kidney disease	No effect
Accelerates aging	No effect
Packaged with	*Packaged with*
Saturated fat	Fiber
Cholesterol	Phytochemicals
Arachidonic acid	Antioxidants

When it is consumed in significant volume, animal protein, not only animal fat, is earning a reputation as a toxic nutrient to humans. More books are touting the benefits of high-protein diets for weight loss and are getting much publicity. Many Americans wish to protect their addiction to high-fat, nutrient-inadequate animal foods. These consumers form a huge market for such topsy-turvy scientific-sounding quackery.

Today the link between animal products and many different diseases is as strongly supported in the scientific literature as the link between cigarette smoking and lung cancer. For example, subjects who ate meat, including poultry and fish, were found to be twice as likely to develop dementia (loss of intellectual function with aging) as their vegetarian counterparts in a carefully designed study.[65] The discrepancy was further widened when past meat consumption was taken into account. The same diet, loaded with animal products, that causes heart disease and cancer also causes most every other disease prevalent in America, including kidney stones, renal insufficiency and renal failure, osteoporosis, uterine fibroids, hypertension, appendicitis, diverticulosis, and thrombosis.[66]

Are Dairy Foods Protecting Us from Osteoporosis?

Dairy products are held in high esteem in America. Most people consider a diet without dairy unhealthy. Without dairy foods, how could we obtain sufficient calcium for our bones? Let's examine this accepted wisdom: is it true, or have we been brainwashed by years and years of misinformation and advertising?

Hip fractures and osteoporosis are more frequent in populations in which dairy products are commonly consumed and calcium intakes are commonly high. For example, American women drink thirty to thirty-two times as much cow's milk as the New Guineans, yet suffer forty-seven times as many broken hips. A multicountry analysis of hip-fracture incidence and dairy-product consumption found that milk consumption has a high statistical association with higher rates of hip fractures.[67]

Does this suggest that drinking cow's milk causes osteoporosis? Certainly, it brings into question the continual advertising message from the National Dairy Council that drinking cow's milk prevents osteoporosis. The major finding from the Nurses'

Health Study, which included 121,701 women ages thirty to fifty-five at enrollment in 1976, was that the data does not support the hypothesis that the consumption of milk protects against hip or forearm fractures.[68] In fact, those who drank three or more servings of milk a day had a slightly higher rate of fractures than women who drank little or no milk.

This does not mean that dairy causes osteoporosis. However, it does suggest that dairy products are not protecting us from osteoporosis as we have been indoctrinated to believe since childhood. On the contrary, studies show fruits and vegetables are protective against osteoporosis.[69]

Osteoporosis has a complex etiology that involves other factors such as dietary acid-alkaline balance, trace minerals, phytochemicals in plants, exercise, exposure to sunlight, and more. Dr. Campbell, head of nutritional research for the China Project, reported, "Ironically, osteoporosis tends to occur in countries where calcium intake is highest and most of it comes from protein-rich dairy products. The Chinese data indicate that people need less calcium than we think and can get adequate amounts from vegetable source plant food." He told the *New York Times* that there was basically no osteoporosis in China, yet the calcium intake ranged from 241 to 943 mg per day (average, 544). The comparable U.S. calcium intake is 841 to 1,435 mg per day (average, 1,143), mostly from dairy sources, and, of course, osteoporosis is a major public health problem here.

To understand the causes of osteoporosis, one

must comprehend the concept of negative calcium balance. Let's say you consume about 1,000 mg of calcium a day. About a third of the calcium ingested gets absorbed. So if you absorb about 300 mg, the remaining 700 mg remains in the digestive tract and passes out with your stool. If, in this same twenty-four-hour period, you excreted 350 mg of calcium in your urine, would you be in a negative or positive calcium balance?

	NEGATIVE BALANCE	POSITIVE BALANCE
Ingested	1,000 mg	500 mg
Absorbed	300 mg	200 mg
Excreted	<u>350</u> mg	<u>100</u> mg
Retained	− 50 mg	+ 100 mg

A negative calcium balance means more calcium is excreted in the urine than is absorbed through digestion. A positive calcium balance means more calcium is absorbed than is excreted. A negative balance over time results in bone loss, as the additional calcium must come from our primary calcium storehouse, our bones.

Epidemiologic studies have linked osteoporosis not to low calcium intake but to various nutritional factors that cause excessive calcium loss in the urine. The continual depletion of our calcium reserves over time, from excessive calcium excretion in the urine, is the primary cause of osteoporosis. Now, let us consider the factors that contribute to this excessive urinary calcium excretion.

**Dietary Factors That Induce Calcium
Loss in the Urine[70]**

animal protein

salt

caffeine

refined sugar

alcohol

nicotine

aluminum-containing antacids

drugs such as antibiotics, steroids, thyroid hormone

vitamin A supplements

Published data clearly links increased urinary excretion of calcium with animal-protein intake but not with vegetable-protein intake.[71] Plant foods, though some may be high in protein, are not acid-forming. Animal-protein ingestion results in a heavy acid load in the blood. This sets off a series of reactions whereby calcium is released from the bones to help neutralize the acid. The sulfur-based amino acids in animal products contribute significantly to urinary acid production and the resulting calcium loss.[72] The Nurses' Health Study found that women who consumed 95 grams of protein a day had a 22 percent greater risk of forearm fracture than those who consumed less than 68 grams.[73]

The most comprehensive epidemiological survey involving hip fractures and food was done in 1992.[74] The authors sought out every peer-reviewed geographical report ever done on hip-fracture incidence.

They located thirty-four published studies of women in sixteen countries. Their analysis showed that diets high in animal protein had the highest correlation with hip-fracture rates, with an 81 percent correlation between eating animal protein and fractures.

The extra calcium contained in dairy foods simply cannot counteract the powerful effect of all the factors listed in the table above. The average American diet is not only high in protein but high in salt, sugar, and caffeine and low in fruits and vegetables. Fruits and vegetables can help buffer the acid load from all the animal protein and reduce calcium loss.[75] So we need to consume a lot more calcium to make up for the powerful combination of factors that induce calcium loss in the urine.

Some researchers believe it is possible to compensate for our high protein intake just by consuming more calcium.[76] This might be the case if the only thing we did to excess was consume a little too much animal protein, but in the context of everything else we do wrong in the American diet and lifestyle, it just doesn't fly.

Drinking more milk is simply not protective. Taking extra calcium supplements may help trim the calcium loss a little and slow the rate of bone loss, but not enough. We need to reduce the other causes, too. We even add vitamin A to milk, and many women take vitamin A supplements, which contributes to more calcium loss.[77]

All these factors help explain why calcium intake does not correlate well with reduced hip-fracture rates around the globe. The Eskimos are a perfect

COUNTRY	ANIMAL PROTEIN INTAKE (APPROXIMATE G/DAY)	HIP FRACTURE RATE (PER 100,000 PEOPLE)
South Africa (blacks)	10.4	6.8
New Guinea	16.4	3.1
Singapore	24.7	21.6
Yugoslavia	27.3	27.6
Hong Kong	34.6	45.6
Israel	42.5	93.2
Spain	47.6	42.4
Netherlands	54.3	87.7
United Kingdom	56.6	118.2
Denmark	58	165.3
Sweden	59.4	187.8
Finland	60.5	111.2
Ireland	61.4	76
Norway	66.6	190.4
United States	72	144.9
New Zealand	77.8	119

example. They consume a huge amount of calcium, over 2,000 mg a day, from all the soft fish bones they eat, yet they have the highest hip-fracture rate in the world because they consume so much animal protein from fish.[78]

The Best Foods for Bones: Fruits and Vegetables

Green vegetables, beans, tofu, sesame seeds, and even oranges contain lots of usable calcium, without the problems associated with dairy. Keep in mind that you retain the calcium better and just do not need as much when you don't consume a diet heavy in animal products and sodium, sugar, and caffeine.

Many green vegetables have calcium-absorption rates of over 50 percent, compared with about 32 percent for milk.[79] Additionally, since animal protein induces calcium excretion in the urine, the calcium retention from vegetables is higher. All green vegetables are high in calcium.

The American "chicken and pasta" diet style is significantly low in calcium, so adding dairy as a calcium source to this mineral-poor diet makes superficial sense—it is certainly better than no calcium in the diet. However, much more than just calcium is missing. The only reason cow's milk is considered such an important source of calcium is that the American diet is centered on animal foods, refined grains, and sugar, all of which are devoid of calcium. Any healthy diet containing a reasonable amount of unrefined plant foods will have sufficient calcium without milk. Fruits and vegetables strengthen bones. Researchers have found that those who eat the most fruits and vegetables have denser bones.[80] These researchers concluded that not only are fruits and vegetables rich in potassium, magnesium, calcium, and other nutrients essential for bone health, but, because they are alkaline, not acid-producing, they do not induce urinary calcium loss. Green vegetables in particular have a powerful effect on reducing hip fractures, for they are rich not only in calcium but in other nutrients, such as vitamin K, which is crucial for bone health.[81]

Deadly Vitamin D Levels

Numerous studies have shown that most Americans are severely vitamin D–deficient, a condition that causes osteoporosis as well as increased heart disease, cancer, and autoimmune disease.

Vitamin D helps maintain healthy levels of calcium in the blood, ensuring that calcium is always available to the body's tissues. It increases calcium absorption in the small intestine, decreases calcium excretion in the urine, and facilitates the release of calcium from bones. A deficiency of vitamin D can cause increased demineralization of bone, leading to weak and soft bones. Strong evidence indicates that three out of four Americans would benefit from vitamin D supplementation with respect to fracture and fall prevention, and possibly other public health targets, such as cardiovascular health, diabetes, and cancer.[82]

The optimal range for vitamin D seems to be between 35 and 50 ng/mL.[83] Almost 80 percent of Americans are below this level. Approximately 50 percent of Americans have a vitamin D level below 20 ng/mL, which is dangerously low. For the past fifteen years, I have been telling people to track their blood levels of vitamin D and to take vitamin D supplements. These recommendations have recently been corroborated by the Food and Nutrition Board of the Institute of Medicine and the American Academy of Pediatrics.

Medical research studies that demonstrate the effectiveness of vitamin D supplements on reducing the risk of bone fractures and cancers depend on doses significantly higher than the standard recommended daily dose of 400 IU.[84] Most people need to take more than 1,000 IU of supplemental vitamin D to achieve adequate blood levels and to get substantial protection against osteoporosis, as well as life-threatening diseases such as cancer and heart disease. Some may need to take even higher doses initially to reestablish optimal blood levels.

Vitamin D is found naturally in very few foods; the primary sources are the sun, fortified dairy products, mushrooms, and supplements. I do not recommend consumption of dairy products, and sun exposure places you at unnecessary risk of skin cancer and wrinkling and aging of your skin. Regardless of the increased risk of skin damage, adequate sunshine is simply not available to our population of indoor workers living in northern latitudes. Taking a daily supplement is your best choice for establishing and maintaining optimal levels of vitamin D.

Got Milk—Or Leave It?

Dairy is best kept to a minimum. There are many good reasons not to consume dairy. For example, there is a strong association between dairy lactose and ischemic heart disease.[85] There is also a clear association between high-growth-promoting foods such as dairy products and cancer. There is a clear association between milk consumption and bladder, prostate, colorectal, and testicular cancers.[86] Dairy fat is also loaded with various toxins and is the pri-

mary source of our nation's high exposure to
dioxin.[87] Dioxin is a highly toxic chemical compound that even the U.S. Environmental Protection
Agency admits is a prominent cause of many types
of cancer in those consuming dairy fat, such as butter and cheese.[88] Cheese is also a powerful inducer
of acid load, which increases calcium loss further.[89]
Considering that cheese and butter are the foods
with the highest saturated-fat content and the major
source of our dioxin exposure, cheese is a particularly foolish choice for obtaining calcium.

Cow's milk is "designed" to be the perfect food
for the rapidly growing calf, but as mentioned above,
foods that promote rapid growth promote cancer.
There is ample evidence implicating dairy consumption as a causative factor in both prostate and ovarian
cancer.[90] In April 2000 the Physicians' Health Study
reported that having 2.5 servings of dairy each day
boosted prostate cancer risk by more than 30 percent.[91] Another controlled study conducted in Greece
has shown a strong association between dairy products and prostate cancer.[92] By analyzing the data, the
authors calculated that if the population of Greece
were to increase its consumption of tomatoes and
decrease its consumption of dairy products, prostate
cancer incidence could be reduced by 41 percent, and
an even greater reduction would be possible in America, where the dietary risk is even higher. Other studies have found that prostate cancer risk was elevated
with increased consumption of low-fat milk, suggest-
ing that the potential threat to prostate health may be
correlated more to dairy protein than dairy fat.[93]

Dairy protein boosts the amount of IGF-1 in the blood. IGF-1 is found in cow's milk and has been shown to occur in increased levels in the blood of individuals consuming dairy products on a regular basis.[94] IGF-1 is known to stimulate the growth of both normal and cancer cells. Case-control studies in diverse populations have shown a strong and consistent association between serum IGF-1 concentrations and prostate cancer risk.[95] One study showed that men who had the highest levels of IGF-1 had more than four times the risk of prostate cancer compared with those who had the lowest levels.[96]

Investigating the link between lactose (milk sugar) and ovarian cancer among the 80,326 women enrolled in the Nurses' Health Study, Dr. Kathleen Fairfield and her associates reported that women who consumed the highest amount of lactose (one or more servings of dairy per day) had a 44 percent greater risk for all types of invasive ovarian cancer than those who ate the lowest amount (three or fewer servings monthly). Skim and low-fat milk were the largest contributors to lactose consumption.[97] Dairy products are just not the healthiest source of calcium.

Perhaps the strongest argument against dairy products in our diet: lots of us are lactose-intolerant. Those lactose-intolerant folks, who don't digest dairy well, are continually barraged with information that makes them believe they will lose their bones if they don't consume dairy products in some way. They may be better off without it.

If you choose to consume dairy, minimize your intake to small amounts. Remember the 90 percent rule: eat 90 percent health-giving whole-plant foods. Dairy may be a part of that 10 percent; however, it is not essential for good health and carries potential health risks.

You do not need dairy products to get sufficient calcium if you eat a healthy diet. All unprocessed natural foods are calcium-rich; even a whole orange (not orange juice) has about 60 mg of calcium.

CALCIUM IN 100 CALORIES OF:

bok choy	775
turnip greens	685
collard greens	539
tofu	287
kale	257
romaine lettuce	194
milk	189
sesame seeds, unhulled	170
broccoli	114
cucumber	107
carrots	81
cauliflower	70
soybeans	59
flaxseeds	48
fish	33
eggs	32
pork chop	4
T-bone steak	3

Government health authorities advise us to consume 1,500 mg of calcium daily. This is a tremendous amount of calcium. So much is recommended because of all the factors mentioned above. Even this high level of calcium will not prevent osteoporosis, but in a population with so many factors that cause osteoporosis, the extra calcium will make the negative balance less negative and partially slow the rate of osteoporosis. However, the only way to prevent osteoporosis and have strong bones is to exercise and to stop the causes of high urinary calcium excretion. *Eat to Live* describes a diet that protects against osteoporosis.

5

Nutritional Wisdom
Makes You Thin

Case Study:
Can you imagine losing 333 pounds? Scott realized that bariatric surgery was not a solution for him and, after much research, embraced Dr. Fuhrman's Eat to Live diet.

Starting in puberty, I put on weight. Even though I was a competitive swimmer, rode my bike everywhere, and played pickup games of football and baseball, I still packed on the pounds.

Eventually I got married and became a stay-at-home dad, which was a privilege but also very isolating and lonely. My weight increased dramatically, yet I denied the seriousness of the problem. One day I woke up and admitted that I had fallen directly into a huge, black pit. In November 2005, I weighed 501 pounds.

I was unable to walk more than a few feet. My knees, lower back, and feet suffered greatly, causing

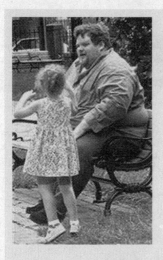
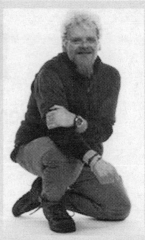

my independence of movement to be completely gone. My wife, who is a nurse, had to help me shower, dress, walk, etc., and consequently I had no self-esteem. She also noticed that I had developed serious sleep apnea. Life was intolerable. Weighing as much as I did, I couldn't move without a lot of pain and exhaustion. I stepped outside my house at the most four to six times a year.

I went to three different surgeons for bariatric surgery consultations but couldn't and wouldn't commit to it. It seemed as though I would be handing my problem over to someone else to fix. This was my problem, and I had to solve it or live with the negative consequences. I chose to solve it.

I discovered Eat to Live and decided to commit to it. After years of trying fad diets to lose weight, I was no longer interested in the D word. Eat to

Live was not about a goal weight. It was about doing what was healthy for my body. I thought the results would follow—and they did! By February of 2009, I had lost 333 pounds and had my health and my life back.

	BEFORE	AFTER
Weight	501 lbs.	168 lbs.
Cholesterol	170	65
Blood pressure	126/72	109/65
Resting heart rate	88	50
Body fat	62%	10%

I started exercising again. For me, biking made complete sense, as it was a way to move around without further destroying what was left of my body. It also reconnected me with all the best parts of my childhood—that sense of adventure and freedom. It was, is, and always will be great for me. That first year I rode approximately 1,400 miles. Last year I rode 19,700 miles, and this year I'm shooting for 25,000. Now, as a family, we do almost all our errands on our bikes. Anywhere we used to go by car, we now take a bike.

When I was morbidly obese, I felt worthless, unclean, stupid, unacceptable, and rejected. Eat to Live gave me a new life. Physically I feel great. My wife even admits that she can't keep up with me now.

Make a sacred pact to commit to this new lifestyle. Do it at any and all costs. This is the only way out.

Now that we've cleared up some popular misconceptions about nutrition, we can go on to analyze food components. After reading this chapter, you will understand how eating lots of nutrient-dense foods will make you lose weight.

Unrefined Carbohydrates Encourage Weight Loss

Our bodies need carbohydrates more than any other substance. Our muscle cells and brains are designed to run on carbohydrates. Carbohydrate-rich foods, when consumed in their natural state, are low in calories and high in fiber compared with fatty foods, processed foods, or animal products.

Fat contains about nine calories per gram, but protein and carbohydrates contain approximately four calories per gram. So when you eat high-carbohydrate foods, such as fresh fruits and beans, you can eat more food and still keep your caloric intake relatively low. The high fiber content of (unrefined) carbohydrate-rich foods is another crucial reason you will feel more satisfied and not crave more food when you make unrefined carbohydrates the main source of calories in your diet.

It is usually the small amount of added refined fat or oils that makes natural carbohydrates so fattening. For example, one cup of mashed potatoes is only 130 calories. Put just one tablespoon of butter on top and you have added another 100 calories.

Protein, fat, and carbohydrates are called *macronutrients*. Vitamins and minerals are referred to as *micronutrients*. All plant foods are a mixture of protein, fat, and carbohydrate (the macronutrients). Even a banana contains about 3.5 percent protein, almost the same as mother's milk. Fruit and starchy vegetables, such as sweet potatoes, corn, and butternut squash, are predominantly carbohydrate but also contain some fat and protein. Green vegetables are about half protein, a quarter carbohydrate, and a quarter fat. Legumes and beans are about half carbohydrate, a quarter protein, and a quarter fat.

One of the principles behind the health and weight-loss formula in this book is not to be overly concerned about the macronutrient balance; if you eat healthful foods, you will automatically get enough of all three macronutrients as long as you do not consume too many calories from white flour, sugar, and oil. So don't fear eating foods rich in carbohydrate and don't be afraid of eating fruit because it contains sugar. Even the plant foods that are high in carbohydrate contain sufficient fiber and nutrients and are low enough in calories to be considered nutritious. As long as they are unrefined, they should not be excluded from your diet. In fact, it is impossible to glean all the nutrients needed for optimal health if your diet does not contain lots of carbohydrate-rich food.

Fresh fruits, beans and legumes, whole grains, and root vegetables are all examples of foods whose calories come mainly from carbohydrate. It is the nutrient-per-calorie ratio of these foods that determines their food value. There is nothing wrong with carbohydrates; it is the empty-calorie, or refined, carbohydrates that are responsible for the bad reputation of carbs.

Understanding the Concept of Caloric Density

Because meats, dairy, and oils are so dense in calories, it is practically impossible for us to eat them without consuming an excess of calories. These calorie-rich foods can pile up a huge number of calories way before our stomachs are full and our hunger satisfied. However, eating foods higher in nutrients and fiber and lower in calories allows us to become satiated without consuming excess calories.

When subjects eating foods low in caloric density, such as fruits and vegetables, were compared with those consuming foods richer in calories, those on meal plans with higher calorie concentrations were found to consume twice as many calories per day in order to satisfy their hunger.[1]

Your body must burn about 23 percent of the calories consumed from carbohydrates to make the conversion from glucose into fat, but it converts food fat into body fat quickly and easily. One hundred calories of ingested fat can be converted to ninety-seven calories of body fat, burning a measly three calories. When you consume oil or animal fat, the fat you eat is easily and rapidly stored by the body.

Converting food fat into body fat is easy; the process doesn't even modify the molecules. Research

MORE BULK MEANS FEWER CALORIES

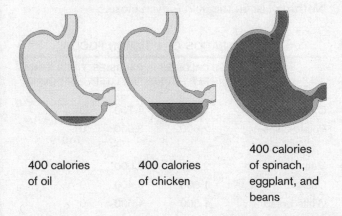

400 calories
of oil

400 calories
of chicken

400 calories
of spinach,
eggplant, and
beans

scientists can actually take fat biopsies off your hips
or waist and tell you where it came from—pig fat,
dairy fat, chicken fat, or olive oil. The fat is still the
same as it was on your plate, but now it is under
your skin. The saying "from your lips to your hips"
is literally true. Fat is also an appetite stimulant—
the more you eat, the more you want.

Foods That Make You Thin

Appetite is not controlled by the weight of the food
but by fiber, nutrient density, and caloric density. It
is even useful to approximate the amount of calories
per volume. Since the stomach can hold about one
liter of food, let's look at how many calories are in a
whole stomachful of a particular food.

It's pretty clear which foods will let you feel full
with the least amount of calories—fruits and vegetables. Green vegetables, fresh fruits, and legumes

again take the gold, silver, and bronze medals. Nothing else in the field is even close.

CALORIC RATIOS OF COMMON FOODS

	CALORIES PER POUND	CALORIES PER LITER	FIBER GRAMS PER POUND
Oils	3,900	7,700	0
Potato chips or french fries	2,600	3,000	0
Meat	2,000	3,000	0
Cheese	1,600	3,400	0
White bread	1,300	1,500	0
Chicken and turkey (white meat)	900	1,600	0
Fish	800	1,400	0
Eggs	700	1,350	0
Whole grains (wheat and rice)	600	1,000	3
Starchy vegetables (potatoes and corn)	350	600	4
Beans	**350**	**500**	**5**
Fruits	**250**	**300**	**9**
Green vegetables	**100**	**200**	**5**

Green vegetables are so incredibly low in calories and rich in nutrients and fiber that the more of them you eat, the more weight you will lose. One of my secrets to nutritional excellence and superior health is the one pound–one pound rule. That is, try to eat at least one pound of raw vegetables a day and one pound of cooked/steamed or frozen green or nongreen nutrient-rich vegetables a day as well. One pound raw and one pound cooked—keep this goal in mind as you design and eat every meal. This may be too ambitious a goal for some of us to reach, but by working toward it, you will ensure the dietary balance and results you want. The more vegetables you eat, the more weight you will lose. The high volume of greens not only will be your secret to a thin waistline but will simultaneously protect you against life-threatening illnesses.

THE NUTRIENT-DENSITY LINE

The nutrient-density scores below are based on identified phytochemicals, antioxidant activity, and total vitamin and mineral content.

Highest nutrient density = 100 points	Lowest nutrient density = 0

100	Dark green leafy vegetables *kale, mustard greens, collard greens, Swiss chard, watercress, spinach, arugula*
95	Other green vegetables *romaine, bok choy, cabbage, Brussels sprouts, asparagus, broccoli, string beans, snow peas, green peas*
50	Non-green nutrient-rich vegetables *beets, eggplant, mushrooms, onions, radishes, bean sprouts, red and yellow bell peppers, radicchio, cauliflower, tomatoes, artichokes, raw carrots*

45   Fresh fruits
*strawberries, blueberries, other berries,
plums, oranges, melons, kiwifruit,
apples, cherries, pineapple, peaches,
pears, grapes, banana*s

40   Beans
*lentils, kidney, great northern, adzuki,
black, pinto, split peas, edamame,
chickpeas*

30   Raw nuts and seeds
*sunflower, pumpkin, sesame, flaxseeds,
almonds, cashews, pistachios, walnuts,
pecans, hazelnuts*

25   Colorful starchy vegetables
*butternut and other squash, sweet
potatoes, corn, turnips*

20   Whole grains/white potatoes
*old-fashioned oats, barley, brown and
wild rice, buckwheat, millet, quinoa,
bulgur, whole grain bread, white
potatoes*

18   Fish

15   Fat-free dairy

15   Eggs

15   Wild meat and fowl

8   Full-fat dairy

6   Red meat

6	Refined grain products
3	Cheese
1	Refined oils
0	Refined sweets
	cookies, cakes, candy, soda

One of the most fascinating areas of research in recent years has been related to the therapeutic value of cruciferous vegetables, which include vegetables in the cabbage family and others such as kale, collards, watercress, arugula, cauliflower, and bok choy. Cruciferous vegetables have the most powerful anti-cancer effects of all foods. Most of the phytonutrients function as antioxidants in your body, meaning they neutralize free radicals, rendering them harmless and reducing cancer risk. The phytonutrients in cruciferious vegetables also activate your body's own antioxidant control system. These unique compounds cycle through the body for three to five days after consumption, offering protection and fueling numerous bodily systems, enabling them to function more effectively.

Vegetables have powerful levels of carotenoids and other nutrients that prevent age-related diseases. For example, the leading cause of age-related blindness in America is macular degeneration. Low carotenoid levels in the macula are now considered a risk factor for macular degeneration.[2] If you eat greens at least five times per week, your risk drops by more than 86 percent. Lutein and zeaxanthin are

LUTEIN AND/OR ZEAXANTHIN IN FOODS[3] (in micrograms)

1 cup cooked kale	28,470
1 cup cooked collard greens	27,710
1 cup cooked spinach	23,940
1 cup cooked Swiss chard	19,360
1 cup cooked mustard greens	14,850
1 cup cooked red bell pepper	13,600
1 cup cooked beet greens	11,090
1 cup cooked okra	10,880
4 cups romaine lettuce	12,770

carotenoids with powerful disease-prevention properties. Researchers have found that those with the highest blood levels of lutein had the healthiest blood vessels, with little or no atherosclerosis.[4]

Nutrient:Weight Ratios Are Misleading

William Harris, M.D., performed an analysis of major food groups titled "Less Grains, More Greens,"[5] though he didn't assign phytochemical activity. Dr. Harris explains in detail why ranking and analyzing foods by nutrient:weight ratios, the nutritional establishment's usual method, is ill-advised and misleading.[6]

People do not eat until a certain weight of food is consumed but rather until they are calorically and nutritively fulfilled. He compares an analysis of spinach with that of spinach with water added (spinach soup) and shows how the weight (added water) does not change the nutrients received. If we analyze the nutrients by weight, we incorrectly think that spinach with water added is much less nutritious.

Furthermore, Harris explains why the food industry, especially the producers of animal products, is opposed to nutrient: calorie analysis. It is because nutrient-per-weight sorting hides how deficient animal foods are in nutrients, especially the crucial anti-cancer nutrients. As Dr. Harris states, nutrient-per-weight sorting is "a great way to keep excess calories, cholesterol and saturated fat in the diet, which is a splendid way to grow an arteriosclerotic, obese, cancer-ridden nation, which is what we have."

EATING TO ENHANCE THE NUTRIENT-PER-CALORIE DENSITY OF ONE'S DIET:

- Causes weight loss that is permanent
- Promotes longevity
- Derails hunger and food cravings
- Increases immune function and disease resistance
- Has therapeutic effects to reverse disease
- Protects against heart disease, stroke, and dementia
- Fuels cellular repair mechanisms protecting against cancer

Fats Are Essential

It is true that most of us eat too much fat, but scientific research is revealing that too little fat can be a problem, too. We have learned that not merely are we consuming too much fat but, more important, we are consuming the wrong fats. Americans consume too much of some bad fats and not enough of other fats that we need to maximize health.

Essential fatty acids (EFAs) are polyunsaturated dietary fats that the body cannot manufacture, so they are required for health. EFAs are important for the structure and function of cell membranes and serve as precursors to hormones, which play an important role in our health. These fats are essential not only in growth and development but also in the prevention and treatment of chronic diseases.[7]

The two primary essential fatty acids are linoleic acid, an omega-6 fat, and alpha-linolenic acid, an omega-3 fat. The body can make other fatty acids, called nonessential fats, from these two basic fats. Linoleic acid's first double bond is at the location of its sixth carbon, so it is called an omega-6 fatty acid, and alpha-linolenic acid's first double bond is on its third carbon, so it is called an omega-3 fatty acid.

Optimal health depends on the proper balance of fatty acids in the diet. The modern diet that most of us eat supplies an excessive amount of omega-6 fat but often too little omega-3 fat. This relative deficiency of omega-3 fat has potentially serious implications. Also, the consumption of too much omega-6 fat leads to high levels of arachidonic acid. Higher levels of arachidonic acid can promote inflammation.

When we have insufficient omega-3 fat, we do not produce enough DHA, a long-chain omega-3

OMEGA-6 FAT	OMEGA-3 FAT
Linoleic acid	Alpha-linolenic acid
▼	▼
GLA (gamma linolenic acid)	EPA (eicospentaenoic acid)
▼	▼
AA (arachidonic acid)	DHA (docosahexaenoic acid)
▼	▼
pro-inflammatory prostaglandins and leukotrienes	anti-inflammatory prostaglandins and leukotrienes

fat with anti-inflammatory effects. High levels of arachidonic acid and low levels of omega-3 fat can be a contributory cause of heart disease, stroke, autoimmune diseases, skin diseases, depression, and possibly increased cancer incidence.[8]

Most Americans would improve their health if they consumed more omega-3 fat and less omega-6 fat. I recommend that both vegetarians and nonvegetarians make an effort to consume 1 to 2 grams of omega-3 fat daily.

ADD A FEW GRAMS OF OMEGA-3 FAT TO YOUR DIET

Flaxseeds	1 tablespoon	1.7 g
Walnuts, English (12 walnut halves)	4 tablespoons	2 g
Soybeans (green, frozen, or raw)	1½ cups	2 g
Tofu	1½ cups	2 g

A diet very high in omega-6 fat makes matters worse; your body makes even less DHA fat. We need enough DHA fat to ensure optimum health. The high level of omega-6 fat competes for the enzymes involved in fatty acid desaturation (conversion to longer-chain fats) and interferes with the conversion of alpha-linolenic acid (omega-3) to EPA and DHA. Therefore, our high fat intake contributes to our DHA fat deficiency.

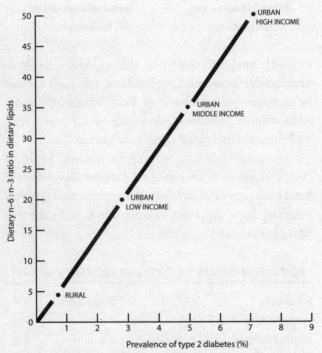

Diabetes is only one of many diseases linked to excessive omega-6 fats.
Source: Simopoulos, A. P. 1999. Essential fatty acids in health and chronic disease. *American Journal of Clinical Nutrition.* 70(3): 560–69.

Our modern diet, full of vegetable oils and animal products, is very high in omega-6 fat and very low in omega-3 fat; the higher the omega-6 to omega-3 ratio, the higher the risk of heart disease, diabetes, and inflammatory illnesses.[9]

Saturated fat, cholesterol, and trans fat also interfere with conversion to DHA. Among the most beneficial effects of a diet rich in plant foods are the low level of saturated fat and trans fat (harmful fats) and the relatively high level of essential fatty acids (beneficial fats). Both meat-based diets and vegetarian diets can be deficient in these healthy fats if they do not contain sufficient green leaves, beans, nuts, seeds, or fish. So, eat less of the fatty foods you usually consume and eat more walnuts, flaxseeds, soybeans, and leafy green vegetables.

The Fat Dictionary

All fats are equally fattening—containing nine calories per gram, compared with four calories per gram for carbohydrates and protein.

ARACHIDONIC ACID is a long-chain omega-6 fat produced by the body, but it is also found in meat, fowl, dairy, and eggs. Products made with excessive amounts of this fatty acid have the potential to increase inflammation and are disease-causing. They may increase high blood pressure, thrombosis, vasospasm, and allergic reaction. They are linked to arthritis, depression, and other common illnesses.

CHOLESTEROL is a waxy fat produced by the body and found in animal foods such as meat, fowl, dairy, and eggs. Eating cholesterol raises blood cholesterol, but not as much as eating saturated fats and trans fats. The amount of cholesterol in plants is so negligible that you should consider them cholesterol-free.

DHA FAT is a long-chain omega-3 fat that is made by the body, but it can also be found in fish such as salmon and sardines. DHA is used in the production of anti-inflammatory mediators that inhibit abnormal immune function and prevent excessive blood clotting. DHA is not considered an essential fat because the body can manufacture sufficient amounts if adequate short-chain omega-3 fats (flaxseeds, walnuts, soybeans, leafy green vegetables) are consumed. However, because of genetic differences in the enzyme activity and because of excess omega-6 fats, many people who do not consume fatty fish regularly are deficient in this important fat.

HYDROGENATED FAT Hydrogenation is a process of adding hydrogen molecules to unsaturated fats, thereby turning these oils, which are liquid at room temperature, into harder, more saturated fats such as margarine. Hardening the fat extends its shelf life so the oil can be used over and over again to fry potatoes in a fast-food restaurant or be added to processed foods such as crackers and cookies. While hydrogenation does not make the fat completely saturated, it creates trans fatty acids, which act like saturated fats. Evidence is accumulating to implicate the harmful nature of these man-made fats in both cancer and heart disease. Avoid all foods whose ingredients contain partially hydrogenated or hydrogenated oils.

MONOUNSATURATED FAT These fats have only one double bond in their carbon chain. They are liquid at room temperature and thought to have health benefits. The supposed health benefits of these fats appear when they are used in place of dangerous saturated fats. But even polyunsaturated oils will lower cholesterol if used in place of saturated fat. Monounsaturated fat is found in avocados, almonds, peanuts, and most other nuts and seeds. Keep in mind that no isolated or refined fat, even these monounsaturated fats, should be considered health food. Oils with the highest percentage of monounsaturated fat include olive, canola, and peanut oils.

POLYUNSATURATED FAT These fatty acids have more than one double bond in their chain. These fats include corn oil, soybean oil, safflower oil, and sunflower oil. They are soft at room temperature. These fats promote the growth of cancer in lab animals more than olive oil (a monounsaturated fat) does.

SATURATED FAT Some naturally occurring fats are called saturated because all of the bonds in their carbon chain are single bonds. These fats are solid at room temperture and are generally recognized as a significant cause of both heart disease and cancer. Saturated fats are found mainly in meat, fowl, eggs, and dairy. Coconut and palm oil are largely saturated and are not desirable. The foods with the most saturated fat are butter, cream, and cheese.

UNSATURATED FAT These fats are a mix of
monounsaturated and polyunsaturated fats. Eating
unsaturated fats lowers cholesterol when substituted for
saturated fats, but excessive amounts may promote
cancer.

There's Something Fishy about Fish Oils

Most of the publicity about the beneficial effects of
essential fats has focused on fish oils, which are rich
in EPA, an omega-3 fat. One problem with fish oils
is that much of the fat has already turned rancid. If
you cut open a capsule of fish oil and taste it, you
will find it tastes like gasoline. Not only are many
people intolerant of the burping, indigestion, and
smelling like a fish, but it is also possible that the
rancidity of the fat places a stress on the liver. I have
noted abnormal liver function in the blood tests of a
few patients who were taking fish oil capsules.
These few patients had their liver function return to
normal when they stopped taking the fish oil.

Recently a lawsuit brought by environmentalists
in California against eight supplement manufacturers or distributors claimed that popular brands of
fish oil supplements contain unsafe and illegal levels
of polychlorinated biphenyls, or PCBs, which are
carcinogenic chemicals.[10] Testing found that levels
of PCBs in popular fish oil supplements varied
wildly, from about 12 nanograms per recommended
dose to more than 850 nanograms in the most contaminated product. The suit claimed that the manu-

facturers were in violation of California law for not disclosing any nonzero PCB levels in their products.

Large amounts of fish oils inhibit immune function.[11] Lowering the function of natural killer cells is not a good thing, as our defenses against infection and cancer diminish. Because of this immune suppression, as well as the toxicity issues, I do not routinely recommend that my patients take fish oil capsules—though there are a few exceptions.

This ability of fish oils to decrease the activity of the immune system makes them useful for some patients with autoimmune illnesses, such as rheumatoid arthritis or inflammatory bowel disease.[12] Some rheumatoid arthritis patients are "fish oil responsive," and many others are not. I often perform a three-month trial of fish oil supplementation to determine a patient's responsiveness. With such patients, the risks of the added oil are minimal compared with the potential benefits, especially if they can avoid toxic drugs. Of course, when using fish oil supplements, consider only the highly purified types, free of PCBs and mercury.

Another case in which fish oils may be useful is the individual who does not convert omega-3 fats into DHA sufficiently. These people may be more prone to depression, allergies, and inflammatory skin disease such as eczema. There are blood tests available for a physician to analyze the fatty acid balance on red blood cell membranes and thereby determine a deficiency of DHA or omega-3 fat. These people often benefit from the addition of fish oils or plant-derived DHA. Laboratory-cultivated DHA made from microalgae is a pure form of DHA without mercury or other toxins. It is well tolerated and does not have a rancid taste or odor.

Does Fish Prevent Heart Disease?

There are two components to a heart attack or stroke. First, you must develop atherosclerotic plaque. This plaque builds up over many years from eating a diet deficient in unrefined plant foods. Almost all Americans have such plaque. Autopsy studies demonstrate atherosclerosis even in the vast majority of American children.[13]

Once this fatty plaque accumulates and partially blocks a coronary artery, a clot can develop in a defect or crack in the surface of the plaque. This clot is called a thrombus, which can enlarge and completely block the vessel, causing a heart attack, or break off and travel upstream, obstructing a more distal coronary site. A traveling thrombus is called an embolus. Emboli and thrombi are the causes of almost all heart attacks and strokes.

Fish contains omega-3 fatty acids (EPA and DHA) that interfere with blood clotting much the same way aspirin does. Once you have significant atherosclerosis, it is helpful to take such anti-clotting agents, especially if you continue a dangerous diet. These fish-derived fats also have some effect on protecting the arterial walls from damage from other fats. For people eating saturated-fat-containing animal products, it is advisable to consume one or two weekly portions of fatty fish, such as sardines, salmon, trout, halibut, or mackerel, and reduce the consumption of other animal products accordingly. Increasing fish intake beyond one or two servings per week has not been shown to offer additional protection.[14]

However, the best way to prevent a heart attack or stroke is to follow a high-nutrient diet with little or no animal products, thereby ensuring that such blockages don't develop in the first place. Then eating fish won't matter. It is true that increasing blood levels of these important fish-derived fats reduces the incidence of heart attacks significantly.[15] However, contrary to popular belief, not only vegetarians but also most others eating diets with adequate plant material get most of their long-chain omega-3 fatty acids from non-fish sources.[16] In fact, the reason the fish-derived fats EPA and DHA are not considered essential fats is that almost all people have enzymes to convert the plant-derived omega-3 fat rapidly into EPA and DHA.[17]

Fish is a double-edged sword, especially because fish has been shown to increase heart attack risk if it is polluted with mercury.[18] Keep in mind that even though men in Finland consume lots of fish, their mortality from coronary heart disease is one of the highest in the world.[19] It seems that the cardioprotective effects of eating a little fish is lost when you eat lots of fish, most likely because lots of fish exposes you to high mercury levels, which can promote lipid peroxidation.[20] Lipid peroxidation occurs when body lipids react with oxygen to cause a compound that plays a major role in the development of diseases such as heart disease, diabetes, and arthritis.

In addition, those who consume fish in the hope of reducing their cardiac risk may be getting more than they bargained for—namely, toxic contaminants, including some that carry a cancer risk.

Fish is one of the most polluted foods we eat, and it may place consumers at high risk for various cancers. Scientists have linked tumors in fish directly to the pollutants ingested along the aquatic food chain, a finding confirmed by the National Marine Fisheries Service Laboratory. In some instances, such as with the PCBs in Great Lakes trout and salmon, it can be shown that a person would have to drink the lake water for one hundred years to accumulate the same quantity of PCBs present in a single half-pound portion of these fish, reported John J. Black, Ph.D., senior cancer research scientist for the Roswell Park Memorial Institute, to the American Cancer Society.[21] From the flounder in Boston Harbor to English sole in Puget Sound, scientists report that hydrocarbon pollution from habitat concentrate in fish. There are high cancer rates around New Orleans, where fresh fish and shellfish are a staple of the local cuisine.

Higher levels of mercury found in mothers who eat more fish have been associated with birth defects, seizures, mental retardation, developmental disabilities, and cerebral palsy.[22] This is mostly the result of women having eaten fish when they were pregnant. Scientists believe that fetuses are much

FISH WITH HIGHEST AND LOWEST MERCURY LEVELS

HIGHEST	LOWEST
tilefish	salmon
swordfish	flounder
mackerel	sole
shark	tilapia
	trout
	cod

Source: Mercury Levels in Commercial Fish and Shellfish.
http://www.fda.gov/food/foodsafety/
productspecificinformation/seafood/
foodbornepathogenscontaminants/methylmercury/
ucm115644.htm.

more sensitive to mercury exposure than are adults, although adults do suffer from varying degrees of brain damage from fish consumption.[23] Even the FDA, which normally ignores reports on the dangers of our dangerous food practices, acknowledges that large fish such as shark and swordfish are potentially dangerous. Researchers are also concerned about other toxins concentrated in fish that can cause brain damage way before the cancers caused by chemical-carrying fish appear.

Fish may also lower the effectiveness of our immune system. Those on high-fish diets have lower blood markers of immune system function, representing a lowered defense against infection and cancer.[24] Another problem with fish is that because fish oils inhibit blood clotting, they increase the likelihood that the delicate vessels in the brain can bleed, causing a hemorrhagic stroke. At the same time fish reduces the risk of heart attacks, it may be increasing the risk of a bleeding problem. Regular fish consumption or fish oil supplements should be avoided if a person has a family history or is at risk of hemorrhagic stroke or other bleeding disorders.

The bottom line: Choose fish over other animal products, but be aware that the place where it was caught and the type of fish matter. Don't accept recreational fish from questionable waters. Never eat high-mercury-content fish. Don't eat fish more than twice a week, and if you have a family history of hemorrhagic stroke, limit it further to only once a month.

Extracted Oils—One Slick Customer

Americans consume large quantities of oil, a refined food processed at high temperatures. When oils are subject to heat, the chemical structure of the essential fatty acids is changed to create toxic derivatives known as lipid peroxides and other toxic and potentially cancer-causing by-products.[25] Clearly, it is best to avoid fried foods and heated oils, not only because they will destroy your chances to achieve a normal weight but also because they are potentially cancer-causing.

Get your fats as nature packaged them. It is best to consume the small amount of fats we need in their original unprocessed, unheated, and natural packages: whole foods. Ground flaxseeds are healthier than flaxseed oil, as they contain valuable fiber, lignans, and other phytonutrients, not just omega-3 fat. Raw sunflower seeds, pumpkin seeds, corn, and avocados are healthy, but their extracted oils may not be. Even cold-pressed oils are subject to the damaging effects of heat and contain lipid peroxides. So I usually recommend to my patients that instead of consuming the oils, they consume a tablespoon of ground flaxseeds daily, or some walnuts, to ensure adequate omega-3 fat intake.

Remember, when you extract the oil from the whole food it was packaged in, you remove it from its antioxidant- and phytochemical-rich protective environment. You turn a moderate nutrient-to-calorie food into a low nutrient-to-calorie food, and at the same time damage the quality of the fat with heat. Romaine lettuce, kale, collards, and Swiss chard are rich in fiber, vitamins, minerals, phytochemicals, vegetable protein, and essential fats— another reason I consider leafy green vegetables the king of all foods.

Your diet should not be fat-free. Indeed, it would be nearly impossible to make this diet fat-deficient, because even green vegetables and beans contain beneficial fats. The focus should be on reducing (or removing) the harmful and processed fats, and instead consuming the healthy fats that are naturally contained in whole natural foods. Nonprocessed fats contained in avocados, sunflower seeds, and almonds, to name just a few sources, can be healthy additions to a wholesome diet of natural foods. Even though these foods have lots of calories, they pack a significant nutritive punch; they are rich in vitamin E and other antioxidants and are not nutrient-depleted the way the oil is when it is extracted, processed, and put in a bottle.

Be aware, however, that unless you are physically very active and slim, you should watch the amount of these relatively fat-rich plant products, as they obviously could interfere with reaching your ideal weight. If you are slim and exercise regularly, you can consume three to four ounces of raw nuts or seeds daily, an avocado, or a little olive oil. Growing children, or an individual who is having difficulty gaining weight, can eat a little more dietary fat, but it still should mostly be fat from the wholesome foods described above.

When you are overweight, you have a good store of fat on your body, so you don't need to worry about not ingesting enough fat. You are not going to become fat-deficient, even if your diet is low in fat. As you lose weight, you will actually be on a "high-fat diet," as you will be utilizing the fat you have around your midsection for energy. The only concern is to maintain a healthy ratio of omega-6 to omega-3 fatty acids, so I advise ingesting one tablespoon of ground flaxseeds every day, if possible. Many like to sprinkle it over fruit or add it to a salad.

Is There an Increased Risk of Stroke from Low-Fat Diets?

There is considerable evidence that while animal fats are definitely associated with an increase in heart disease, more fat may offer protection against hemorrhagic stroke.[26] Of course, recent investigations have shown the strong protective effects of

fruits and vegetables, but some data suggests t...
fat, even animal fat, offers some protection to the
smaller intracerebral vessels that cause hemorrhagic
strokes.[27]

There are two main types of strokes: ischemic
and hemorrhagic. Almost all heart attacks and the
vast majority of strokes are associated with ischemia
(lack of blood flow) from blood clots. The small percentage of strokes that are hemorrhagic (approximately 8 percent) result not from a cholesterol-laden
vessel leading to a clot but from a rupture of a small
artery in the brain as a result of years and years of
high blood pressure.[28] Some of these small, fragile
blood vessels in the brain possibly become more
resistant to rupture when they are more diseased
with fat. It is entirely possible that in certain cases,
the same diet that leads to abnormal clot formation
and causes 99 percent of heart attacks and over 90
percent of strokes may help the small intracerebral
vessels resist the tendency to rupture from years of
uncontrolled hypertension that results from a high-
salt diet. This is in no way a legitimate excuse to eat
more animal products. It makes more sense to eat the
healthful anti–heart attack diet and keep your blood
pressure down by not consuming much added salt.

The data is so confusing because many of the
studies group all types of strokes together, when
they are in fact very different diseases with completely different causes. Considering ischemic (or
embolic) strokes, the data from both human and rat
studies illustrates the importance of adequate essential omega-3 fat intake, including an increased

omega-3:omega-6 ratio.[29] These omega-3 fats are the same ones that protect against heart attacks, which are also of an ischemic nature. Keep in mind, saturated fat intake has consistently been associated with an increase in strokes in general because most strokes are of the ischemic (embolic) variety.[30]

Finally, to make things even more confusing, some monounsaturated fat intake offers a degree of protection against strokes and does not have the cholesterol-raising and other negative effects of saturated fats.[31] The studies showing the nutritional value of monounsaturated fats lend support to the Mediterranean diet and those advocating a diet rich in olive oil.

Obviously, some omega-6 fat is still essential and necessary for normal disease resistance. My view is that thin individuals should consume more monounsaturated fats from wholesome high-fat vegetation such as avocados, raw nuts, and seeds. Heavier people, because of their higher risk of heart disease, diabetes, and cancer, as well as the very limited occurrence of hemorrhagic stroke in the overweight, should limit their intake of these fats. Since heavier people have more stored fat on their body, they do not benefit from a higher intake of dietary fat the same way thin individuals do. As the overweight lose weight, they are already on a high-fat diet, consuming their stored body fat.

Let me remind you that the best fats are the monounsaturated fats and essential fats (omega-3 and omega-6) present in whole, natural plant foods, including avocados, and raw nuts and seeds. Studies continue to show that consumption of raw nuts protects against both heart attack and stroke, without the risks of increasing heart disease and cancer, as is the case with the high consumption of animal-origin fats.[32] When the fats you consume are from whole foods rather than oil, you gain nature's protective package: a balance of vitamins, minerals, fibers, and phytonutrients.

Nuts and Seeds Protect against Cardiovascular Death

Raw nuts and seeds are packed with nutrients. Lignans, bioflavonoids, minerals, and other antioxidants protect the fragile freshness of the nut and seed fats, and plant proteins and plant sterols naturally lower cholesterol.

Perhaps one of the most unexpected and novel findings in nutritional epidemiology in the past five years has been that nut and seed consumption offers such strong protection against heart disease. Several clinical studies have observed beneficial effects of diets high in nuts (including walnuts, peanuts, almonds, and other nuts) on blood lipids.[33] A review of twenty-three intervention trials using nuts and seeds convincingly demonstrated that daily consumption decreases total cholesterol and LDL (bad) cholesterol.[34] Not only do nuts and seeds lower LDL cholesterol, but they also raise HDL (good) cholesterol. Interestingly, they can help normalize a dangerous type of LDL molecule—the small, dense LDL particles that are damaging to blood vessels, particularly to the endothelial cells lining the blood vessels.[35]

When specifically compared with changes in known risk factors, such as lowering blood glucose or cholesterol levels, eating nuts and seeds has been found to decrease cardiovascular death and increase life span.[36] To date, five large studies (the Adventist Health Study, the Iowa Women's Health Study, the Nurses' Health Study, the Physicians' Health Study, and the CARE Study) have examined the relationship between nut and seed consumption and the risk of atherosclerotic heart disease. All found a strong inverse association.

Based on the data from the Nurses' Health Study, it was estimated that substituting the fat from one ounce of nuts for the equivalent energy from the carbohydrate in an average diet was associated with a 30 percent reduction in heart disease risk. The substitution of nut fat for saturated fat was associated with a 45 percent reduction in risk.

The Physicians' Health Study added much more to the story. The most fascinating, and perhaps most important, finding is that nuts and seeds do not just lower cholesterol and protect against heart attacks. Components of nuts and seeds also seem to have anti-arrhythmic and anti-seizure effects that dramatically reduce the occurrence of sudden death.[37] The Physicians' Health Study followed 21,454 male participants for an average of seventeen years. Researchers found a lower risk of sudden cardiac death and other coronary heart disease end points after controlling for known cardiac risk factors and other dietary habits. When compared with men who rarely or never consumed seeds or nuts, those who consumed two or more servings per week reduced the risk of sudden cardiac death by about 50 percent. Sudden cardiac death is not a heart attack, but rather a life-threatening cardiac arrhythmia called ventricular fibrillation or ventricular tachycardia. People who have heart disease do not always die of a heart attack; they can die of an irregular heartbeat that prevents the heart from pumping properly.

Eat Seeds and Nuts Instead of Oil for Healthy Weight Loss

Epidemiologic studies indicate an inverse association between frequency of nut and seed consumption and body mass index. Interestingly, their consumption may actually suppress appetite and help people get rid of diabetes and lose weight.[38] In other words, populations consuming more nuts and seeds are likely to be slim, and people consuming less seeds and nuts are more likely to be heavier. Well-controlled nut-feeding trials, designed to see whether eating nuts and seeds resulted in weight gain, showed the opposite: eating raw nuts and seeds promoted weight loss, not weight gain. Several studies have also shown that eating a small amount of nuts or seeds actually helps dieters feel satiated, stay with the program, and have more success achieving long-term weight loss.[39]

By contrast, refined oil, which contains 120 calories per tablespoon, is fattening and can sabotage weight loss. Plus, it does not have any protective effects on the heart. The secret here is to forgo the oil and instead make salad dressings, dips, and sauces by blending in seeds and nuts.

The healthiest diet for all ages is one that includes some healthy fatty foods. This same diet will also prevent and reverse disease. Even for people who are overweight, I recommend one ounce of raw, unsalted seeds or nuts per day, such as sesame seeds, sunflower seed, flaxseeds, pumpkin seeds, walnuts, pistachio nuts, or almonds.

Trans Fat: A Wolf in Sheep's Clothing

Trans fats do not exist in nature. They are laboratory-designed and have adverse health consequences. They interfere with the body's production of beneficial fatty acids and promote heart disease.[40] As trans fatty acids offer no benefits and only clear adverse metabolic consequences, when you see the words *partially hydrogenated* on the side of a box, consider what's inside poisonous and throw it in the trash.

Trans fats are surely cancer-promoting and raise your cholesterol as much as saturated fat.[41] Considering that they also reduce HDL (good) cholesterol, trans fats may be even more atherogenic than saturated fatty acids.[42] Convincing evidence from the Nurses' Health Study and others indicates that trans fats are as closely associated with heart attacks as the fats in animal products.[43]

The amount of trans fats used in foods has significantly decreased in recent years. Many food manufacturers have reformulated their products to reduce or eliminate trans fats. Food manufacturers now must indicate trans fat content on their products' nutritional labels. Beware that levels of less than 0.5 gram per serving can be listed as 0 grams trans fat, making it possible for a person eating multiple servings of a food labeled free of trans fat to still consume a significant amount.

The Fatty Conclusion

There is no question that a high-fat diet increases the risk of many cancers. This has been demonstrated in hundreds of animal and human studies. It's not only the amount of fat but also the type of fat that is linked to increased risk (just like the type of protein). It gets complicated, so here are the main points:

1. Any extracted oil (fat) can promote cancer because consuming even the healthier fats, such as olive oil, in excess adds too many empty calories. Excess calories have toxic effects, contributing to obesity, premature aging, and cancer.

2. Excess omega-6 fatty acids promote cancer risk, while omega-3 fats, which are harder to come by, tend to lower risk. Omega-6 fats are found in polyunsaturated oils such as corn oil and safflower oil, whereas omega-3 fatty acids are abundant in seeds, greens, and some fish.

3. The most dangerous fats for both heart disease and cancer are saturated fats and trans fatty acids, listed as "partially hydrogenated" on food labels. You would be foolish not to

182   Joel Fuhrman, M.D.

avoid these fats. Trans fats may raise breast cancer risk by more than 45 percent.[44]

4. Whole natural plant foods (whole grains, greens, nuts, and seeds) supply adequate fat. Eating an assortment of natural foods will ensure that you are not deficient in fat. For those who require more DHA fats, flaxseeds, hemp seeds, chia seeds, walnuts, and plant-derived DHA supplements are the healthiest and cleanest sources.

Remember, a low-fat diet can be worse than a higher-fat diet if it has more saturated fat or trans fat and if it contains an excessive amount of refined carbohydrates.

Note that lean meat or fowl, which contains 2 to 5 grams of fat per ounce, contains less fat, less saturated fat, and fewer calories per ounce than cheese, which has 8 to 9 grams of fat per ounce. Cheese has much more saturated fat (the most dangerous fat), about ten times as much saturated fat as chicken breast. Cheese is the food that contributes the most saturated fat to the American diet. Most cheeses are more than 50 percent of calories from fat, and even low-fat cheeses are very high-fat foods.

Americans have this fetish with watching fat and forgetting everything else we know about nutrition. Fat is not everything. If the fats you consume are healthy fats found in raw seeds, nuts, and avocados, and if your diet is rich in unrefined foods, you needn't worry so much about the fat—unless you are overweight.

	PERCENTAGE OF CALORIES FROM FAT	PERCENTAGE OF FAT THAT IS SATURATED FAT
Cream cheese	89	63
Gouda cheese	69	64
Cheddar cheese	74	64
Mozzarella cheese	69	61
Mozzarella cheese, part skim	56	64
Kraft Velveeta Spread	65	66
Kraft Velveeta Light	43	67
Ricotta, whole milk ·	68	64
Ricotta, part skim	51	62

The take-home message regarding fat is this: Avoid saturated fats and trans fats (hydrogenated fats) and try to include some foods that contain omega-3 fat in your diet.

Giving Up the Myths about Protein—Like Changing Your Religion

Remember those "Basic Four" food group charts we all saw in every classroom in elementary school? Protein had its own box, designated by a thick steak, a whole fish, and an entire chicken. Dairy foods had their own special box as well. A healthy diet, we were taught, supposedly centered on meat and milk. Protein was thought to be the most favorable of all nutrients, and lots of protein was thought to be the key to strength, health, and vigor. Unfortunately, cancer rates soared. As a result of scientific investigations into the causes of disease, we have had to rethink what we were taught. Old habits die hard; most Americans still cling to what they were taught as children. There are very few subjects that are more distorted in modern culture than that of protein.

Keep in mind that we do need protein. We can't be healthy without protein in our diet. Plant foods have plenty of protein. You do not have to be a nutritional scientist or dietitian to figure out what to eat, and you don't need to mix and match foods to achieve protein completeness. Any combination of natural foods will supply you with adequate protein, including all eight essential amino acids as well as nonessential amino acids.

It is unnecessary to combine foods to achieve protein completeness at each meal. The body stores and releases the amino acids needed over a twenty-four-hour period. About one-sixth of our daily protein utilization comes from recycling our own body tissue. This recycling, or digesting our own cells lining the digestive tract, evens out any variation from meal to meal in amino acid "incompleteness." It requires no level of nutritional sophistication to get sufficient protein, even if you eat only plant foods.

It is only when a vegetarian diet revolves around white bread and other processed foods that the protein content falls to low levels. However, the minute you include unprocessed foods such as vegetables, whole grains, beans, or nuts, the diet becomes protein-rich.

Green Grass Made the Lion

Which has more protein—oatmeal, ham, or a tomato? The answer is that they all have about the same amount of protein per calorie. The difference is, the tomato and the oatmeal are packaged with fiber and other disease-fighting nutrients, and the ham is packaged with cholesterol and saturated fat.

Some people believe that only animal products contain all the essential amino acids and that plant proteins are incomplete. False. They were taught that animal protein is superior to plant protein. False. They accept the outdated notion that plant protein must be mixed and matched in some complicated way that takes the planning of a nuclear physicist for a vegetarian diet to be adequate. False.

I guess they never thought too hard about how a rhinoceros, hippopotamus, gorilla, giraffe, or elephant became so big eating only vegetables. Animals do not make amino acids from thin air; all the amino acids originally came from plants. Even the nonessential amino acids that are fabricated by the body are just the basic amino acids that are modified slightly in some way by the body. So the lion's muscles can be composed of only the protein precursors and amino acids that the zebra and the gazelle ate. Green grass made the lion.

I see twenty to thirty new patients per week, and I always ask them, "Which has more protein—one hundred calories of sirloin steak or one hundred calories of broccoli?" When I tell them it's broccoli, the most frequent response I get is, "I didn't know

PROTEIN CONTENT OF COMMON FOODS IN
INCREASING ORDER OF PROTEIN PER CALORIE

	PROTEIN (GRAMS)	CALORIES	PROTEIN PER CALORIE	PERCENT PROTEIN
One banana	1.2	105	0.01	5
One cup of cooked brown rice	4.8	220	0.02	9
One corn on the cob	4.2	150	0.03	11
One baked potato	3.9	120	0.03	13
One cup of regular pasta	7.3	216	0.03	14
One 6-oz. fruit yogurt	7.0	190	0.04	15
Two slices of whole wheat bread	4.8	120	0.04	16
One Burger King cheeseburger	18.0	350	0.05	21
Meat loaf with gravy (Campbell's)	14.0	230	0.06	24
One cup of frozen peas	9.0	120	0.08	30
One cup of lentils (cooked)	16.0	175	0.09	36
One cup of tofu	18.0	165	0.11	44
One cup of frozen broccoli	5.8	52	0.11	45
One cup of cooked spinach	5.4	42	0.13	51

Note: Green vegetables have the most protein per calorie of all the above.

broccoli had protein in it." I then ask, "So where did you think the calories in broccoli come from? Did you think it was mostly fat, like an avocado, or mostly carbohydrate, like a potato?"

People know less about nutrition than any other subject. Even the physicians and dietitians who attend my lectures quickly answer, "Steak!" They are surprised to learn that broccoli has about twice as much protein as steak.

When you eat large quantities of green vegetables, you receive a considerable amount of protein. Remember, one ten-ounce box of frozen broccoli contains more than 10 grams of protein.

How Much Protein Do We Need?

Over the years the amount of protein recommended by authorities has gone up and down like a yo-yo. It wasn't until nitrogen-balance studies became available that we could actually measure protein requirements.

Today the recommended daily allowance (RDA) is 0.8 mg/kg body weight, 45 or about 44 grams for a 120-pound woman and 55 grams for a 150-pound man. This is a recommended amount, not a minimum requirement. The assumption is that about 0.5 mg/kg is needed, and then a large safety factor was built into the RDA to almost double the minimum requirement determined by nitrogen-balance studies. Still, the average American consumes over 100 grams of protein daily—an unhealthy amount.

Only 10 percent of the total calories consumed by the average person needs to be in the form of protein. In fact, as little as 2.5 percent of calories from protein may be all that is necessary for the average person.[46] Regardless of the many opinions on adequate or optimal protein intake, most plant foods, except fruit, supply at least 10 percent of calories from protein, with green vegetables averaging about 50 percent. High-nutrient diets that are plant-food-predominant, like the one I recommend, supply approximately 40 to 70 grams of protein daily in the range of 1,200 to 1,800, calories per day. That is plenty of protein.

Furthermore, the outdated notion of "high biological value" protein is based on essential amino acid profiles that grant eggs a 100 percent score based on the nutritional needs of rodents. It should not be surprising that the growth needs of rats are not quite the same as those of humans. For example, birds and rats have high requirements for methionine and cystine, the sulfur-containing amino acids. The sulfur-containing amino acids are important when growing feathers and fur. More recently, the essential amino acid profiles have been updated to reflect more closely the needs of humans. Human breast milk, for example, is lacking if we are considering the nutritional requirements of baby rats, but ideal when looking at human requirements.

Today, protein scores are computed differently from in the past. They are based on human needs, not rats', and soy protein earns a higher score than beef protein.[47]

Using a computer dietary-analysis program, I tried to compose a natural-foods diet deficient in any required amino acid. It was impossible. Almost any assortment of plant foods contained about 30 to 40 grams of protein per 1,000 calories. When your caloric needs are met, your protein needs are met automatically. Focus on eating healthy natural foods; forget about trying to get enough protein.

What about the athlete, weight lifter, or pregnant woman? Don't they need more protein? Of course an athlete in heavy training needs more protein. I was on the U.S. World Figure Skating Team in the early 1970s. I often exercised more than five hours daily. Besides all the grueling work on the ice, I did plenty of weight lifting and running. With all that exercise, I needed more protein, but I needed lots more of everything, especially calories. When you take in more food, you get the extra protein, extra fat, extra carbohydrates, and extra nutrients that you need. I loaded up the backseat of the car with huge amounts of fruits, vegetables, raw nuts, and whole grains. I ate lots of food and took in more protein (and everything else) in the process. Your protein needs increase in direct proportion to your increased caloric demands and your increased appetite. Guess what? You automatically get enough. The same is true during pregnancy.

When you meet your caloric needs with an assortment of natural plant foods, you will receive the right amount of protein—not too much, not too little.

Putting the RDAs into Perspective

The RDAs are levels set by our government for various nutrients considered to be desirable for good health. But are they correct? Are these levels appropriate, and will even higher levels of certain nutrients benefit us? Difficult questions to answer, but first we must consider how the RDAs were derived.

The RDAs were first developed when the government began questioning the nutritional value of military rations distributed to our soldiers during World War II. Later, our government's Food and Nutrition Board looked at the foods they expected most people to eat. By analyzing the average diet, they came up with a suggested minimum and then added an upward adjustment to theoretically ensure optimal health.

The RDAs are biased in favor of the conventional level of intake. They are not based on how people should eat to maintain optimal health; rather, they have been formulated to represent how we do eat. They characterize the conventional diet: high in animal products; lots of dairy products and fat; and low in fiber, antioxidants, and other nutrients, such as vitamin C, that are rich in plant foods. The RDAs reflect a diet that caused all the problems in the first place.

So we see a tendency to keep RDAs for plant-based nutrients low while keeping RDAs for animal-based nutrients high. Take, for example, the most ridiculous recommendation from the RDA— that for vitamin C. Any diet utilizing an abundance of unrefined natural plant foods offers a significant amount of vitamin C. The diets I recommend, and consume myself, contain between 500 and 1,000 mg of vitamin C each day, just from food. If you consumed a diet only half as good as I recommend, you would still consume between 250 and 500 mg of vitamin C each day. The RDA of 60 merely reflects the inadequacy of the American diet and how impossible it would be to get enough vitamin C if you ate a diet so low in natural plant foods.

You can take 1,000 mg of vitamin C in the form of a pill to make up for how deadly deficient your diet is, but then you would be missing all the other plant-derived antioxidants and phytochemicals that come in the same package as the vitamin C. The government must hold the RDA ridiculously low because it would be inconsistent with the other absurd dietary suggestions and make it impossible to achieve such levels without supplementation.

Most of the dietary recommendations from our government have been discarded and updated over time. Such recommendations, such as the "Basic Four" food group guide, have always been at least ten years behind current science and strongly influenced by food manufacturers. The current RDAs should meet the same fate; they are based on outmoded nutritional opinions that do not stand up to scientific scrutiny. Last, and most important, is that thousands of phytonutrients lack RDAs. There are subtle nuances and nutritive interactions that create disease resistance from the synergy of diverse substances in natural foods. Like a symphony orchestra whose members play in perfect harmony, our body depends on the harmonious interaction of nutrients, both known and unknown. By supplying a rich assortment of natural foods, we best maximize the function of the human masterpiece.

Remember the two main messages of this chapter. First, when food is refined and the macronutrients are removed from nature's natural packaging, they assume disease-causing properties. Second, green vegetables ran away with the title and legumes and fresh fruits took home a distant silver and bronze in the nutrient-density Olympics.

6

Breaking Free of Food Addiction

Case Study:
Isabel lost eighty pounds and has kept it off for over four years!

Every once in a while, I feel amazed. I was so depressed and felt so hopeless the day that I ordered Eat to Live. *Now it's like "Wow, I'm doing this, and I love it!"*

I was tired, unhappy, and mad at myself for continuously failing to lose weight and keep it off. I was thirty-one and had had weight issues for as long as I could remember. I'm only five feet tall but weighed 203 pounds. My back hurt, I had migraine headaches and acne, and I was a couch potato. I dreaded dressing up to go anywhere because I didn't have anything pretty to wear and didn't want anyone to see me obese. I would have locked myself in my house if I could have. I was tired of

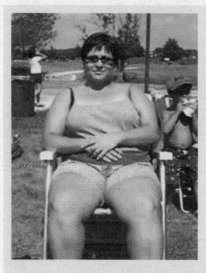
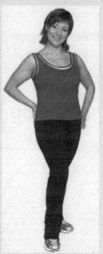

the stares and people making fun of me. I was always the "big girl," and there always seemed to be someone around to remind me of it.

I tried so many different diets, but nothing ever stuck. I read the book and was impressed by Dr. Fuhrman's scientific research and knowledge, plus everything made a lot of sense. I started to follow his nutritional guidelines right away, and by that summer I had lost fifty pounds. Things really clicked when I stopped focusing on numbers. I stopped setting weight goals and freaking out if I didn't lose weight fast enough. I trusted that each day I ate according to the Eat to Live guidelines, I was getting healthier, and I "let" my body do its thing.

My current weight loss is now eighty pounds, and my overall body fat has been reduced from 47 percent to 25 percent. I feel fantastic, and my blood tests are great. I look younger—actually some people don't even recognize me! I feel like a new woman.

I rarely get migraines now. I have fewer lower back issues. I am no longer an emotional eater. I have less leg pain due to a pesky varicose vein that threatened to pop out. My skin has cleared up, and I have better mental clarity. My self-esteem and self-confidence have improved.

I now have energy to be active. I can do things that I had absolutely no desire to try before. I became a certified personal trainer, because now that I feel great, I want to help others feel better.

Eat to Live really DOES *work. If anyone is struggling or contemplating, just go for it! Do as much as you can and* NEVER *give up. Here are my tips for success:*

- *Forget the scales and deadlines.*
- *Get into a routine. Get regular exercise.*
- *Join the Member Center at DrFuhrman.com for support.*
- *Don't be afraid to say no at social gatherings. Your health should come before pleasing others.*

An Important Discovery

Hunger is an experience that many people fear. It seems absurd that fear of starvation could exist in the most overfed population in human history. However, our obsession with food and eating is undeniable. People often react with abject fear when contemplating going without food for even short periods of time. Continuous eating not only undermines healthy weight loss, it is just plain unhealthy. Eating the wrong (low-nutrient) foods leads to what I call "toxic hunger" and the desire to overconsume calories. When we do not meet our micronutrient needs, we do not feel well unless our digestive tract is continuously at work. Toxic hunger overrides the natural instinct that controls appetite and leads to a dramatic increase in calorie consumption.

I have observed that a diet style sufficiently high in micronutrients can decrease sensations leading to food cravings and overeating behaviors. The sensations commonly and traditionally considered to be "hunger," and even reported in medical textbooks as such, disappear for the majority of individuals after eating this micronutrient-rich diet. A new sensation, which I call "true hunger," arises instead. Understanding the science and human physiology behind this important distinction is important.

Everybody You Know Is a Food Addict

When our bodies have become acclimated to a noxious or toxic agent, it is called addiction. Indulging in the addiction is mildly pleasurable, but if we stop taking the substance, such as nicotine or caffeine, we feel ill as the body mobilizes cellular wastes and attempts to repair the damage caused by the exposure. This is called withdrawal. If you drank four cups of coffee or caffeinated soda every day, you would get a withdrawal headache when you tried to stop the habit. To feel better, you could take more caffeine (or other drugs) or eat food more frequently, which would help, because eating and digesting retards detoxification or withdrawal. Similarly, toxic hunger is heightened by the consumption of caffeinated beverages, soft drinks, and processed foods. It occurs predominantly after digestion ceases and the digestive tract is empty, and it can make a person feel extremely uncomfortable if he or she does not eat or drink a caloric load (to inhibit detoxification) for relief.

Symptoms of Toxic Hunger

- headaches
- fatigue
- nausea
- weakness
- mental confusion and irritability
- abdominal and esophageal spasm
- fluttering and cramping in the stomach

The confusion is compounded because when we eat the same heavy or unhealthful foods that are causing the problem to begin with, we feel better while the detoxification process is halted or delayed. This makes becoming overweight inevitable, because if we stop digesting food, even for a short time, our bodies will begin to experience symptoms of detoxification or withdrawal from our unhealthful diet. To counter this, we eat heavy meals that require a long period of digestion, or we eat too often and keep our digestive tract busy and overfed almost all the time to lessen the discomfort from our stressful diet style.

> In the *anabolic* phase, we digest and store the calories for future use.
>
> In the *catabolic* phase, we burn the stored calories.

Our body cycles between periods of digestion-assimilation (anabolic phase) and utilization of the stored calories (catabolic phase), which begins when the digestive process ends. During the anabolic phase, the absorbed glucose is stored in the liver and muscle tissues as glycogen, to be broken down and utilized at a later time when we are not eating and digesting. During the catabolic phase, we "live off" the nutrients stored in the anabolic phase. The breakdown of stored glycogen is called glycolysis, and it is during this process that our body swings into heightened detoxification activity.

When we are breaking down our body fats and glycogen stores, the body is exposed to more released cellular toxins, and elimination and detoxification are increased accordingly. This elimination of toxins can cause discomfort, especially when our tissues have an excessive toxic burden. These uncomfortable symptoms are not caused by "lower blood sugar," though the symptoms occur in parallel with low blood sugar. When our diet is low in phytochemicals and other micronutrients, we build up more intracellular waste products. It is well accepted in the scientific literature that toxins such as free radicals, advanced glycation end products (AGEs), and lipid A2E build up in human tissues with diets low in antioxidants and other micronutrients and that these substances contribute to disease.[1]

It has been noted that overweight individuals developed more oxidative stress (as a result of free-radical damage) when fed a low-micronutrient-containing meal compared to normal-weight individuals. Increased peroxidases and aldehydes, derived from damaged lipids and proteins, were measurable in the urine.[2] This indicates that people prone to obesity experience more withdrawal symptoms, directing them to overconsume calories. It is a vicious cycle that both promotes the problem and prevents its resolution. Subjects fed healthier diets did not build up these inflammatory markers.[3] When we consume excess animal proteins (which create excess nitrogenous wastes) and don't eat sufficient phytochemical-rich vegetation, we exacerbate the buildup of metabolic waste products in our body.[4]

THE BLOOD SUGAR CURVE

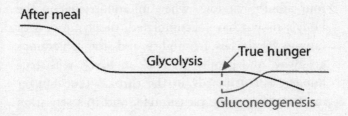

As the hours go by and we have not eaten, glycogen stores are utilized for energy (glycolysis). Glycolysis occurs after digestion ceases and is a perfectly comfortable state not accompanied by symptoms in a healthy individual eating a healthy diet. As we continue to burn off the glycogen stores, true hunger eventually kicks in, signaling the need for calories before gluconeogenesis begins. Gluconeogenesis is the breakdown of muscle tissue that occurs to supply the body with glucose when there is no glycogen left. The body cannot make the glucose it needs to fuel the brain from stored fats, but it can make glucose from amino acids derived from muscle tissue. True hunger is protective of our muscle mass and gives us a clear signal to eat before gluconeogenesis begins.

True Hunger or Toxic Hunger?

What I have observed and quantified with thousands of individuals is that the drive to overconsume calories is blunted by high micronutrient consumption. The symptoms that were thought to be hypoglycemia or even hunger, which occur as soon as glycolysis begins, simply disappear after eating very healthfully for a few months. After that two- to four-month window, when micronutrients in the body's tissues have accumulated, the symptoms of fatigue, headaches, irritability, and stomach cramps go away, and people get back in touch with true hunger, felt primarily in the throat. True hunger makes eating more pleasurable, and this sensation better directs us to a more appropriate amount of calories for our body's biological needs.

In our present toxic food environment, many have lost the ability to connect with the body signals that tell us how much food we actually need. Nature has given our bodies the beautifully orchestrated ability to signal precisely how much to eat to maintain an ideal weight for long-term health. I have documented this process, demonstrating that this otherwise poorly studied phenomenon is real. It has resulted in thousands of people losing dramatically large amounts of weight. Hundreds have lost more than a hundred pounds, some more than three hundred pounds, without surgical interventions and with lasting success. Healthful eating is more effective than portion control for long-term weight control. It modifies and diminishes the sensations of toxic hunger, enabling overweight individuals to be more comfortable eating fewer calories.

True hunger signals when our bodies need calories to maintain our lean body mass. If you ate food only when experiencing true hunger, you could not become overweight to begin with. If you have a significant layer of fat around your waist, it means you have regularly consumed food in response to toxic hunger or have eaten recreationally. The body does not store large amounts of fat when fed a wholesome natural diet and given only the amount of food demanded by true hunger.

True hunger is felt in the throat, neck, and mouth, not in the stomach or head. It is not uncomfortable to feel real hunger; it makes food taste better when you eat, and it makes eating so much more pleasurable. There is nothing fluttering or bouncing around, it is not painful, and you know when you feel it that it is a normal reaction that signals a need for food. It tells you that the body is physiologically ready to digest food and the digestive glands have regained their capacity to secrete enzymes appropriately. The result is that you feel better and do not overeat.

Symptoms of True Hunger

Enhanced taste sensation
Increased salivation
Gnawing throat sensation

True hunger requires no special food to satisfy it. It is relieved by eating almost anything. You can't crave some particular food and call it hunger; a craving by definition is an addictive drive, not something felt by a person who is not an addict. Remember, almost all Americans are addicted to their toxic habits. A disease-causing diet is addicting. A health-supporting diet is not. You do not have to carry around a calculator and a scale to figure out how much to eat. A healthy body will give you the correct signals. To achieve an ideal weight and consume the exact amount of calories to maintain a lean body mass that will prolong your life, you must get back in touch with true hunger. Eat when hungry and don't eat when not hungry.

How to Achieve a State of True Hunger

1. Do not eat when not hungry.
2. Do not snack, unless you are sure it is true hunger.
3. Do not overeat. Don't eat until you feel full or stuffed.
4. Do not eat a big dinner.
5. Don't eat after dinner. Instead, clean the kitchen, brush and floss, and stay away from food. Look forward to how good food will taste the next morning when you are hungry again.
6. Discontinue or wean off caffeine, salt, alcohol, sweets, butter, cheese, processed foods, soft drinks, smoking, and illegal and legal drugs (if safe to do so).

More frequent eating has been shown to lead to more calories consumed by the end of the week.[5] In addition, in scientific studies reduced meal frequency increased the life span of both rodents and monkeys, even when the calories consumed each week were the same in the group fed more frequently and the group fed less frequently.[6] The body needs time between meals to finish digesting, because when digestion has ended, the body can more effectively detoxify and promote cellular repair. To maximize health, it is not favorable to be constantly eating and digesting food.

Wait until you feel hungry to eat. Try to eat less at dinner so you are hungry for three meals per day. Get your body into a regular schedule, eating three meals per day, without overeating at any one meal. If you do not feel hungry for the next meal, delay eating or skip the meal entirely. Next time, eat much less until you get better skilled at eating the appropriate amount so that you feel hungry in time to eat again at the next mealtime. It is permissible to eat two meals a day instead of three if you are hungry for only two meals. For most people who exercise regularly, three meals with no snacking is the norm. We actually require less food than most people realize. Once we get rid of the perverted toxic hunger, our central nervous system can accurately measure and give us the right signals for maintaining our ideal weight on the right amount of calories. You will eventually develop the skill of knowing the right amount of food to eat at each meal, because it relieves your hunger, you feel satisfied (but not full), and you are hungry again in time for the next meal.

You May Feel Poorly at First

Try to stop a sugar addict from eating sweets or take the colas, pizza, and burgers away from a fast-food addict, and wow, do they feel ill. This is called withdrawal. When we stop doing something harmful to ourselves, we feel sick as the body attempts to repair the damage caused by longtime exposure to noxious substances, reduces tolerance, mobilizes cellular wastes, and deals with empty receptor sites. If you quit smoking, even when there is not a molecule of nicotine left in your body, you may still feel ill as your body is actively engaged in the repair of damage caused by the offensive substance. All of a sudden the long-term smoker finds he is feeling worse from having stopped smoking, not better. The nicotine may be gone, but he starts coughing more and bringing up mucus. As a degree of health returns, the body becomes less and less tolerant of the abnormal noxious irritants that have built up over time. Because of the restored ability to repair damaged cells, inflammation may increase temporarily as the tissues become more reactive to the waste products that were retained there. Inflammation serves a corrective function here as the body's immune system reacts protectively to remove noxious substances and restore cellular function.

Toxic food works the same way. After moving on to a truly healthful diet, the body's enhanced self-repair mechanisms bring about symptoms, sometimes even brief low-grade fevers, emotional instability, fatigue, and headaches. Don't be alarmed if during the first week or two of healthy eating, you feel worse and the desire to use food to curtail discomfort is heightened. This usually passes within the first four days.

Why Diets Fail

The American press, diet books, and even most of the scientific research community are thoroughly confused about nutrition and dieting. Almost every article on the topic discusses some magic food, supplement, metabolism booster, or ratio of fat, carbohydrate, and protein that can solve all your weight problems. Research articles continue to test diets low in fat, high in fat, low in carbohydrates, and high in carbohydrates, and the media continue to report the successes and failures of these diets. It goes on and on in circles, but trying to micromanage carbohydrate, fat, or protein intake will not increase your health and longevity. Even worse, that sort of dieting encourages temporary fluctuations in caloric intake, leading to unsustained changes in body weight, often called yo-yo dieting. These diets hardly work and are bad for your health because it is not healthy to lose and gain weight over and over. They demonstrate that any diet that does not address micronutrient quality is not very effective.

What you are learning here is different, as it is not some perfect ratio of fat, carbohydrate, or protein that will lead you to your ideal weight and superior health. Sure, we need to eat less fat, less protein, and fewer carbohydrates, the only three sources of calories in food. Obviously, we need some calories, but we want to make sure that the fat, protein, and carbohydrates that we choose to eat are whole foods and as nutrient-dense as possible. The healthiest way to eat, and the way to make you naturally and automatically desire fewer calories, is to understand the concept of nutrient density, to eat healthfully to remove your food addictions, and to allow the body to reprogram your tastes. Eating pleasure is enhanced because you eat when hunger is present. You will find that your taste preferences adapt to what is eaten regularly, and improved nutrition enhances the taste apparatus.

Although diet books are everywhere, it is estimated that more than 75 percent of all Americans are overweight.[7] Investigations report such a sweeping and rapid increase of obesity globally that it is considered a serious medical epidemic, affecting a significant portion of the world's population.[8] The World Health Organization (WHO) estimates that the spread of processed food and American fast food worldwide has made obesity and the diseases of low-nutrient, high-calorie eating bigger contributors to premature death worldwide than starvation. WHO has stated:

"Households should select predominantly plant-based diets rich in a variety of vegetables and fruits, pulses or legumes, and minimally processed starchy staple foods."[9]

Because being overweight or obese dramatically increases the risk of all the major causes of death, the spread of America's toxic food industry may be the most serious health issue facing the modern world. Ideal body weight and overall health are inseparable. A weight-loss program can be considered successful only if the weight loss is permanent and safe and it promotes overall health. Temporary weight loss is of little or no benefit, especially if it compromises your health. The confusing diet wars and opposing opinions among diet authors are paralyzing the potential to improve the health of millions of suffering individuals.

In the classic portion-controlled (calorie-counting) diet, it is likely that the body will not get adequate fiber or nutrients. The body will have a compounded sensation of hunger, cravings, and addictive withdrawal, which for most is simply overwhelming. This dieting philosophy invariably results in people losing weight then gaining it back. Calorie counting simply doesn't work in the long run. A diet based on portion control and calorie counting generally permits the eating of highly toxic, low-nutrient foods and then requires us to fight our addictive drives in the attempt to eat less. This combination undernourishes the body, resulting in uncontrollable and frequent food cravings, along with a heightened desire for concentrated calories. This low micronutrient intake in conjunction with withdrawal symptoms can lead to perverted cravings, such as the desire to eat junk food, drink alcohol, or take drugs. Cravings are not the result of hunger; they are the result of toxic habits. Anyone seeking to adopt a healthy diet must accept that there will be a period (generally six weeks or less) during which the body will attempt to detoxify. You may feel ill during this time, and true hunger may be absent the entire time. Without an adequate education in superior nutrition and solid principles to stick to, dieters flounder and fail, bouncing from one diet to another, always losing a little and regaining, frequently regaining more than they lost.

Misinformation works hand in hand with self-deception. Countless diets advertise that you can eat all the foods you love and still lose weight. Consequently, why would anyone want to completely revamp his or her diet? It seems as though it would be far easier to eat less of something that you love than it would be to switch to eating something that you may not currently like. The problem is that in practice, eating less of the same things has been proven not to work. Studies have shown that portion-control diets result in significant weight loss that is maintained over five years for fewer than three people out of one hundred.[10]

It is merely a matter of time before those trying to keep their portions small increase the amount of food they are eating. The amount of fiber in these diets is insufficient, and the nutrient density is poor. These diets restrict calories, but because the food choices and meal plans are so calorie-dense, dieters must eat tiny portions in order to lose weight. These choices don't satisfy their desire to eat, and they wind up craving food and becoming frustrated. When dieters can't stand eating thimble-size portions anymore and finally eat until satisfied, they put weight on with a vengeance. These diets are founded on weak science and perpetuate nutritional myths. To become healthy, disease-resistant, and permanently thin, you can't escape the necessity of eating large amounts of nutrient-rich, healthy food.

Are You Dying to Lose Weight?

Many of the most heavily promoted and bestselling diet books are also among the most dangerous. Some of the more popular books and websites promote high-protein, low-carbohydrate dietary patterns, emphasizing how dangerous it is to ingest white flour, sugar, and corn syrup. Of course I agree with the dangers of consuming high-glycemic junk, but I think it is time to put these high-protein diets to bed. There should be no controversy here. High-protein diets are not life span favorable, they do not offer the anti-cancer protection inherent in a diet much richer in plant-derived micronutrients, and they are not cardioprotective. In fact, even when they result in some weight loss, they can still raise LDL cholesterol and cause or permit the advancement of heart disease.[11] The mild degree of weight-loss success they offer a minority of people, from the removal or reduction of dangerous, low-nutrient carbohydrates, is simply not good enough.

The popularity of these books is evidence that people are looking for a way to lose weight without having to curtail their dangerous love affair with rich, unhealthful foods. They preach what people want to hear: you can eat lots of fat, cholesterol, and saturated fat and still lose weight. This illicit romance can lead to tragic consequences.

High-protein-diet gurus typically promote the idea that their recommended diet is the healthiest. They would have their devotees believe there is a worldwide conspiracy of more than 3,500 scientific studies involving more than 15,000 research scientists reporting a relationship between the consumption of meats, poultry, eggs, and dairy products and the incidence of heart disease, cancer, kidney failure, constipation, gallstones, diverticulosis, and hemorrhoids, just to name a few health problems. The point here is not to be confused about nutrition and health by misinformation; we need to strive to eat far fewer animal products and more high-nutrient plant foods. Many of these diets have people afraid to eat healthful fresh fruits because they contain carbohydrates. Fruit consumption, however, shows a powerful dose-response association with a reduction in heart disease, cancer, and all-cause mortality.[12]

Due to its emphasis on eating more animal products and fewer carbohydrates, the popular Atkins diet is a prototype of dietary misinformation. Tragically, an otherwise healthy sixteen-year-old girl died after following the Atkins diet for three weeks. More recent popular diets are also dangerous. I consider the South Beach diet one of the most dangerous diets because the three phases encourage people to go on and off a ketogenic diet, which can cause electrolyte shifts leading to life-threatening cardiac arrhythmias.[13] There was a tremendous explosion in sudden cardiac deaths in young and middle-aged women that occurred in parallel with the period of popular enthusiasm for these carbohydrate-restricted, high-protein, ketogenic diets. This was first reported at the American Heart Association's forty-first annual conference in 2001 after a national surveillance study was performed by Dr. Zheng and his colleagues at the Centers for Disease Control (CDC).[14] Similar deaths were seen in the past related to liquid high-protein diets.[15] A coincidence? I doubt it; this should not be taken lightly.

The medical literature has shown that ketogenic diets can cause a pathological enlargement of the heart called cardiomyopathy, which is reversible, but only if the diet is stopped in time.[16] In *The South*

Beach Diet, written by a cardiologist, the reader is led through a series of dietary phases that cycle back and forth between weight regain and carbohydrate restriction. Allowing one's weight to fluctuate up and down is risky. It can lead to heart problems and increase the presence of the most dangerous type of vulnerable atherosclerotic plaque, increasing heart attack risk. When you have a cardiologist recommending weight cycling and recurrent ketogenic carbohydrate restriction to vulnerable heart patients, it is not just irresponsible but illustrative that incorrect dietary advice can become deadly.

As discussed in chapter four, high levels of animal protein show a strong correlation with higher cancer incidence. Hundreds of scientific studies have documented the link between animal products and certain cancers:

- Increased risk of epithelial and lung cancer[17]
- Increased risk of pancreatic cancer[18]
- Increased risk of colon cancer[19]
- Increased risk of stomach and esophageal cancer[20]
- Increased risk of bladder and prostate cancer[21]
- Increased growth of mammary tumors[22]

Although it would be wrong to say that animal foods are the sole cause of cancer, it is now clear that increased consumption of animal products combined with decreased consumption of fresh products has the most powerful effect on increasing one's risk for various kinds of cancer. Most medical researchers agree that meat consumption is an important factor in the etiology of human cancer.[23] In fact, reducing animal protein in the diet may be the most important dietary intervention one can take to reduce cancer risk.[24] High-protein weight-loss diets promoting high-animal-product and low-plant-product (carbohydrate) consumption are not only unhealthy; they could be fatal.

Short-Term Benefits, Long-Term Dangers!

Besides all the dangers reviewed here, it should be clear that eating meat actually correlates with weight gain, not weight loss, unless you radically cut carbs from your diet to maintain a chronic ketosis.[25] Researchers from the American Cancer Society followed 79,236 individuals over ten years and found that those who ate meat more than three times per week were much more likely to gain weight as the years went by than those who tended to avoid meat.[26] The more vegetables the participants ate, the more resistant they were to weight gain.

If increasing one's risk of heart attack and cancer isn't enough of an argument against high-protein diets, the science is conclusive that they also cause kidney damage, kidney stones, and gout.[27] Many people develop kidney problems at a young age under the high-protein stress. Due to the accumulated research, the American Kidney Fund's medical advisory panel issued a press release stating that high-protein weight-loss diets can result in irreversible scarring in the kidneys. This is also observed in bodybuilders who consume excess protein in an attempt to pack on more muscle. The only treatments are dialysis and kidney transplantation. This research shows that kidney function is impacted even in healthy athletes. That should send a message to anyone who is on a high-protein weight-loss diet.[28]

Overweight individuals are likely to have some kidney damage already, since almost 25 percent of people over age forty-five, especially those with diabetes or high blood pressure, have a degree of kidney impairment. Researchers have concluded, "The potential impact of protein consumption on renal function has important public health implications given the prevalence of high protein diets and use of protein supplements."[29] Diabetics are at increased risk of kidney disease and are extremely sensitive to the stress a high-protein diet places on the kidney.[30] In a large, multicentered study involving 1,521 patients, most of the diabetics who ate too much animal protein had lost over half of their kidney function, and almost all the damage was irreversible.[31]

Blood tests that monitor kidney function typically do not begin to detect problems until more than 90 percent of the kidneys have been destroyed.

A Diet of Nutritional Excellence

There is an important take-home message here—and that is to understand how critical a life-or-death issue nutrition is. We must get this right. Humans are primates, and all other primates eat a diet of predominantly natural vegetation. If primates eat some animal products, it is a very small percentage of their total caloric intake. Modern science shows that most common ailments in today's world are the result of nutritional ignorance. However, we can eat a diet rich in phytochemicals from a variety of natural plant foods that will afford us the ability to live a long and healthy life.

I always try to emphasize the benefits of nutritional excellence. With a truly healthy diet, you can not only expect a drop in blood pressure and cholesterol and a reversal of heart disease, but your headaches, constipation, indigestion, and bad breath should all resolve. Eating for nutritional excellence enables people to reverse diabetes and to gradually lose their dependence on drugs. You can expect to reach a normal weight without counting calories and dieting, as well as achieve robust health and live a long life free of the fear of heart attacks and strokes.

Nutritional excellence, which involves eating plenty of vegetables, fruits, and beans, does not have to exclude all animal products, but it has to be very rich in high-nutrient plant foods (which should make up well over 80 percent of your caloric intake). No more than 10 percent of your total calories should come from animal foods. There is insufficient data at this point to suggest that there is a clear longevity advantage to adhering to a vegan diet (one that is entirely free of animal foods). However, the scientific literature suggests that there is a longevity advantage to dropping your animal-food consumption to as little as one or two servings per week. The most consistent finding in the nutritional literature based on every epidemiological study is that as fruit and vegetable consumption increases, chronic diseases and premature deaths decrease.

My Eat to Live dietary approach has already been tested and shown to be the most effective diet style for lowering cholesterol, as reported in the medical journal *Metabolism*.[32] A recent study also showed that participants who followed my plan for two years lost more weight and kept it off better than those following diets previously studied.[33]

Longevity and disease protection should be the ultimate goals of dietary advice; you can lose weight snorting cocaine and smoking cigarettes. When you settle for second-class nutritional advice, you doom yourself not only to a shorter life but also to a poor quality of life in your later years. Humans can survive long enough to reproduce with varying diet styles, but we can use nutritional science to greatly extend the potential of human health and enable a quality life expectancy. We can do better than our parents and better than our ancestors. We have an unprecedented opportunity in human history to live longer and better than ever before. The high-protein, high-animal-product promoters, who appeal to those people with that dietary preference, mutilate the nutritional science to promote their agenda, destroy life-enhancing opportunities for millions, and perpetuate needless premature deaths.

Eat to Live means the weight-loss benefits are only the tip of the iceberg. Thousands of scientific studies are demonstrating the potential of foods to extend your life span and offer dramatic protection against cancer. What makes Eat to Live unique among diet styles is that it encourages the consumption of nutrient-rich produce, particularly those foods with dramatic health benefits. The result is that these disease-protective biochemical nutrients reduce food cravings, remove food addictions, and curtail overeating behavior. Without this knowledge, and without the attention to nutrient quality, diets are doomed to fail.

You can't get to an ideal level of dietary protection, which includes enough of these fruit and vegetable super-foods, unless you significantly reduce your consumption of animal products, processed foods, oils, flours, and sweeteners. This leaves caloric space and stomach space for a sufficient amount of highly protective foods. This is what Eat to Live is all about. When you eat sufficient volumes of beneficial foods in delicious and satisfying ways, you will not have room for the other foods that are not health-promoting, and you will eventually lose your desire for them.

The chicken, pasta, and olive oil diet is the perfect formula for mediocre health and a poor life expectancy. Chicken, oil, and pasta are all low-nutrient foods. Not grain-based, meat-based, or corn-based, a nutritarian diet is based on high-nutrient plant foods of varying colors. I coined the word *nutritarian* to represent a person whose dietary focus is on eating healthful, nutrient-rich foods. A nutritarian recognizes that nutrient-rich produce has disease-preventive, therapeutic, and life-extending properties.

What if all Americans:

- ate a large bowl of green salad daily
- had a large serving of steamed greens daily
- ate a cup of beans daily
- had at least an ounce of raw seeds and nuts daily
- ate at least three fresh fruits daily
- had some tomatoes, peppers, onions, mushrooms, herbs, and garlic daily

Can you imagine what would happen to our nation's growing health-care costs; our epidemic of obesity, cancer, and diabetes; and our suffering economy, overburdened with out-of-control medical costs, if all Americans did these things?

Eat to Live isn't for everyone. Some people may decide to ignore the life-enhancing information presented here. A multitude of health promoters offer diets, nutritional supplements, surgical procedures, and even drugs with the promise of weight loss without changing the way you eat. This promise alone is enough to keep people from doing the work to change; it gives the subconscious a way out. The subconscious mind is not logical. Many of these diets have been debunked, but that doesn't damage their allure.

Breaking Up Is Hard to Do

Occasionally, I meet someone who tells me, "I read *Eat to Live*. I know that it makes sense. But I can't eat like that." Or, "I read your book, but I could never be a vegetarian." Most often it turns out that the person didn't read the book in its entirety, just skimmed it. These individuals fear that healthful dietary changes will remove all the pleasure from their lives.

Habits are hard to break, no question about it. Some people cannot be convinced by all the best science in the world that it is better to eat healthy foods. Nothing short of disease, fear, or pain (and often all three) will motivate them to change. Toxic eating can be just as addictive as smoking or taking drugs. The same steps are necessary to overcome the addiction. The first step is to recognize that you have a problem and that it is an addiction. Knowledge can help defeat addictions. It also helps to have a support system of others to reinforce the reality that any temporary suffering incurred as a result of change will bring about a much more pleasurable and happier life.

Addictive behavior can seem like an effective way to escape sadness, loneliness, and fear because it brings momentary pleasure. It is difficult to break old, addictive eating habits and form new, healthy ones. One of the difficulties is the immense power of addiction, which makes the human mind anxious to rationalize and justify bad habits. As a result, people often fail before they even attempt to change. They either use denial about the vital necessity of change— the need to improve their health and happiness— or they simply give up without even trying, thinking that change is too difficult. Keep in mind, part of you (your intellect) wants to change and be healthy. It wants the suffering caused by your bad habits to end. But part of you (part of your subconscious) does not want to change. It wants to avoid conflict and the discomfort that comes with withdrawal from your addictive bad habits. That part of you wants to pretend that things are just fine the way they are, thank you, and it can come up with some mighty convincing reasons why you should not follow the Eat to Live plan. Here are some common ones:

- It's too radical a change.
- There's not enough protein.
- I will get too thin and my skin will wrinkle.
- My family won't eat this way.
- It is too difficult to eat this way on the road.
- There is nothing to eat in a restaurant.
- I've tried dieting before, and I know I'll just gain all the weight back.
- I really don't like vegetables.

Addictions affect our ability to think rationally; they prejudice our judgment in favor of maintaining the addiction. That is why it is so difficult even to decide to change, much less actually change. Those addicted to rich, heart attack–causing foods are more than happy to believe the lie that a low cholesterol level is not desirable and readily parrot high-protein enthusiasts who spread the myth that low cholesterol is dangerous. Many people addicted to animal foods would embrace the belief that the earth is flat if they could use it to justify their consumption of fatty meats, butter, and cheese.

The modern food and drug industry has converted a significant portion of the world's people to a new religion—a massive cult of pleasure seekers who consume coffee, cigarettes, soft drinks, candy, chocolate, alcohol, processed foods, fast foods, and concentrated dairy fat (cheese) in a self-indulgent orgy of destructive behavior. When the inevitable results of such bad habits appear—pain, suffering, sickness, and disease—the addicted cult members drag themselves to physicians and demand drugs to alleviate their pain, mask their symptoms, and cure their diseases. These revelers become so drunk on their addictive behavior and the accompanying addictive thinking that they can no longer tell the difference between health and health care.

The benefits of a diet based on nutritional excellence accrue over time, and achieving them takes some effort. But Eat to Live does not have to be an all-or-nothing decision on day one. Incremental improvements bring benefits, too, and change can take place over time. Healthy foods taste fantastic, but you may have to rehabilitate your taste buds and take some time to learn new cooking techniques and recipes to appreciate them.

Instead of searching for weight-loss gimmicks and tricks, adopt a resolution to be healthy. Focusing on your health, not on your weight, will eventually result in long-term weight loss. Eating a healthy diet, one that is rich in an assortment of natural plant fibers, will help you crave less and feel satisfied without overeating. Other diet plans fail because they cater to modern American tastes, which include too many processed foods and animal products to be healthy. Stop measuring portions and trying to follow complicated formulas. Instead, eat as many vegetables, beans, and fresh fruits as possible, and less of everything else. Don't succumb to those other plans, which are an insult to your body as well as your intelligence.

7

Eat to Live Takes On Disease

Case Study:
Ronnie was in a downward spiral of unhealthy eating,
binge drinking, and depression. He started
Eat to Live and gained a new life!

I weighed over 300 pounds. After quadruple
bypass surgery, feeling that I had been fixed, I went
back to smoking two to four packs of cigarettes a
day, and drinking heavily, and eating fried foods
galore in massive quantities. Once again, my health
went south and my weight went up rapidly. I tried
the occasional diet plan (Atkins, Ornish), only to
watch my health deteriorate further.

I ended up in the hospital again. This time doc-
tors placed three stents, but within a few weeks I
was having chest pains again. I decided to look for
help, found Dr. Fuhrman on the Internet, and
started reading Eat to Live.

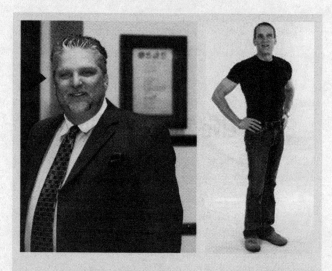

I began my journey pegging the scale out at 300 pounds. I was motivated to get my weight and health under control. I committed to Dr. Fuhrman's high-nutrient diet style. Within the first seven months I lost 110 pounds. After twelve months, I had arrived at my ideal weight with a total weight loss of 140 pounds!

My chest pains completely ceased. I stopped all medications and as a result have been able to save over $600 a month in out-of-pocket pharmaceutical expenses.

After a year of Eat to Live, my progress was as follows:

	JULY 2008	JULY 2009
Weight	300 lbs*	160 lbs
Blood pressure	161/110 (on meds)†	115/70 (no meds)

Waist	58"	34"‡
BMI	41.5 (morbidly obese)	21.7 (healthy)
Total cholesterol	228 (on meds)§	132 (no meds)
Triglycerides	312	63
LDL	148	75

*Ronnie weighed more, but 300 pounds was his scale's limit.
†300 mg of Avapro and 200 mg of Toprol XL for high blood pressure.
‡He now wears a size smaller pants than he did in high school.
§20 mg of Lipitor for high cholesterol.

We are living among an addicted population of compulsive eaters, creating allergic and sickly individuals. Eat and live like most Americans and you will eventually suffer from an assortment of ailments—like most Americans.

Good health is not merely the absence of disease. Good health assumes protection from disease in the future and can be predicted only by a healthy lifestyle and diet. You cannot buy your health; you must earn it through healthy living. Visiting physicians, acupuncturists, chiropractors, homeopaths, naturopaths, osteopaths, and other health providers cannot make you healthy. You can receive *symptomatic* relief for your condition, but treatments do not make you healthy.

For most people, illness means putting their fate in the hands of doctors and complying with their recommendations—recommendations that typically involve taking drugs for the rest of their lives while they watch their health gradually deteriorate. People are completely unaware that most illnesses are self-induced and can be reversed with aggressive nutritional methods.

Both patients and physicians act as though everyone's medical problems are genetic or assumed to be the normal consequence of aging. They believe that chronic illness is just what we all must expect. Unfortunately, the medical-pharmaceutical business has encouraged people to believe that health problems are hereditary and that we need to swallow poisons to defeat our genes. This is almost always untrue. We all have genetic weaknesses, but those weaknesses never get a chance to express themselves until we abuse our body with many, many years of mistreatment. Never forget, 99 percent of your genes are programmed to keep you healthy. The problem is that we never let them do their job.

My clinical experience over the past twenty years has shown me that almost all the major illnesses that plague Americans are reversible with aggressive nutritional changes designed to undo the damage caused by years of eating a disease-causing diet. The so-called balanced diet that most Americans eat causes the diseases Americans get.

These conditions, and many others, can be effectively prevented or treated through superior nutrition. As their medical problems gradually melt away, patients can be slowly weaned off the medications they have been prescribed.

Food Is the Cure

Patients are told that food has nothing to do with the diseases they develop. Dermatologists insist that food has nothing to do with acne, rheumatologists insist that food has nothing to do with rheumatoid arthritis, and gastroenterologists insist that food has nothing to do with irritable and inflammatory bowel disease. Even cardiologists have been resistant to accept the accumulating evidence that atherosclerosis is entirely avoidable. Most of them still believe that coronary artery disease and angina require the invasive treatment of surgery and are not reversible with nutritional intervention. Most physicians have no experience in treating disease naturally with nutritional excellence, and some uninformed physicians are convinced it is not possible.

Dietary-Caused Illnesses with High Prevalence

acne	allergies	angina
appendicitis	arthritis	asthma
atherosclerosis	colonic polyps	constipation
diabetes (adult)	diverticulosis	esophagitis
fibromyalgia	gallstones	gastritis
gout	headaches	hemorrhoids
high blood pressure	hypoglycemic	indigestion
irritable bowel	symptoms	lumbar spine
syndrome	kidney stones	syndromes
macular	musculoskeletal pain	osteoporosis
degeneration	stroke	uterine fibroids
sexual dysfunction		

Not only are common disorders such as asthma associated with increased body weight and our disease-causing diet, but in my experience these diseases are also curable with superior nutrition in the majority of cases.[1] Asthma is an example of a disease considered irreversible that I regularly watch resolve with better nutrition.

My patients routinely make a complete and *predictable* recovery from these illnesses, predominantly through aggressive dietary changes. I am always delighted to meet new patients who are ready to take responsibility for their own health and well-being.

You can watch a new you being made by the wisdom of your body, and this new you will result in all your systems and organs, including your brain, functioning better. Depression, fatigue, anxiety, and allergies are also related to our improper diet. The brain and immune system are able to withstand stress better when our body is properly nourished.

I am neither a research scientist nor a writer by profession. I am a practicing physician who sees at least five thousand patients a year. I work with these patients, educating them and motivating them to do more than others have asked them to do. The results I see with my patients are *thrilling*. Diseases that are considered irreversible I see reversed on a daily basis.

Predictable Disease Reversal Is the Rule, Not the Exception

The overwhelming majority of my patients with high blood pressure are able to normalize their readings and eventually go off their medication. The majority of my patients with angina can end their symptoms of coronary artery disease in the first few months on the diet I prescribe. Most of the rest make a recovery, but it takes longer. The point is, they do recover.

More than 90 percent of my Type II diabetics are able to discontinue their insulin within the first month. More than 80 percent of my chronic headache and migraine sufferers recover without medication, after years of looking for relief with various physicians, including headache specialists.

Some people, especially other physicians, may be skeptical. There are so many exaggerated and false claims made in the health field, especially by those selling so-called natural remedies. Nevertheless, it is wrong to underestimate the results obtainable through appropriate but rigorous nutritional intervention. Even many of my patients with autoimmune illnesses (such as lupus, rheumatoid arthritis, asthma, and hyperthyroidism) are able to recover and throw away their medications. The results are so spectacular that I am subjected to skepticism and even periodic expressions of anger from other physicians.

When one of my patients who had a severe case of rheumatoid arthritis went back to her previous physician, a rheumatologist, and told him she was now well and did not require any medication, he replied, "It must just be that you are resting more." She said, "I'm not resting more. In fact, I am more active than ever because my pain is gone, and I stopped the drugs." He replied, "It's just a temporary remission;

you'll be back soon with another crisis." She never went back.

On the positive side, more and more physicians are becoming interested in nutritional intervention. Such care is clearly more cost-effective than traditional interventions, reduces health-care expenditures, and saves lives. Nothing is more emotionally rewarding for a physician than to watch patients actually get better. How can this not catch on?

An American Has an *Avoidable* Heart Attack Every 30 Seconds

Heart disease is the number one killer in the United States, accounting for more than 40 percent of all deaths. Each year approximately 1.25 million Americans suffer a heart attack or myocardial infarction (MI); more than 400,000 of them die as a result.[2] Most of these deaths occur soon after the onset of symptoms and well before victims are admitted to a hospital.

Every single one of those heart attacks is a terrible tragedy, as it could have been avoided. So many people die needlessly because of wrong, weak, and practically worthless information from the government, physicians, dietitians, and even health authorities such as the American Heart Association. Conventional guidelines are simply insufficient to offer real protection against heart disease.

If you are an American over the age of forty, your chance of having atherosclerosis (hardening) of your blood vessels is over 95 percent. You may think,

"Heart disease won't happen to me!" But I have news for you: it has already happened, and your chance of dying from a heart attack because of your atherosclerosis is about 40 percent. Your exercise program and your Americanized low-fat diet won't help you much, either. You need to do more.

Quick Quiz: Heart Disease

1. **Percentage of children between the ages of four and eleven who already have signs of heart disease?**[3]
   A. None
   B. 10 percent
   C. 40 percent
   D. More than 75 percent

2. **Percentage of female heart attack victims who never knew they had heart disease and then die as a result of their first heart attack?**[4]
   A. None
   B. 10 percent
   C. 25 percent
   D. More than 75 percent

3. **Percentage of heart disease patients who undergo angioplasty and then have their treated arteries clog right back up again within six months?**[5]
   A. 5 percent
   B. 10 percent
   C. 25 percent
   D. None of the above

Answers: 1. D   2. C   3. C

American Heart Association Recommendations Are Dangerous

The typical dietary advice, represented by the American Heart Association's guidelines, is still a dangerous diet. It is not likely to protect you from having a heart attack and does not allow heart disease to reverse itself. Moderation kills. The fact is that such dietary advice still allows heart disease to advance in the overwhelming majority of patients.

> **WARNING: Do not merely comply with these overly permissive recommendations of the American Heart Association, or you will most likely die of a heart attack.**
>
> • Total fat intake should be restricted to 25 to 35 percent of total calories.
> • Cholesterol intake should be less than 300 mg daily.
> • Salt intake should not exceed 1,500 mg of sodium daily.

Just to highlight a small difference between the American Heart Association guidelines and my recommendations: my diets have less than 300 mg of cholesterol *per week!* More than a dozen studies have demonstrated that the majority of patients with coronary artery disease who follow an American Heart Association Therapeutic Lifestyle Changes (TLC) diet have their condition worsen.[6] No study has ever shown that the patients who follow an American Heart Association diet can reverse or stop the worsening of coronary artery disease.

In contrast, numerous studies have documented that heart disease is reversible for the majority of patients following a vegetarian diet.[7] Most often these diets, such as the Ornish program, are not even optimal diets, as they do not sufficiently limit processed grains, salt, and other low-nutrient-density processed foods. Nevertheless, they are still effective for most patients.

The medical literature continues to refer to the diet recommended by the National Cholesterol Education Program as "low-fat." By worldwide standards it should be called a high-fat diet, but more important, it should be called a low-nutrient-density diet—one with a dangerously low level of plant-derived nutrients. As a result of following this almost worthless advice, heart disease patients usually eat a diet that derives over 80 percent of its calories from processed foods and animal products.

No matter how poorly they eat most patients claim that they are already on a healthful diet. They believe that eating a chicken-and-pasta-based diet is in some way healthy merely because they eat less red meat. Yet chicken is almost as dangerous for the heart as red meat; switching from red meat to white meat does not lower cholesterol.[8] Such conventional diets simply do not lower cholesterol sufficiently and do not contain adequate heart-protective factors such as fiber, antioxidants, folate, bioflavonoids, and other phytochemicals.

Another real problem with these so-called low-fat diets is that they are often low in fiber and phytochemical-rich vegetation and may not be carefully designed to include enough of the cardioprotective fats. For example, multiple studies have shown the protective effects of consuming walnuts, which are rich in omega-3 fatty acids. A study of 34,192 California Seventh-Day Adventists showed a 31 percent reduction in the lifetime risk of ischemic heart disease in those who consumed raw nuts frequently.[9] Numerous further studies have confirmed the significant role that walnuts, and nuts overall, play in protection against heart disease.[10] The ideal diet for heart disease reversal, then, is almost free of saturated fat, trans fat, and cholesterol; rich in nutrients and fiber; and low in calories, to achieve thinness. However, it should contain sufficient essential fatty acids, so it is important to add a small amount of nuts and seeds, such as walnuts and flaxseeds.[11]

Dramatically Lower Your "Bad" Cholesterol without Drugs

Some studies published in the past have concluded that dietary changes alone are insufficient to alter plasma lipid levels.[12] The message reported in both the lay and medical media is that low-fat diets don't work. This reinforces the concept that there is not much we can do to alter our genetics, except maybe take drugs. Sadly, the diets offered by nutritional authorities are not aggressive enough to offer true protection or to expect predictable recovery in patients with heart disease. These so-called heart-healthy diets are not anything like my dietary recommendations.

The concern that some medical authorities have

regarding "low-fat" diets is that these diets may lower your HDL and raise your triglycerides.[13] This is true. Lowering fat intake is not the principal step necessary to achieve a cardioprotective diet. It is not sufficient merely to lower your fat intake. If all you do is cut back on fat, you may see little benefit and possibly raise your triglycerides.

However, triglyceride levels increase on low-fat diets only when the diets *are high in refined foods, low in fiber, and unsuccessful in weight reduction*.[14] My observations have been corroborated by other studies.[15] Researchers have compared a high-vegetable-and-fruit diet (like the one recommended in this book) with a grain-based, low-fat diet. Study participants who ate the high-vegetable-and-fruit diet experienced a 33 percent drop in their bad cholesterol (LDL)—a reduction that is greater than that achieved with most cholesterol-lowering drugs.[16] This reduction is dramatically greater than for subjects eating a grain-rich Mediterranean diet or the modern low-fat diet recommended by the American Heart Association.

I rarely ever see triglycerides rise when patients are placed on my nutrient-dense, high-fiber, low-fat diet. For 95 percent of patients, triglycerides drop dramatically. This is also because my patients do not overeat; they lose weight because they feel satisfied from all the fiber in the natural foods and because the diet has such a high nutrient-per-calorie density. We watch the triglyceride problem melt away as they lose the unwanted pounds; triglycerides drop precipitously with weight loss.

The conclusion of the nutrition committee of the American Heart Association is something we all agree on:

> There is overwhelming evidence that reduction in saturated fat, dietary cholesterol, and weight offer the most effective dietary strategies for reducing total cholesterol, LDL-C levels, and cardiovascular risk. Decreases in saturated fat should come at the expense of total fat because there is no biological requirement for saturated fat.[17]

So the main difference between my recommendations and those of the American Heart Association is that I adhere more rigorously to these conclusions than they do. You must do what is necessary to achieve the results desired. If you water down the recommendations to make them more politically or socially acceptable, you sell out the people who want real help and are willing to do what is necessary to protect themselves. An example of the results possible with such aggressive dietary intervention is the patient above.

The results I see with my patients are consistently more spectacular than with other dietary interventions because my advice is generally more rigorous and takes into account the nutrient-per-calorie density of foods to devise a plant-based diet that is maximally effective.

Some studies from other parts of the world also show fairly impressive results utilizing what they

Case Study: Cliff Johnston

Cliff is a chiropractic physician. His father died of heart disease at age forty-seven. Cliff is now forty-five years old. Guess what *he* was headed for? Luckily, he became my patient and was able to get appropriate advice in time.

	8/6/96	9/11/96	% CHANGE
Cholesterol	401	170	−58
Triglycerides	1,985	97	−95
GGT	303	55	−82
Glucose	136	89	−35

The GGT is a parameter of liver function, and the elevated level reflected a degree of fatty infiltration in the liver, negatively affecting its function. The elevated glucose showed the beginning of diabetes. Both were resolved when I placed him on an appropriate diet.

I had originally asked him to wait two months to have his blood redrawn, but he was so enthusiastic and feeling so great because his weight went from 206 to 178 in the one-month period that he came back four weeks early. Can you imagine losing twenty-eight pounds in one month while eating as much food as you like? This is a lot of weight to lose in one month, and is not typical.

call "anti-atherogenic" vegetarian diets, as illustrated by a Russian study where all types of lipid abnormalities were found to improve significantly.[18]

Heart Attack Counterattack

Two things are necessary to predictably reverse heart disease: one is to become thin and superbly nourished, and the other is to get your LDL below 100. Reversal of heart disease then occurs. If one expects to diminish atherosclerotic plaque over time and stabilize the plaque so the chance of having a heart attack significantly decreases, I insist that he or she must strive to achieve the following parameters of normalcy:

- The patient must achieve a normal weight or become thin (less than one inch of abdominal fat in women, and less than three-quarters of an inch in men), or be in the process of steadily losing weight toward this goal.
- The patient must achieve normal cholesterol. My definition of normal is an LDL cholesterol below 100 (most authorities are now using this benchmark). Drugs are rarely needed to attain this level when an aggressive nutritional approach is taken. An LDL below 100 earned as a result of nutritional excellence is much more protective than an LDL below 80 as a result of medication. When you achieve a favorable cholesterol level with proper nutrition, you promote a whole cascade of favorable effects, such as lower levels of inflammation; reduction of fat deposits all over the body, including inside the blood vessels; lower blood pressure; and reduced propensity of blood to clot.

- The patient's diet must be nutrient-dense. Animal products and detrimental fats must be avoided to prevent the after-meal fat surge.[19] Refined carbohydrates should also be avoided to prevent the after-meal glucose surge and to control triglycerides.

- Blood pressure must return to within the normal range, below 130/85, or be slowly improving and moving toward this minimal goal. The normalization of blood pressure as medications are gradually discontinued represents the reversal of atherosclerosis and is an important criterion to predict cardiac safety. The person who has removed his or her cardiac risk no longer requires blood pressure medication to maintain normal blood pressure readings. The vessels have become more elastic through nutritional intervention.

Angioplasty and Bypass Surgery Can Be Avoided

My vigorous, nutritionally centered reversal treatment should be started in every patient diagnosed with coronary artery disease before elective revascularization procedures are considered. My experience has shown that most patients will pursue an aggressive regimen when it is supported by a knowledgeable and involved physician who provides sustained guidance and support. After spending adequate time with a doctor reviewing all the risks of the conventional approach and discussing how reversal is possible with aggressive nutritional management, how many patients do you think would choose to have their chests split open with bypass surgery?

Even if you are lucky enough to have no postoperative complications from bypass, some degree of brain injury occurs in almost every patient from the time spent hooked up to the heart-lung machine. On neuropsychological testing six months later, about 20 percent still show deterioration.[20] Brain injury can range from subtle degrees of intellectual impairment or memory loss to personality changes and permanent brain damage.[21]

Even if you do fine after angioplasty, stent placement, or bypass, atherosclerosis develops at a faster rate in those arteries that were subject to bypass or angioplasty—the plaque grows faster after surgery. Approximately 25 percent of arteries treated by angioplasty clog up again within four to six months.[22] This is called restenosis.

Restenosis is an iatrogenic (physician-caused) disease. Because restenosis involves scarring, it does not behave like native atherosclerosis and does not respond as favorably or as predictably to lifestyle modifications later on. In other words, because of the changes made to the atherosclerotic plaque by the angioplasty treatment, the blockages are less responsive to nutritional intervention when they return. Many patients are worse off after treatment, not better. If they had followed my coronary artery disease reversal plan instead, they would be watching their heart get healthier each week.

Stenting attempts to reduce this high risk of restenosis but has not solved the problem.[23] Stents are tiny wire-mesh tubes that are laced in the narrowed segment of arteries that were stretched by balloon angioplasty. A stent may also cause vascular instability or inflammation where the stent ends and the native plaque begins, thus increasing the risk for coronary thrombosis.[24] It would be good to remind patients that revascularization procedures do not influence the underlying disease, because the rest of the coronary vasculature, with diffuse, nonangiographical noticeable atherosclerosis, is still there posing a risk for future cardiac events, whether the procedure is done or not.

Heart attacks most commonly occur when plaque of a lipid-rich segment ruptures. These vulnerable areas of plaque are not necessarily those that are seen as significantly narrowed on catheterization. Heart attacks still occur in the minimally narrowed segments, areas that may appear normal on catheterization and stress testing.

Most of an Iceberg Is Hidden Underwater

Normal stress test results or cardiac catheterization results do not mean you do not have atherosclerosis. You can have a heart attack the day after you are told your vessels are clear. These tests show only advanced disease.

Massive atheromas (fatty deposits) lurking within the vascular wall—outside the view of angiography (cardiac catheterization)—account for two-thirds of myocardial infarctions.[25] Most heart attacks occur at sites invisible to the tests done by cardiologists.[26]

This is why invasive cardiac procedures relieve pain but do not have an impressive record of reducing the risk of future heart attacks.

Only strong risk-factor control, with aggressive nutritional intervention, can reverse diffuse disease, avoiding the high probability of that heart attack occurring down the road. Your survival depends on risk-factor management—quitting smoking and lowering your weight, blood pressure, glucose, cholesterol, and insulin levels as a result of careful nutrition—not the procedures done by the interventional cardiologist or cardiac surgeon. Only then will beneficial changes occur in the plaque composition, promoting healing of the blood vessel's lining that will stabilize the vessel wall and substantially reduce the risk of a heart attack.

You are deluding yourself if you think chelation or drugs alone will reverse your condition while you remain overweight and nutritionally malnourished. Chelation will not dissolve your atherosclerosis as claimed. The studies done on this therapy are not impressive.[27] In spite of chelation, patients generally continued to deteriorate unless they changed their diet, lost weight, and lowered their cholesterol. In other words, changes not related to chelation.

The areas of vulnerable plaque that cause heart attacks have a large fatty core of cholesterol. Removing the lipid from the plaque can make it smaller and more resistant to rupture. Use common sense; chelation could no more suck fatty substance out of a coronary artery than it could suck the fat off your left hip. There is no way chelating agents can selectively remove the lipids in atheromas.

These atheromas that form on the inside of our blood vessels are fatty tumors with a fibrous cap. They shrink and become more resistant to rupture proportionally to, and as a result of, weight reduction, caloric restriction, nutritional excellence, and aggressive lipid lowering. The most impressive results of shrinking and removing atheromas occur after the person has lost all excess body fat. Body fat is designed for energy storage. Atheromas are more difficult to remove; they resolve after other fat storage sites have been depleted. Fortunately, the same body that created the atheromas has the ability to disintegrate them.

Many of my patients were advised by other physicians to undergo angioplasty or bypass. When they refused, they were referred to my office and chose aggressive nutritional management. Without exception, they have all done well; chest pain has resolved in almost every case (only one went to repeat angioplasty because of a recurrence of chest symptoms); and none has died from cardiac disease.

A typical patient is John Pawlikowski. I see patients like him almost every day. John's story is not unusual—but a miracle to him nevertheless. John came to me with a history of steadily worsening angina. His chest pains were increasing. His stress thallium test suggested multivessel coronary artery disease. He underwent a cardiac catheterization, which revealed a 95 percent stenosis of the left anterior descending artery, and the left circumflex had diffuse disease. He had normal heart function. His cholesterol was 218, he weighed 180 pounds, and he was on two blood pressure medications.

Within a few weeks of following my diet, John's chest pain ceased and he stopped taking nitroglycerin tablets for chest pain relief. In two months his weight dropped to 152—a loss of twenty-eight pounds in eight weeks—and his stress test normalized. Today, sixteen years later, he still weighs 150 pounds, following the same diet. He is well, with no heart problems, and is physically fit; his blood pressure runs about 120/70. He is eighty-eight years old and requires no medication.

JOHN'S LABORATORY REPORTS

	6/6/94	5/5/99	% CHANGE
Cholesterol	218	161	−26
Triglycerides	140	80	−43
HDL	48	65	35
LDL	144	80	−44
Cholesterol:HDL ratio	4.7	2.4	−49

Revascularization procedures may be necessary in rare circumstances, such as triple vessel disease with reduced cardiac output or an injured (stunned) heart muscle. However, I am convinced that aggressive nutritional therapy with the addition of nutritional supplements (and, if needed, medication) will provide a more favorable outcome for the majority of patients than angioplasty, stent placement, and bypass.

One might argue, where are the adequate studies that prove this? But where are the studies to prove revascularization will give a better outcome with a stable patient, without a reduction in cardiac output? The benefits of revascularization procedures for patients with good cardiac function have not been convincingly demonstrated, and there is considerable evidence to suggest that the adverse outcomes outweigh the potential benefits. Furthermore, these dubious results are measured against patients who refuse revascularization and then follow the normal (worthless) dietary recommendations. When we factor in the results I see with very aggressive nutritional management, it seems likely that many patients would be at lower risk if they avoided invasive cardiac procedures and surgery. Fortunately, I am not the only physician in America with this opinion, but sometimes it sure seems as if I am.[28]

Rarely will you find a cardiologist who advises aggressive nutritional therapy before angioplasty or bypass. And physicians who offer medical interventions are usually satisfied if blood pressure is below 140/90 and cholesterol level is under 200. Those levels are not sufficiently normal to offer true protection.

Your Doctor Lied: You Do Have High Blood Pressure and High Cholesterol

Studies clearly demonstrate that the higher one's cholesterol level, the higher the risk of heart disease; conversely, the lower one's cholesterol level, the lower the risk. For true protection, do not be satisfied until your LDL cholesterol is below 100. There is nothing particularly magical about the number 200—heart disease risk continues to decrease as one's cholesterol decreases below this level. The average cholesterol level in China is 127. The Framingham Heart Study showed that participants with cholesterol levels below 150 did not have heart attacks.[29] In fact, most heart attacks occur in patients whose cholesterol runs between 175 and 225. That is the average cholesterol range among Americans, and the average American has heart disease. Do you want to be average, or do you want to be healthy?

I know you were told that if your blood pressure is below 140/90, it is normal. Unfortunately, this is not true, either. It is *average*—not *normal*. This number is used because it is the midpoint of adult Americans older than sixty. The risk for strokes and heart attacks starts climbing at 115/70.

In societies where we do not see high rates of heart disease and strokes, we do not see blood pressure increase with age.[30] Almost all Americans have blood pressure that is unhealthfully high. At a minimum, we should consider blood pressure higher than 125/80 abnormal.

Numerous scientific investigations have shown that the following interventions have some degree of effectiveness in lowering blood pressure:[31]

- Weight loss
- Sodium restriction
- Increased potassium intake
- Increased calcium and magnesium intake

- Alcohol restriction
- Caffeine restriction
- Increased fiber intake
- Increased consumption of fruits and vegetables
- Increased physical activity or exercise

Studies have shown controlling sodium intake and weight loss to be effective in reducing blood pressure, even in the elderly.[32] How can you integrate these interventions into your lifestyle? It's simple. Eat many more fruits, vegetables, and legumes; eat less of everything else; and engage in a moderate amount of exercise. High blood pressure is relatively simple to control.

Though it took a full two years, Rhonda Wilson dropped her weight from 194 to a slim 119. She was also able to come off blood pressure medication as a result of her newfound commitment to a healthful lifestyle. When she first came to me, she was on two medications to control her high blood pressure. These two medications were not sufficient, as her blood pressure was still excessively high. Rhonda did not see normal blood pressure readings for a long time and was not able to stop her blood pressure medication until she became relatively thin. Her story illustrates a common dilemma. It is not unusual for some people to lose some weight, yet still have high blood pressure. Some individuals develop high blood pressure and diabetes even from a small amount of excess body fat. For these individuals, it is even more important to maintain an ideal weight.

I encourage my patients to do what it takes to normalize their blood pressure so they do not require medication. Prescribing medications for high blood pressure has the effect of giving someone a permission slip. Medication has a minimal effect in reducing heart attack occurrence in patients with high blood pressure because it does not remove the underlying problem (atherosclerosis), it just treats the symptom. Patients given medication now falsely believe they are protected, and they continue to follow the same disease-causing lifestyle that led to the problem to begin with, until the inevitable occurs—their first heart attack or stroke. Maybe if high blood pressure medications had never been invented, doctors would have been forced to teach healthful living and nutritional disease causation to their patients. It is possible that many more lives could have been saved.

Only You, Not Your Physician, Must Take Full Responsibility

Do not expect to receive valuable health advice from your typical doctor. Physicians usually do not help; they rush through their patient appointments, especially in the current HMO climate, because they are paid so poorly for each visit and are pressured to see as many patients as possible each day. Your physician is likely doing just as poorly as you are and eating just as unhealthfully or worse. After reading this book, you could improve his health and reduce his risk of premature death more than he could help yours. Even when physicians offer their full time and effort, their recommendations are invariably too mild to have a significant benefit.

Drs. Randall S. Stafford and David Blumenthal, of Massachusetts General Hospital in Boston, reviewed the records of more than 30,000 office visits to 1,521 U.S. physicians of various specialties and found that doctors measured patients' blood pressure during 50 percent of the visits. However, doctors tested their patients' cholesterol levels only 4.6 percent of the time. Physicians offered patients advice on how to lose weight in 5.8 percent of the visits, and suggestions on how to quit smoking 3 percent of the time. On average, doctors gave patients advice on dietary and other changes that can help lower cholesterol in 4.3 percent of the visits, and advice on exercise in 11.5 percent of the visits. When records were reviewed for those who had cardiovascular disease, the typical (almost worthless) dietary counseling and exercise were usually never even mentioned.[33] Obviously, we have a long way to go.

Diabetes—The Consequence of Obesity

More than twenty million Americans have diabetes.[34] As our population grows fatter, this figure is climbing. Diabetes is a nutritionally related disease—one that is both preventable and reversible (in the case of Type II diabetes) through nutritional methods.

Diabetes can take a severe toll—causing heart attacks and strokes, as well as other serious complications. More than 80 percent of adults with Type II diabetes die of heart attacks and strokes.[35] The statistics are even more frustrating when you watch people gain weight, become even more diabetic, and develop attendant complications, all while under the care of their physicians.

> As our country's weight has risen, diabetes has increased accordingly. The worldwide explosion in diabetes parallels the increase in body weight.

Patients are told to learn to live with their diabetes and to learn to control it because it can't be cured. "No, no, and no!" I say. "Don't live with it, get thin and get rid of it, as many of my patients have!"

There are basically two kinds of diabetes: Type I, or childhood-onset diabetes, and Type II, or adult-onset diabetes. In Type I, which generally occurs earlier in life, children incur damage to the pancreas—the organ that produces and secretes insulin—so they have an insulin deficiency. In Type II, the most common type, the individual produces near-normal levels of insulin, but the body is resistant to it, so the level of blood sugar, or glucose, rises. The end result is the same in both types—the individual has a high glucose level in his or her blood.

Both types of diabetes accelerate the aging of our bodies. Diabetes greatly promotes the development of atherosclerosis and cardiovascular disease, and it ages and destroys the kidneys and other body systems. Diabetes is the leading cause of blindness in adults and is the leading cause of kidney failure.

We witness today a huge number of Type II diabetes patients with terrible complications, such as amputations, peripheral neuropathy (painful nerve damage in the legs), retinopathy (the major cause of blindness in diabetics), and nephropathy (kidney damage); complications of Type II diabetes are just as bad as those of Type I diabetes.[36]

Diabetics, regardless of type, have higher levels of triglycerides and increased levels of LDL cholesterol than the general population. Diabetics have more than a 400 percent higher incidence of heart attacks than nondiabetics. One-third of all patients with insulin-dependent (Type I) diabetes die of a heart attack before age fifty. This acceleration of the atherosclerotic process, and the resulting high mortality rate, is present in both types of diabetes.[37]

By simple logic, you would expect that any dietary recommendations designed for diabetics would at least attempt to reduce the risk of heart attack, stroke, or other cardiovascular event. Unfortunately, the nutritional advice given to diabetics is to follow the same diet that has proved not to work for heart disease patients. Such a diet is risky for all people, but for the diabetic it is exceptionally hazardous—it is deadly. The combination of refined grains, processed foods, and animal products guarantees a steady stream of available customers for hospitals and emergency rooms.

When Type I patients take a more aggressive and progressive nutritional approach, they can prevent many of the complications that befall diabetics. They can expect a normal life span, because it is the interaction between diabetes and the disease-causing modern diet that results in such dismal statistics, not merely being diabetic. Type I diabetics will still require some insulin, but often I find my Type I diabetic patients requiring about half as much insulin as they did prior to adopting my lifesaving program. Their sugars don't swing wildly up and down, and since they are using less insulin, they have less chance of developing potentially dangerous hypoglycemic episodes.

Type II diabetics adopting this approach can become undiabetic and achieve wellness and even excellent health. They can be diabetes-free for life! Almost all my Type II diabetic patients are weaned off insulin in the first month. Thanks to their excellent nutrition, these patients have much better (lower) blood sugars than when they were on insulin. The horrors of diabetes about to befall them are aborted.

I have also observed patients who came to me with diabetic retinopathy and peripheral neuropathy gradually improve and eventually resolve their conditions. Dr. Milton Crane reported similar findings in his patients: seventeen out of twenty-one patients who adopted a plant-rich vegan diet obtained complete relief from their peripheral neuropathy.[38]

Insulin for Type II Diabetes Makes Things Worse

Insulin works less effectively when people eat fatty foods or gain weight. Diets containing less fat improve insulin sensitivity, as does weight loss.[39] An individual who is overweight requires more insulin, whether he or she is diabetic or not. In fact, giving overweight diabetic people even more insulin makes them sicker by promoting weight gain. They become even more diabetic. How does this process work? Our pancreas secretes the amount of insulin demanded by the body. A person of normal weight with about a third of an inch of periumbilical fat will secrete X amount of insulin. Let's say this person gains about twenty pounds of fat. His body will now require more insulin, almost twice as much, because fat on the body blocks the uptake of insulin into the cells.

If the person is obese, with more than fifty pounds of excess fat, his body will demand huge loads of insulin from the pancreas, even as much as ten times more than a person of normal weight needs. So what do you think happens after five to ten years of forcing the pancreas to work so hard? You guessed it—pancreatic poop-out.

The pancreas begins to secrete less insulin, in spite of the huge demands of the body. Eventually, with less insulin available to move glucose from the bloodstream into the cells, the glucose level in the blood starts to rise and the person gets diagnosed with diabetes. In most cases, these individuals are still secreting an excessive amount of insulin (compared with a person of normal weight), just not enough for them. When they eat a less taxing diet and lose weight, they don't need the extra insulin to control the sugars.

What this means is that typical Type II diabetes

is caused by overweight in individuals who have a smaller reserve of insulin-secreting cells in the pancreas. In the susceptible individual, even ten to twenty pounds of excess weight could make the difference. Losing the extra weight enables these individuals to live within the capabilities of their body. Most Type II diabetics still produce enough insulin to maintain normalcy as long as they maintain a thinner, normal weight.

Following my program is the most important thing a diabetic individual can do to extend his or her life span. It has been known for years that intentional weight loss improves diabetics' blood sugars, lipids, and blood pressure. One study documented a significant increase in life expectancy, with an average of 25 percent reduced premature mortality when diabetic individuals dropped their body weight. Other studies have come to similar conclusions.[40] Imagine the results when a program of nutritional excellence achieves the weight loss.

Insulin is a dangerous drug for Type II diabetics. These are people who are overweight to begin with. Insulin therapy will result in further weight gain, accelerating their diabetes. A vicious cycle begins that usually causes patients to require more and more insulin as they put on the pounds. When they come to see me for the first time, they report their sugars are impossible to control in spite of massive doses of insulin, which they are now combining with oral medication. It is like walking around with a live hand grenade in your pocket, ready to explode at any minute.

Don't Merely Control Your Diabetes—Get Rid of It for Good

As my patients begin the program I usually cut their insulin in half. The insulin is then gradually phased out over the next few days or weeks, depending on their response and how advanced their condition was when they started. Most patients can stop all insulin within the first few days. The warning I give to patients and their physicians adopting this program is not to underestimate how effective it can be. If the medications, especially insulin, are not dramatically reduced, a dangerous hypoglycemic reaction—driving the blood sugar level too low—can occur from overmedication. It is safer to undermedicate and let the glucose levels run a little high at first, then add back a little medication if necessary. This will minimize the risk of hypoglycemia. Since this diet is so powerfully effective in reversing diabetes and other diseases of nutritional neglect, it is essential that you work closely with a doctor who can help you adjust your medication dose downward in a careful fashion.

Note: No diabetic patient on medication should make dietary changes without the assistance of a physician, as adjusting the medication will be necessary to prevent hypoglycemia, or excessively lowering the blood sugar level.

I typically continue or begin Glucophage (metformin) or other similar drugs. The newer medications that do not interfere with weight loss are safer than the older oral medications diabetics used in the past. Eventually, as more weight is lost, these patients can have normal glucose levels without any medication. They become nondiabetic, though diabetes can recur should they adopt a more stressful and girth-growing diet.

Gerardo Petito's case exemplifies the outcome I see with other diabetic patients on a regular basis. Gerardo stated that his main reason for coming to me was that he wanted to control his diabetes better. On his first visit, on January 18, 2000, he was taking three medications: Accupril 20 mg for blood pressure and two medications for diabetes, Glucophage 500 twice daily and fifteen units of insulin twice daily. He had been on insulin for seven years. His fasting glucose in the morning had been running around 175 with this regimen. His blood pressure was 140/85 and he weighed 256 pounds.

After a lengthy discussion, Gerardo agreed to follow my dietary advice. I instructed him to cut back his insulin dose to ten units the evening of the visit and to five units the following morning; after that, he was to take no more insulin.

When Gerardo came back for his second visit two weeks later, he weighed 237, a loss of nineteen pounds in just two weeks. His glucose in the morning was averaging 115, and his blood pressure was down to 125/80. Other than checking his blood test and doing an EKG for the record, I made no changes in his program. He was enjoying the diet and following my advice to the letter.

At Gerardo's third visit the next month, he

weighed 221, a loss of thirty-five pounds in fifty-two days. He had just returned from a cruise, where he continued to follow his healthful diet. His morning glucose was averaging around 80 (completely normal), so I stopped the Glucophage. His blood pressure was 88/70, so I discontinued the Accupril.

Ten months after Gerardo's first visit, he weighed 190, a loss of sixty-six pounds, his cholesterol was 134, and his blood pressure was 112/76. His hemoglobin A1C, a measure of diabetic control, was 5.3, in the nondiabetic range. He was on no medication.

Rather than controlling his blood pressure and diabetes, he chose to follow my advice and get rid of his medical problems altogether.

Advice for the Diabetic Patient

The general advice given in this book is sufficient for most diabetics. The most important goal is how much weight you lose, not whether your glucose is a little higher or lower in the short run. Follow my guidelines for aggressive weight loss in the next chapter. If you follow my program to the letter, it will not be necessary to make your diet complicated by following diabetic food exchanges and counting calories. Most people do not have to measure portions, either. Your goals are the same as the patient with coronary artery disease: get thin and aggressively treat your risk factors. With time, your body will normalize your numbers. Keep the following guidelines in mind:

1. Refined starches such as white bread and pasta are particularly harmful; avoid them completely.
2. Do not consume any fruit juice or dried fruits. Avoid all sweets, except for fresh fruit in reasonable quantities. Two or three fruits for breakfast is fine, and one fruit after lunch and dinner is ideal. The best fruits are those with less sugar—grapefruit, oranges, kiwifruit, strawberries and other berries, melons, and green apples.
3. Avoid all oil. Raw nuts are permitted, but only one ounce or less.
4. The name of your diet is the "greens and beans diet"; green vegetables and beans should make up most of your diet.
5. Limit animal-food intake to no more than two servings of fish weekly.
6. Try to exercise regularly and consistently, like dispensing your medication. Do it on a regimented schedule, preferably twice daily. Walking stairs is one of the greatest exercises for weight loss.

As the information in this book becomes your prescription for health, you can avoid heart attacks and strokes. If this diet were adopted by the general public, these illnesses would become rare and diabetes would practically disappear from our society.

The Eat to Live Formula Lowers Triglycerides

Some physicians and nutritionists believe that individuals suffering from obesity, diabetes, and elevated triglycerides may have good results in losing weight and controlling their high triglycerides and elevated glucose with a high-protein, low-carbohydrate diet. They believe this because it has been observed that high-carbohydrate diets can raise triglyceride levels.

I agree that a diet high in *refined* carbohydrates is not advised and will worsen this condition. However, I want to make it absolutely clear that these patients can achieve spectacular results without the added dangers of a diet high in animal protein and saturated fat. They merely need advice on how to modify the plant-based diet for their condition. They do so by eating a relatively high-protein plant-based diet that reduces the amount of low-fiber carbohydrates. The diet is heavy in beans, raw vegetables, and cooked greens. The results are invariably impressive.

Headaches, Hypoglycemia, and Hunger

It's almost incredible to believe, but almost all patients with headaches and hypoglycemia get well permanently following the formula for health in this book. I believe it has very much to do with *detoxification*.

The body can heal itself when the obstacles to healing or stressors are removed. The reason people can't ever make complete recoveries is that they are addicted to their bad habits and unhealthful ways of eating and drinking.

Imagine if you were drinking ten cups of coffee daily. If you stopped drinking coffee, you would feel ill; you might get headaches, feel weak, even get the shakes. Fortunately, this would resolve slowly over four to six days, and then you would be well.

So, if you were this heavy coffee drinker, when do you think you would feel the worst? Right after eating, upon waking up in the morning, or when delaying or skipping a meal?

You are correct if you answered either upon first waking up or when delaying or skipping a meal. The body goes through withdrawal, or detoxification, most effectively when it is not busy digesting food. A heavy meal will stop the ill feelings, or you'll feel better if you just drink another cup of coffee, but the cycle of feeling ill will start all over again the minute the caffeine level drops or the glucose level in your blood starts to go down.

Delaying a meal brings about symptoms most people call "hunger." These symptoms include abdominal cramping, weakness, and feeling ill—*the same as during drug withdrawal*.

This is not hunger. Our dietary habits, especially eating animal-protein-rich foods three times a day, are so stressful to the detoxification system in our liver and kidneys that we start to get withdrawal, or detoxification, symptoms the minute we aren't busy processing such food.

Real hunger is not that uncomfortable. True hunger is mediated by the hypothalamus in the brain. The hunger-related activity of the hypothalamus correlates best with an increased sensation of need in the mouth and throat area.[41]

You could feel better by drinking a cup of coffee every three hours, evenly spaced out, to keep your caffeine blood levels constant. Or you could take medications such as Fioricet, Cafergot, Excedrin, Esgic, Fiorinal, Migranal, Wigraine, and others whose active ingredients are narcotics, barbiturates, ergotamines, or caffeine; or you can just get some amphetamines or cocaine from the alley behind the liquor store. Either way, I hope you understand that temporarily feeling better does not mean getting well. Putting toxic drugs in your body can only compromise your health and lead to further dependence and suffering. In order to detoxify, you need to feel worse, not better; then after the withdrawal symptoms are completed, you will truly become well.

Feeling better can mean becoming sicker. Feeling worse (temporarily) may mean getting well.

In medical school my classmates and I learned from a researcher that animal protein places a detoxification stress on the liver and that the nitrogenous wastes generated are toxic. These metabolic toxins (about fourteen of them) rise in the bloodstream and accompany the rise in uric acid after a meal rich in animal protein. Withdrawal from these toxins can cause uncomfortable symptoms in susceptible individuals, symptoms that many call hypoglycemia.

The word *hypoglycemia* means "low glucose in

the bloodstream." It gives people the impression that the low glucose level itself is the cause of the problem.

Certain uncommon medical conditions (such as insulin-secreting tumors), excessive diabetic medication, and other rare illnesses can cause hypoglycemia and even hypoglycemic coma, but I am referring to those people with reactive hypoglycemia. They feel ill when they delay eating, but they do not have a serious medical condition, nor do their blood sugars drop dangerously low. Most people carrying this diagnosis do not have fasting glucoses below 50; when their blood is drawn when they delay eating and feel extremely ill, the blood sugar is usually not low enough to account for their feeling so ill. There seems to be no correlation between the severity of the symptoms and their low glucose levels, but they feel uncomfortable if they try to stop treating themselves with high-protein diets.

It is a massive oversimplification to think that a lower level of glucose in the blood is the sole cause of this problem. I find that the people with the most troublesome symptoms do not even have low glucose levels.

Many doctors learn during their training that if the liver is compromised, such as in cirrhosis, the patient cannot effectively remove these toxins and may consequently feel mentally affected, confused, and even psychotic unless they are fed a low-protein diet, generating a lower level of nitrogenous wastes. For this reason, it is standard medical care to feed a patient with advanced liver disease a low-protein diet.

Most Americans are protein-toxic. Like the patient with cirrhosis (but less so), they are toxic because their body detoxification system struggles under the excessive nitrogen load in addition to all the salt, caffeine, sweets, trans fats, and other noxious chemicals we consume. So the stomach empties and we feel ill, not hungry. Most people are too toxic to feel hungry. Detoxification symptoms appear first. Most people are driven to eat because it is time to eat or because they feel detoxification discomfort. *Most Americans have never felt* true hunger *in their entire overfed existence.*

Many people come into my office with a diagnosis of hypoglycemia, meaning they feel ill when they delay eating. They are often told to eat a diet with frequent feedings of high-protein food. I insist that this diet is the precise cause of the condition, not the remedy; it is no more a remedy than putting them on a cup of coffee every hour. Sure, they will feel better temporarily, but if they want to make a complete and lasting recovery, they must unscramble their thinking. They must put up with about one week of not feeling so great, but then they can be set free from their discomfort and their addiction to bad habits and a toxic diet.

When I first begin treating patients with hypoglycemic symptoms, I continue them on snacks between meals and use some raw nuts and beans at each meal. They are forbidden to consume any refined carbohydrates such as bread, pasta, sweets, or fruit juice, to prevent swings in insulin. In some individuals, insulin levels swing up too high and then too low merely because they are eating refined sugars and refined grains, and not natural, unrefined food. These individuals are just sensitive to the junk food eaten by most Americans. The notoriously unreliable glucose tolerance test, in which patients consume about 100 grams of glucose, duplicates eating a huge quantity of junk food. Even normal people can feel ill from this experience.

Invariably, within two or three weeks their symptoms diminish and they gain the ability to delay eating without feeling ill. They can then follow the same diet I recommend for everyone without feeling any ill effects.

If you have this condition, you must also avoid alcohol, coffee, tea, artificial flavorings, and food additives. Fresh fruit does not need to be restricted.

Headache Sufferers Rejoice

Recurrent headaches are not much different. They are almost always the result of nutritional folly and, like other reasons that keep doctors' offices busy, are completely avoidable.

The relationship between food triggers and migraines has been the subject of much debate, with varying results from medical researchers. Headache specialists such as Seymour Diamond, director of the Diamond Headache Clinic at Columbus Hospital in Chicago, report that about 30 percent of patients can identify food triggers.[42]

My experience in treating migraine and severe-headache patients with a more comprehensive nutritional approach has shown that 90 to 95 percent of patients are able to remain headache-free after the first three-month period. These patients avoid common migraine triggers, but also in the healing phase they adhere to a strict natural-food vegan diet of primarily fruits and vegetables rich in natural starches, such as squash and brown rice. These patients must avoid all packaged and processed foods, which are notorious for containing hidden food additives, even though they are not disclosed on the labels. They also avoid all added salt.

I believe I obtain such impressive results not merely because of avoiding triggers but because the patient becomes healthier and is able to process toxins more effectively. Additionally, when animal-product consumption is significantly lowered or removed from the diet, the liver is not faced with breaking down this heavy toxic load and can perform its normal detoxification function more effectively.

Very often in the initial phase of my program, when patients are on a diet with a lower level of tissue irritants, a headache will be precipitated. In other words, it is possible that the patient will initially feel worse, not better. I encourage such patients not to take medication during this initial phase, if at all possible. Instead, I recommend that they drape a cold washcloth over their forehead and lie down in a dark room to rest. The prescribed diet, very low in sodium and animal protein, resolves the headaches in the large majority of patients. If it does not, not all is lost, because some fasting usually clears up the problem in most of the remaining headache sufferers.[43]

My patients begin by following a diet along the lines of the one described on the next page. They are instructed not to take any medication after the first week; after that time they are encouraged to control their pain with ice, hot showers, and pressure bands. They will never recover if they don't first detoxify themselves of their addiction to pain medications. These medications may offer pain relief, but they perpetuate the headache at the same time. Drugs that are used for headaches, such as acetaminophen (Tylenol), barbiturates, codeine, and ergotamines, all cause headaches to recur on a rebound basis as these toxins begin to wash out of the nervous system. Even a little aspirin can cause a chronic daily-headache syndrome.[44]

15 COMMON MIGRAINE TRIGGERS

sweets	dairy and cheese	salted or pickled foods
fermented foods	chocolate	vinegar
pizza	smoked meats	alcohol
monosodium glutamate	nuts	food additives
	hydrolyzed protein	baked goods
yeast		

The first phase of the anti-headache diet is followed strictly for two weeks. Then if the person is headache-free, I expand the diet to include a wider variety of fruits and begin to add beans in the second phase. I usually have the patient avoid nuts for the first few weeks because these bother some people. All dairy and yeast should be avoided as well.

Phase One Anti-Headache Diet
with a Greater Than 90 Percent Cure Rate

Breakfast

Melon, apple, or pear

Oatmeal and water, no sweetener

Yeast-free whole grain bread

Lunch

Large green salad, with one teaspoon of olive oil

One starchy vegetable or grain—corn, sweet potato,
brown rice

Grapes, pear, or apple

Dinner

Large green salad with tomatoes, with one teaspoon
of olive oil

One steamed green vegetable—string beans, asparagus,
artichokes, broccoli, zucchini

One starchy vegetable or grain—butternut or acorn
squash, potato, millet, whole wheat pasta

Tomato sauce (unsalted) permitted

Autoimmune Diseases and All the Rest

If dangerous drugs were the only way for a person
to gain relief from suffering, we would be forced to
accept the drawbacks of conventional therapy for
autoimmune illnesses. The reality is, however, that
dietary and nutritional interventions work for autoimmune diseases such as rheumatoid arthritis.

Caring for such patients has been a major portion of my work as a physician for the past twenty years. I have seen scores of rheumatoid arthritis, lupus, and connective tissue disease patients recover completely through these interventions. Many of my patients have also made complete recoveries from allergies and asthma. Not every patient obtains a complete remission, but the majority are able to avoid the use of medication.

The key to treating autoimmune illnesses is to obey the H = N/C formula. Only then can the immune system begin to normalize its haywire circuitry.

Research studies from around the world confirm that this approach is effective.[45] While more research is needed in this area, all the studies that have been done are predictably positive and document improvement in blood inflammatory markers, as well as patient symptoms. I see this occur on a daily basis.

Here are the main ways to increase the possibility of obtaining remission or improvement in patients with autoimmune diseases:

1. A strict plant-based (vegan), dairy-free, wheat-free, and gluten-free diet is usually necessary; a lower-protein diet is helpful.
2. A high nutrient-per-calorie density with caloric restriction sufficient to obtain a normal weight is essential.
3. Arachidonic acid and DHA levels should be checked with an essential fatty acid profile. If the fatty acid balance is abnormal, supplementation with omega-3 fatty acids to achieve sat-

isfactory balance may be necessary. Ground flaxseeds, pure plant-derived DHA, or in some cases high-potency fish oil can be used.

4. Therapeutic fasting can be an extremely effective adjunct to control the autoimmune response and reset the hyperactive immune system to a more normal (lower) level of activity. Do not fast if you are are dependent on multiple immunosuppressive drugs, such as methotrexate and Imuran, as it is not safe to fast while on such medication. It is essential that patients contemplating this therapy be properly supervised by a physician. Those interested in learning more about therapeutic fasting for autoimmune illness should read my book *Fasting and Eating for Health*. Physicians can request medical journal articles, including case studies that I wrote about this therapy along with comprehensive medical references, from me via my website (DrFuhrman. com) or office.

5. Undertaking food elimination and challenge can uncover hidden food sensitivities. Most of the offending foods have already been eliminated—animal products, wheat, and dairy—but many patients find other foods that can worsen their condition as well. These foods are not routinely uncovered with allergy testing. It usually requires a short period of fasting and then the gradual introduction of only one new food each day, eliminating any food that causes an increase in

pain over the fasted state. I would like to repeat this to make it clear—the elevated levels of IgG and IgE against various foods on allergy tests are indeed common in patients with rheumatoid arthritis and other autoimmune diseases; however, there is not an adequate clinical correlation between those foods and the foods we find to be aggravating the symptoms. Other researchers have noted the same thing.[46] I usually instruct patients to save their money and forgo those tests.

Diet Is the First Line of Defense

Working with patients with autoimmune diseases such as connective tissue disease, myositis, rheumatoid arthritis, and lupus is very rewarding. These patients were convinced that they could never get well and are usually eternally grateful to be healthy again and not require medication. I regularly get notes and letters, such as these unsolicited comments:

"After three months I am off all drugs."

—Richard Arroni

"I would like to shout, Dr. Fuhrman did it."

—Fred Redington

"Six months ago I prayed I would die, now I'm ready to live again."

—Jennifer Fullum

"Thank you for saving my life."

—Harriet Fleming

An aggressive nutritional approach to autoimmune illnesses should always be tried *first* when the disease is in its infancy. Logically, the more advanced the disease is, and the more damage that has been done by the disease, the less likely the patient will respond. My experience with inflammatory diseases such as rheumatoid arthritis is that some patients are more dietary-sensitive than others and that some patients have very high levels of inflammation that are difficult to curtail with natural therapy. Nevertheless, the majority benefit—and since the conventional drugs used to treat these types of illnesses are so toxic and have so many risky side effects, the dietary method should be tried first. Modern drugs often contribute to the disability and misery of patients with an autoimmune illness and increase cancer risk. Studies show that the long-term outcome is poor after twenty years of taking such medication.[47] A study in the *British Journal of Rheumatology* showed the major drugs to treat rheumatoid arthritis, such as azathioprine, cyclophosphamide, chlorambucil, and methotrexate, increase the likelihood that the person will die of cancer.[48]

Patients who use drugs that suppress the immune system forgo some protection that the immune system offers against infection and cancer. These individuals need a superior diet, even if they can't stop all medication.

So many of the patients I see, especially the ones who have made recoveries, are angry at their former physicians who did not even suggest nutrition before starting them on medication. These individuals are usually so "sick of being sick," they will do anything to get well. They don't find the diet restrictive and show enthusiasm and determination to recover their health. It is terrifically exciting to see such patients make recoveries and eliminate the need for medication.

Diseases Resolve or Improve with Nutritional Excellence

Other conditions that also respond exceptionally well to dietary modification include menstrual complaints and irritable bowel syndrome.

Researchers testing similar diets to the one I recommend have noted that a low-fat vegetarian diet increases sex-hormone-binding globulin as it reduces estrogen activity.[49] This not only reduces one's risk of breast cancer but also significantly reduces the pain and bloating associated with menstruation.

I also see a large number of patients with irritable bowel syndrome. Some feel better within three days of following this diet, although others take a few weeks or longer to adjust to the comparatively large amount of fiber. Both animal products and flour products are triggers for bowel symptoms in many individuals.[50] British researchers have documented that increased production of methane and other gaseous products representing increased fermentation in the colon from meats, dairy products, and refined grains correlate with bowel complaints. However, there are other mechanisms by which a natural-food diet high in nutrients and fiber reestablishes normal gut motility and tone. It can take time to undo a lifetime of wrong eating; most of my patients need three months to see improvement. Of course, sometimes diets have to be modified for individual uniqueness. In such cases, working with a knowledgeable physician is helpful.

Most chronic illnesses have been earned from a lifetime of inferior nutrition, which eventually results in abnormal function or frequent discomfort. These illnesses are not beyond our control, they are not primarily genetic, and they are not the normal consequence of aging. True, we all have our weakest links governed by genetics; but these weak links need never reveal themselves unless our health deteriorates. Superior health flows naturally as a result of superior nutrition. Our predisposition to certain illnesses can remain hidden.

Certainly, this method of healing is not for everybody. Some would prefer to eat conventionally and take whatever medication is indicated for their condition. That is their inalienable right. However, it is also the right of sick and suffering individuals who seek a natural approach to be aware of how effective aggressive nutritional interventions can be. I would like to take these patients down the streets of Manhattan for a ticker-tape parade to spread the word: You don't have to be sick. Remember, health is your greatest wealth!

8

Your Plan for Substantial Weight Reduction

Case Study:
Emily lost one hundred pounds and took years off her body. In just two months, her blood pressure and cholesterol stats reflected healthy numbers.

When I first started the journey to get my health back, I was obese and depressed, and I knew I was very ill. It was an effort just to get out of bed in the morning. I knew that if I was ever going to succeed, I had to have something simple and concrete to follow.

I had dieted in the past and always felt deprived and miserable, but for the first time, I was eating lots of good-quality food and feeling great doing it! Within the first month I dropped twenty pounds, and my cholesterol dropped from 214 to 145. That solidified my desire to commit to Dr. Fuhrman's nutritional wisdom for the rest of my life.

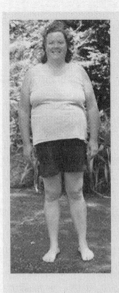
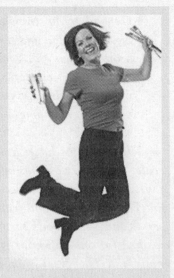

After reading Eat to Live, *I knew I had my answer. I kept copies of the Six-Week Plan with me at all times and used it to guide all my decisions.*

- *Those first couple of weeks I didn't feel like eating romaine lettuce, collard greens, or Brussels sprouts. I followed the plan.*
- *I was heavily addicted to salt, creamy cottage cheese, ranch dressing, cheddar cheese, and crunchy peanut butter. I followed the plan.*
- *I craved diet cola, diet pudding, and my usual bedtime snack of a large bowl of cereal and milk. I followed the plan.*
- *My son became seriously ill and life suddenly became an out-of-control roller coaster. I followed the plan.*

- He had to be transferred to a hospital in another state, and I had to find my way around a new city. I followed the plan.
- The hospital cafeteria food looked comforting and inviting and the candy in the gift shop called out my name. I followed the plan.

Three months later, back home, I got on the scale. I was forty pounds lighter, and, more important, I was no longer addicted to toxic foods. I now craved fresh greens and fruits. Diet soda, diet desserts, and salty foods tasted disgusting to me. I walked for one-half hour every morning and evening and felt great. My body was thoroughly refreshed after a good night's sleep, and my brain fog had completely disappeared.

When I started my journey, I weighed 226 pounds, and now I weigh 126 pounds. That's a total weight loss of one hundred pounds, which I've kept off! That's a big deal for me, because in the past, I would gain weight back immediately after quitting a diet. This is for life!

What have we learned so far? First, eating foods with too few nutrients is bad for your health. Second, a large amount of animal products in your diet correlates with a vast number of diseases. Last, unrefined plant foods offer the best protection against disease. The question is, how can we translate this data into a health program that will help us achieve a healthy weight, maximize our well-being, and let us enjoy meals at the same time? That is, in part, what the rest of this book will answer. The first part of this chapter describes exactly what I want you to do for the next six weeks of your life. The rest of the chapter shows how you can incorporate these principles into the rest of your life in a practical and sensible way—the Life Plan—with more flexibility than the Six-Week Plan, including both vegetarian and non-vegetarian options. The life plan is a nutritarian diet. I coined the term *nutritarian* to describe someone who strives for more micronutrients per calorie in their diet style. A nutritarian understands that food has powerful disease-protecting and therapeutic effects and seeks to consume a broad array of micronutrients via their food choices.

The Six-Week Plan

Get ready for the most exciting six weeks of your adult life. If you follow my program precisely for the next six weeks, your body will undergo a remarkable transformation and you will be witness to its miraculous self-healing ability. With no compromise for these first six weeks, you will unleash a biochemical and physiological makeover that will change you forever. You will be thrilled with how easily your weight drops and the subtle changes you experience in your physical and emotional well-being. Maybe even more meaningful than the weight loss, you will feel better than you have in years. Your nose won't feel stuffed, your allergies can disappear, and your constipation will go away. Most people quickly find they are no longer aware that their digestive tract even exists, as they no longer experience stomachaches, cramping, and intestinal discomfort. You will no longer require headache remedies, pain pills, digestive aids, and other drugs that attempt to alleviate the suffering caused by unhealthy eating. I always like to compare the health of my patients after this initial six-week intervention with how they felt when they first came in with their typical complaints of diabetes, high blood pressure, and high cholesterol and triglycerides. The results are remarkable when their weight, blood pressure, and blood tests are rechecked. I encourage people to do a scientific test: do this very strictly for just six weeks and see how much weight you lose. Most get so excited with the results during the six-week "trial" that they are motivated to keep going. Results encourage change, and results motivate. The stricter you are, the more quickly your taste will change.

The Six-Week Plan includes none of those optional, low-nutrient foods described later in this chapter. Whether you have a serious medical condition or not, your body will undergo an energizing and healing transformation. It will overcome food addictions and get the physiological housecleaning it has been yearning for. It will be hard, initially, but the immediate results will help keep you focused.

I know many of you have not succeeded with diets in the past or have been disappointed with your rate of progress. Such will not be the case here. Your life is too important. Your ideal weight is within reach. Give this diet a true test and do as I recommend. See how much weight you lose, how far down you can get your lipids (cholesterol and triglycerides), and how many symptoms such as headache, gastritis, indigestion, and nasal congestion disappear. Once you see the incredible results, you will be so pleased that you will feel comfortable with only occasional deviation from this ideal diet. Eat to live for the first time in your life and give yourself this life-changing opportunity.

The Six-Week Plan gives your body time to adjust to this new way of eating. At the beginning the weight comes off quickly, but as you approach your target weight, your weight loss will slow down. Your taste buds will change. They will actually become more sensitive to the subtle flavors in natural foods, and six weeks is sufficient time for any symptoms arising from the new diet to subside. Results beget results. After you have lost about twenty-five pounds, you will feel like exercising more and be thrilled to see even more spectacular results when you go to the gym and sculpt the body you have always dreamed of.

It is not unusual for my patients to lose one pound per day over the first ten to fourteen days on this plan. Sometimes more. One patient, George, who came to me with high blood pressure, lost eight pounds in the first three days. Much of that was probably water weight from cutting out all the salt in his diet; nevertheless, his blood pressure came down and he continued to lose weight over the next few months at a rate of about ten pounds per month. He had a little turkey on Thanksgiving and made a few other minor deviations from the plan, but he found the diet easy. He used some of my recipes and recommended products and soon lost the full hundred pounds he needed to take off.

Raw Vegetables (Including Salad)

These foods are to be eaten in unlimited quantities, but think big. Since they have a negative caloric effect, the more you eat, the more you lose. Raw foods also have a faster transit time through the digestive tract and result in a lower glucose response and encourage more weight loss than their cooked counterparts.[1] The object is to eat as many raw vegetables as possible, with a goal of one pound (sixteen ounces) daily. Meeting this one pound goal is not that hard to do. A small head of romaine lettuce is 6 to 8 ounces, a medium tomato or bell pepper weighs about 4 to 6 ounces, Include raw vegetables such as snow peas, red bell peppers, carrots, raw peas, tomatoes, cucumbers, and sprouts. The entire pound is less than 100 calories of food, and when you chew very well and spread this out between meals, you may find it easy to consume this amount each day.

Cooked Vegetables

Eat as many steamed or cooked green vegetables as you can. Cooked non-green nutrient-dense vegetables such as eggplant, mushrooms, peppers, onions, tomatoes, carrots, and cauliflower are unlimited as well. My saying, "The more you eat, the more weight you will lose," also applies here. Again, the goal is one pound per day. If you can't eat this much, don't force yourself, but the idea is to completely rethink what your idea of a portion is; make it huge. One of the keys to your success is to eat a decent portion of food; so when you eat these greens, try to eat a much larger portion than you might have in the past. A serving of 11/2 cups of cooked kale weighs 7 ounces, 2 cups of cooked broccoli or Brussels sprouts weighs 11 ounces, and 2 cups of cauliflower weighs 9 ounces.

Go for variety in your cooked vegetables by using string beans, broccoli, artichokes, asparagus, zucchini, kale, collards, cabbage, Brussels sprouts, bok choy, okra, Swiss chard, turnip greens, escarole, beet greens, spinach, dandelion greens, broccoli raab, cauliflower, peppers, mushrooms, onions, and tomatoes.

> Remember that eating one pound of green vegetables and one pound of raw vegetables a day is an average goal to shoot for, but you should eat only the amount of food that is comfortable for you. Some people may do better with more or less.

Beans or Legumes

Beans or legumes are among the world's most perfect foods. They stabilize blood sugar, blunt the desire for sweets, and prevent mid-afternoon cravings. Even a small portion can help you feel full, but in the Six-Week Plan I encourage you to eat at least one full cup daily.

Beans contain both insoluble and soluble fiber and are very high in resistant starch. While the benefits of fiber are well-known, resistant starch is proving to be another highly desirable dietary component. Although it is technically a starch, it acts more like fiber during digestion. Typically, starches found in carbohydrate-rich foods are broken down into glucose during digestion, and the body uses that glucose as energy. Much like fiber, resistant starch "resists" digestion and passes through the small intestine without being digested. Because of this, some researchers classify resistant starch as a third type of fiber.

Beans are the best food source of resistant starch. Overall, the starch in beans is about evenly divided between slowly digested starch and resistant starch, although the amount of resistant starch can vary depending on the type of bean and the preparation method. This means that a significant amount of the carbohydrate calories listed for the beans is not absorbed.

Resistant starch offers many additional unique health benefits. It:

- Aids weight loss and digestive health
- Helps prevent constipation
- Helps to maintain lower blood sugar levels
- Reduces the risk of developing diabetes and heart disease
- Reduces the risk of colon cancer

Legume or bean intake is an important variable in the promotion of long life. An important longitudinal study showed that a higher legume intake is the most protective dietary factor affecting survival among the elderly, regardless of their ethnicity. The study found that legumes were associated with long-lived people in various food cultures, including the Japanese (soy, tofu, natto), the Swedes (brown beans, peas), and Mediterranean peoples (lentils, chickpeas, white beans).[2] Beans and greens are the foods most closely linked in the scientific literature with protection against cancer, diabetes, heart disease, stroke, and dementia.

Consider beans your preferred high-carbohydrate food. They can be flavored and spiced in interesting ways, and you can eat an unlimited quantity of them. Eat some beans with every lunch. Among your choices are chickpeas, black-eyed peas, black beans, cowpeas, split peas, lima beans, pinto beans, lentils, red kidney beans, soybeans, cannellini beans, pigeon peas, and white beans.

Fresh Fruit

Eat at least four fresh fruits per day, but no fruit juice. Shred or cut up apples and oranges and add them to your salad for flavor; they will help you feel full. Clementines are a nice addition to a green salad. Pineapple is good with vegetables and can be cooked with tomatoes and vegetables for a Hawaiian-flavored vegetable dish. On the Six-Week Plan, no fruit juice is permitted, except for small quantities

EAT TO LIVE

The Six-Week Plan

UNLIMITED

Eat as much as you want:

all raw vegetables (goal: 1 lb. daily)

cooked green and non-green nutrient-rich vegetables
(goal: 1 lb. daily; non-green nutrient-rich vegetables
are eggplant, mushrooms, peppers, onions, tomatoes,
carrots, cauliflower)

beans, legumes, bean sprouts, and tofu (goal: 1 cup
daily)

fresh fruits (at least 4 daily)

LIMITED

Cooked starchy vegetables or whole grains:

butternut and acorn squash, corn, white potatoes, rice,
sweet potatoes, bread, cereal (not more than one
serving, or 1 cup, per day)

raw nuts and seeds (1 oz. max. per day)

avocado (2 oz. max. per day)

dried fruit (2 tablespoons max. per day)

ground flaxseeds (1 tablespoon max. per day)

OFF-LIMITS

dairy products

animal products

between-meal snacks

fruit juice

oils

for salad dressings and cooking. Juicing fruits allows you to quickly consume three times the calories without the fiber to regulate absorption. The nutrient-per-calorie ratio is much higher for the whole food. Frozen fruit is permissible, but avoid canned fruit because it is not as nutritious. If you need to use canned fruit as a condiment (mandarin oranges, pineapple), make sure it is unsweetened.

Dried fruits should be used only in very small amounts for sweetening. Exotic fruits are interesting to try and will add variety and interest to your diet. Some of my personal favorites are blood oranges, persimmons, and cherimoyas. Eat a variety of fruits; try to include many of the following: apples, apricots, bananas, blackberries, blueberries, clementines, grapes, kiwifruit, kumquats, mangoes, melons, nectarines, oranges, papayas, peaches, pears, persimmons, pineapples, plums, raspberries, starfruit, strawberries, and tangerines.

Starchy Vegetables and Whole Grains

These two food categories are grouped together because either can be the culprit for those who have difficulty losing weight. While wholesome high-carbohydrate foods are a valuable addition to a disease-prevention diet, they are more calorically dense than the nonstarchy vegetables. Therefore, cooked high-starch vegetables and whole grains should be limited to one serving daily on the Six-Week Plan. Diabetics, those who want to lose weight more rapidly, and those who have difficulty losing weight no matter what they do may want to restrict these foods altogether, at least until they have arrived at their target weight. Eating lots of greens makes it difficult to overconsume high-starch vegetables. You just won't have room for that much. Examples of starchy vegetables include corn, sweet potatoes, white potatoes, butternut squash, acorn squash, winter squash, chestnuts, parsnips, rutabagas, turnips, water chestnuts, yams, and pumpkins. Grains include barley, buckwheat (kasha), millet, oats, quinoa, brown rice, and wild rice. On some days, you may choose to have a cup of oatmeal or other whole grain at breakfast. On other days, save your serving of starch for dinner.

One final note: soaking whole grains, such as brown rice, buckwheat, and quinoa, for a day before cooking them increases their nutritional value.[3] Certain phytonutrients and vitamins are activated as the grain starts to germinate. These include powerful chemopreventive phenols that inhibit the growth of abnormal cells.[4] A twenty-four-hour soak induces the early stage of germination, but you will not see the sprouts. Soaking a day ahead also shortens cooking time.

Nuts and Seeds

Nuts and seeds contain 150 to 200 calories per ounce. Eating a small amount—one ounce or less— each day, however, adds valuable nutrients and healthy unprocessed fats. Nuts and seeds are ideal in salad dressings, particularly when blended with fruits and spices or vegetable juice (tomato, celery, carrot). Always eat nuts and seeds raw because the roasting process alters their beneficial fats. Commercially packaged nuts and seeds are often cooked in hydrogenated oils, adding trans fats and sodium to your diet, so these are absolutely off the list. If you find that you tire of eating nuts and seeds raw, try lightly toasting them at home—this process does not deplete their beneficial properties and adds some variety for pleasure. Among the raw nuts and seeds you can add to your diet are almonds, cashews, walnuts, black walnuts, pecans, filberts, hickory nuts, macadamias, pignolis, pistachios, sesame seeds, sunflower seeds, pumpkin seeds, hemp seeds, chia seeds, and flaxseeds.

Spices, Herbs, and Condiments

Use all spices and herbs, except for salt. When using condiments, a little mustard is okay, but pickled foods contain too much salt and should be avoided. If you love to use ketchup or tomato sauce, you may find a lower-calorie, unsweetened ketchup at the health-food store and a tomato sauce made with no oil. Better yet, make your own tomato sauce with onion and garlic but no oil or salt.

Ten Easy Tips for Living with the Six-Week Plan

1. **Remember, the salad is the main dish: eat it first at lunch and dinner.**

You have the tendency to eat more of whatever you eat first because you are the hungriest. Raw foods have high transit times; they fill you up and encourage weight loss. You can't overeat on them. Successful, long-term weight control and health, as you know by now, are linked to your consumption of raw greens. They are the healthiest food in the world. Many of my patients with obesity or diabetes eat lettuce with every meal, including breakfast. They might have iceberg lettuce with their fruit breakfast, a mixed baby greens salad at lunch, and a romaine-based salad at dinner. You can eat more than a pound if you like, but don't fret if you are too full and can't eat the whole pound. It is merely a goal; just relax and enjoy eating.

2. Eat as much fruit as you want but at least four fresh fruits daily.

Eat as many fruits as you would like with your meals. Four fruits are about 250 calories, but here it is okay to splurge, even during the Six-Week Plan, particularly if you have a sweet tooth. Finish lunch or dinner with watermelon, a whole cantaloupe, or a box of blueberries or strawberries. The best dessert is fresh fruit or blended frozen fruit. Eating lots of fresh fruit is satisfying and filling and helps win you over to the Eat to Live way.

3. Variety is the spice of life, particularly when it comes to greens.

Variety is not merely the spice of life, it makes a valuable contribution to your health. The nice thing is that you never have to be concerned about overeating raw vegetables, salads, or cooked greens.

There are a variety of foods that you can use to make vegetable salads, including the following: lettuce (including romaine, bib, Boston, red leaf, green ice, iceberg, arugula, radicchio, endive, frisée), watercress, celery, spinach, cucumbers, tomatoes, mushrooms, broccoli, cauliflower, peppers, onions, radishes, kohlrabi, snow peas, carrots, beets, cabbage, and all kinds of sprouts.

Even more vegetables can be eaten cooked. They include broccoli, kale, string beans, artichokes, Brussels sprouts, bok choy, spinach, Swiss chard, cabbage, asparagus, okra, zucchini, and collard, mustard, and turnip greens. These vegetables can be flavored in various ways. Greens are always great with mushrooms, onions, garlic, and stewed tomatoes. If you don't have time to cook, just defrost a box of frozen green vegetables. Throw a box of frozen artichoke hearts, asparagus, or peas on your salad. This is less than 150 calories of food. Cooked greens are very low in calories but give you the nutritional power of ten pounds of other foods. Frozen greens such as broccoli and peas are nutritious and convenient—they are flash-cooked and frozen soon after being picked and are just as nutritious as fresh.

4. Beware of the starchy vegetable.
For the Six-Week Plan, limit cooked high-starch grains and vegetables to one cup a day. One cup of a high-starch vegetable would be one corn on the cob, one small- to medium-size baked potato, or one cup of brown rice or sweet potato. Fill up on

the raw vegetables and cooked green vegetables first. However, most of your starch consumption should come from colorful starchy vegetables— such as butternut or acorn squash, corn, turnips, parsnips, rutabagas, and sweet potatoes—rather than starchy grains.

All whole grains should be considered high-starch foods. If you do use bread, a thin whole wheat pita is a good choice for sandwiches because it is less bread and can hold healthful fillings such as vegetables, eggplant, and bean spreads. When you eat grains, use whole grains such as brown or wild rice, and use them in place of a cooked starchy vegetable at dinner. Refined starchy grains (such as bread, pasta, and white rice) and white potatoes should be even more restricted than the vegetable-based starches, which are more nutri-ent-dense. Restricting the portion size of rice, potatoes, and other cooked starchy vegetables to one serving is not necessary for everybody to lose weight on the Life Plan, only for those whose metabolism makes it difficult to lose weight. Many can still achieve an ideal body weight by cutting out refined starches only, such as white bread and pasta, without having to limit starchy vegetables to merely one serving. Your diet should be adjusted to your metabolic needs and activity level.

5. Eat beans or legumes every day.
Beans are a dieter's best friend. On the Six-Week Plan the goal is to eat an entire cup of beans daily; you may have more than one cup if you choose.

Beans are a powerhouse of superior nutrition. They reduce cholesterol and blood sugar. They have a high nutrient-per-calorie profile and help prevent food cravings. They are digested slowly, which has a stabilizing effect on your blood sugar and a resultant high satiety index. Eggplant and beans, mushrooms and beans, greens and beans are all high-nutrient, high-fiber, low-calorie main dishes. Throw a cup of beans on your salad for lunch. Eat bean soup. Scientific studies show a linear relationship between soup consumption and successful weight loss.[5] As a weight-loss strategy, eating soup helps by slowing your rate of intake and reducing your appetite by filling your stomach.

6. Eliminate animal and dairy products.

For the Six-Week Plan, eliminate animal products completely or, if you must include them, use only lean fish (flounder, sole, or tilapia) once or twice a week and an egg omelet once a week. No dairy products are permitted in the Six-Week Plan.

7. Have a tablespoon of ground flaxseeds every day.

This will give you those hard-to-find omega-3 fats that protect against diabetes, heart disease, and cancer.[6] The body can manufacture EPA and DHA from these omega-3 fats for those of us who do not consume fish. An additional source of omega-3 fat might be a few walnuts or soybeans. Edamame, those green soybeans in the freezer section of most health-food stores, taste great and are a rich source of omega-3 fat. I also recommend a nutritional supplement containing DHA, especially for those who are poor DHA converters (which can be determined via a blood test). Vegetable-derived (from microalgae) DHA is a good choice.

8. Consume nuts and seeds in limited amounts, not more than one ounce per day.

Pecans, walnuts, sunflower seeds, and other nuts and seeds may be rich in calories and fat, but scientific studies consistently report that nuts and seeds offer disease protection against heart attack, stroke, and cancer and also help lower cholesterol.[7] They can be used in larger amounts once you reach your ideal weight. Raw nuts and seeds are ideal foods for kids, athletes, and those who want to gain weight. One ounce of nuts is about 200 calories and can fit into a cupped hand, so do not eat more than this one handful of nuts per day. They are best used in salads, salad dressings, and dips, because when eaten with greens, they greatly enhance the absorption of nutrients from the green vegetables. You should never snack on nuts and seeds; they should be part of a meal.

9. Eat lots of mushrooms all the time.

Mushrooms make a great chewy replacement for meat. Exploring their variety is a great way to add interesting flavors and textures to dishes. Store them in paper bags, not plastic, as too much moisture speeds spoilage. Try adding them to beans, seasoned with herbs and lemon juice. Even though they are a fungus and not a real vegetable, mushrooms contain a variety of powerful phytochemicals and have been linked to decreased risk of chronic diseases, especially cancer.

Onions Add Fast Flavor to Foods

Dried onion powder can be quickly added to any salad dressing, soup, or vegetable dish. Red onions or scallions, sautéed in a little water or raw and sliced extra thin, make great flavor enhancers for salads and vegetable dishes. Leeks are in the onion family, too. Using just the white part and the lower lighter green part, slice and simmer them or roast them with other vegetables.

10. Keep it simple.

Use the basic skeleton plan below to devise menu plans so you will know what to eat when there is no time to decide.

Simplify, Simplify, Simplify

Breakfast: fresh fruit
Lunch: salad, beans on top, and more fruit
Dinner: salad and two cooked vegetables (1 lb.), fruit dessert

You do not have to prepare fancy recipes all the time. If you're going to be out for a while, just grab some leftover vegetables; lettuce and tomato on whole grain bread or stuffed into a whole wheat pita pocket; and a few pieces of fruit. Wash and dry plenty of heads of romaine lettuce on the weekend or when you have the time.

"The best prescription is knowledge."

—Dr. C. Everett Koop

The Life Plan

Losing weight will do you no good unless you keep it off. When you adopt a nutritarian diet style as a longevity plan, slimness will be a by-product of your new commitment to excellent health. Once the Six-Week Plan is over, you will move on to the Life Plan, which offers more choices. This is a critical juncture. You have lost a great deal of weight; you don't want to revert to your previous unhealthy diet. You need to decide not only how to maintain the benefits you have achieved but how to change your diet forever. Many of my patients have found a good balance by following the 90 percent rule.

The 90 Percent Rule

For longevity and weight loss, the Life Plan diet should aim to be made up of at least 90 percent unrefined plant foods. My most successful patients treat processed foods and animal foods as condiments, constituting no more than 10 percent of their total caloric intake.

The obvious corollary to the principle of consuming a large quantity of nutrient-dense foods is that you should consume smaller quantities of low-nutrient foods. Therefore, if you want to follow a nutritarian diet style to achieve dramatic health and longevity benefits, you must not have significant amounts of animal foods, dairy, or processed foods in your diet. If you desire these foods, use them occasionally or in very small amounts to flavor a vegetable dish. After the Six-Week Plan, if you want to add animal products back into your diet, then add a little white-meat chicken or turkey once a week, and beef even less frequently. In this manner, you can alternate: one night with a small serving of animal product and the next night a vegetarian dinner. Use animal products primarily as condiments—to add flavor to soups, vegetables, beans, or tofu—not as the main dish.

If after the first six weeks you choose to reintroduce dairy back into your diet, use fat-free dairy only (skim milk, nonfat yogurt). You can add an unsweetened fat-free yogurt or soymilk yogurt to your fruit breakfast, but do not eat fruit-flavored yogurt, as it contains sugar. Your total animal-product consumption (beef, poultry, fish, dairy products) should be limited to twelve ounces or less per week. Keep a close eye on your weight with both these additions.

How does this work out in terms of calorie consumption? The accepted wisdom is that the "average" woman should consume fewer than 1,600 calories daily, and a man fewer than 2,300 calories. To hold to the 90 percent rule, I recommend women not consume more than 150 calories per day of low-nutrient food, or about 1,000 calories weekly. Men should not consume more than 200 calories of low-nutrient food daily, or about 1,400 calories weekly.

In real life, this means that if you choose to have a bagel for lunch, you use up your 150-calorie allotment of low-nutrient food for the day. If you put one tablespoon of olive oil or a few ounces of animal food on your salad for lunch, then you should have only plant foods for dinner, with no added oils, pasta, or bread. Using the 90 percent rule, you are allowed to eat almost any kind of food, even a small cookie or candy bar, as long as all your other calories that day are from nutrient-dense vegetation.

---

100 Calories of Low-Nutrient Foods Equals:

- 2½ teaspoons of olive oil
- ½ bagel
- 1/2 cup of pasta
- 1 small cookie
- 2 ounces of broiled chicken or turkey breast
- 3 ounces of fish
- 1½ ounces of red meat
- 1 thin slice of cheese
- 1 cup of 1 percent or skim milk

In general, the Life Plan dictates that you eat not more than one or two items of low-nutrient foods daily. Everything else must be unrefined plant foods. The number of calories consumed will vary from person to person. Those who exercise or who are naturally thin can eat more than those who exercise less and have a weight problem. Therefore, the number of calories permitted from these low-nutrient foods should decrease as your total caloric intake goes down. For those who have a lot of weight to lose, eat less than 100 calories per day of low-nutrient foods.

Most people are addicted to the foods they grew up with. They feel deprived if their diet denies them the foods they love. With the Life Plan these food loves will become condiments or rewards for special occasions. You will be surprised how much more you will enjoy a healthier diet once you become accustomed to a different way of preparing foods and eating. It will take time; there will be a period of adjustment.

The USDA Food Guide Pyramid that most people are familiar with is designed around the foods Americans choose to eat already. Its goal is to improve the poor eating habits of Americans, but it fails. The USDA pyramid does not encourage the consumption of nutrient-dense plant foods. Anyone following the USDA guidelines, eating six to eleven daily servings of refined grains (breads, cereals, pastas) and three to five servings of animal products and dairy, is certain to obtain insufficient antioxidants and phytochemicals, depriving himself or herself of the opportunity to maximize prevention against common diseases. However, I do not recommend a grain-based diet. Potatoes, rice, and even whole grains do not contain the phytochemical power of fruits and vegetables. As I showed earlier, a high intake of refined grains in the diet is linked to common cancers. A high intake of fruits has the opposite effect. Fruits protect powerfully against cancer.[8]

My food pyramid represents a nutritarian diet style emphasizing high-nutrient foods as the base of the pyramid. These nutrient-dense foods provide

THE LIFE PLAN: DR. FUHRMAN'S FOOD PYRAMID

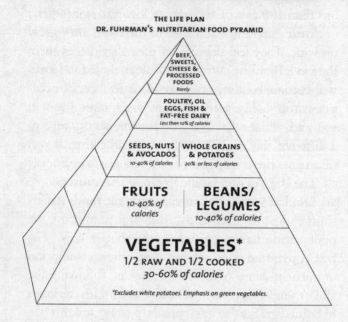

THE LIFE PLAN
DR. FUHRMAN'S NUTRITARIAN FOOD PYRAMID

BEEF,
SWEETS,
CHEESE &
PROCESSED
FOODS
Rarely

POULTRY, OIL
EGGS, FISH &
FAT-FREE DAIRY
Less than 10% of calories

SEEDS, NUTS
& AVOCADOS
10-40% of calories

WHOLE GRAINS
& POTATOES
20% or less of calories

FRUITS
10-40% of calories

BEANS/
LEGUMES
10-40% of calories

VEGETABLES*
1/2 RAW AND 1/2 COOKED
30-60% of calories

Excludes white potatoes. Emphasis on green vegetables.

the majority of calories, while other foods contribute only a minimal amount.

Going for Broke: Serious Health Conditions Require Serious Intervention

Before coming to my office, most of my patients failed to achieve the results they sought. They experienced either a worsening of their heart condition or weight gain no matter what program they chose, even those who followed a vegetarian diet. In my care, these same patients are able to achieve impressive results for the first time, because they "do it" 100 percent. For some, "trying" is definitely not good enough; it doesn't work. The 10 percent of optional calories of low-nutrient foods is just that, optional; you might find that you feel better and don't need to include even that much. If you want to lose weight more rapidly; if you have a particularly slow metabolic rate, diabetes, or cardiovascular disease; or if you are a health and longevity enthusiast, kiss even these 150 (low-nutrient) calories good-bye and make the Six-Week Plan your Life Plan. Considering what a struggle it is to make a 90 percent change, it is not much harder to do it all the way.

I will now turn to the most commonly asked questions I hear in my office.

What if I Fall off the Diet?

Since the goal is to eat at least 90 percent of your diet from nutrient-dense plant foods, if you fall off the plan in one area, make up for it in another. If you accomplish the goal stated above—eating all the recommended amounts of green vegetables, beans, and fruits—you will have consumed fewer than 1,000 calories of nutrient-dense food, with more than 40 grams of fiber. By consuming so many crucial nutrients and fiber, your body's drive to overeat is blunted.

Do you see the difference between these recommendations and those of more traditional authorities who recommend eating less food to lose weight? With my program you are encouraged to eat more food. Only by eating more of the right food can you successfully be healthy and well nourished and feel satisfied. On this plan you consume more than ten times the phytochemicals and ten times the fiber that most Americans consume. Keep in mind that it is the undiscovered nutrients in whole natural foods that offer the greatest protection against cancer.

Is This a Low-Calorie Diet?

Yes. Excess calories don't just make you overweight—they shorten your life. This diet style enables people to feel satiated with 1,000 to 2,000 calories per day, whereas before it took 1,600 to 3,000. The simple trick is to receive lots of nutrient bang for each caloric buck.

Of course, those who are considerably active or involved with exercise or sports need more calories, but that's okay—they will have a bigger appetite and need more food to satisfy their hunger. They will get more protein and other nutrients needed for exercise by consuming more food, not a different diet.

Some people can lose weight merely by switching their calories to a healthier plant-based cuisine while maintaining approximately the same caloric consumption. Chinese consume more calories than do Americans, yet are about 25 percent thinner than Americans. This is because the modern American diet receives about 37 percent of its calories from fat, with lots of sugar and refined carbohydrates. The combination of high fat and high sugar is a metabolic disaster that causes weight gain, independent of the number of calories.

Other people are not able to lose weight as easily. They need the entire package: the metabolic benefit of the natural plant foods, along with the satiety that results from both the greater bulk of my "unlimited" foods and the consequent nutrient fulfillment. These patients need even fewer calories. The good news is that they can be satisfied with fewer calories permanently. The Eat to Live plan has both these benefits, making it a powerful weight-normalization plan as well as the healthiest possible diet.

The menus, recipes, and strategies for eating explained in this book also make it possible to achieve the current dietary guidelines of the National Heart, Lung, and Blood Institute of the National Institutes of Health (NIH) for those desiring to lose weight. According to these guidelines, women should choose a diet with fewer than 1,200 calories a day and men one with fewer than 1,600.[9]

A computer analysis of many different diets has shown that the Eat to Live plan is the only way to meet the National Institutes of Health guidelines for calories while at the same time supplying adequate nutrients and fiber content. Even the dietary menus for 1,200-calorie and 1,600-calorie diets published in the National Institutes of Health's guide for physicians do not meet the RDAs, because the traditional American food choices are too low in nutrients. The NIH diets are too low in important nutrients such as chromium, vitamin K, folate, and magnesium, whereas the Eat to Live plans and suggested menus more than meet all RDAs within the NIH's caloric limits.

How Do I Know How Many Calories
I Should Eat?

Don't worry about it. Try to follow my rules for a
longevity diet and just watch the weight fall off. If
you were never able to lose weight in the past, be
happy with about one to two pounds per week. If
you are not losing weight as fast as you'd like, write
down what you eat and how much, to see if you are
really consuming a whole pound of raw vegetables a
day and an entire pound of steamed green vegetables
a day. If you are an overweight female following my
guidelines and losing about one to two pounds per
week, you are probably consuming about 1,100 to
1,400 calories a day. You can count calories if you
want, but it is not necessary; you will feel sated
and content on fewer calories than you were eating
before.

My observations over the years have convinced
me that eating healthfully makes you drop unwanted
pounds efficiently, independent of caloric intake. It's
as if the body wants to get rid of unhealthy tissue
quickly. I have seen this happen time and time again.
Eating the exact same diet, many patients drop
weight quickly and easily and then automatically
stop losing when they reach an ideal weight. Time
and time again, I have seen individuals who were not
overweight nonetheless lose weight after the switch.
In a few months, however, they gravitated back to
their former weight as their health improved. It is as
if the body wanted to exchange unhealthy tissue for
healthy tissue.

What if My Family Does Not
Want to Eat This Way?

Nobody should be made to eat healthfully. Encourage your family to learn about what you are doing and to read this book so that they can help support you. The key is for them to learn what you are doing out of love and respect for you, not because you are trying to force this way of eating down their throats. That will be their decision later. The best way to help other people is by setting an example. Lose the weight, get in great health, and wait for your friends and family to ask how you did it. Very few people object to the presence of healthy foods as long as you do not take away their comfort foods. You can always make healthful meals for yourself and some extra food for the rest of the family. Over time it will get easier. Keep in mind that some people require more time to make changes.

My patient Debra Caruso faced this dilemma. Her teenage son and daughter told her they were definitely not going to eat this way. Debra knew they could all afford to lose weight. There was so much junk food in the house that it was even tempting her. Yet Debra lost more than fifty pounds that first year. Luckily, she had a loving and supportive husband who tried his best to help in any way he could. The first thing he did was buy an extra refrigerator that they kept in the garage. Debra and her husband had a family meeting to enforce the rule that any unhealthy food would be kept in one cupboard and in the refrigerator in the garage. If the teenagers wanted something other than the food prepared by their mom, they could make it themselves and clean up after themselves. She agreed to cook their favorite main dishes, whatever they wanted, twice a week. Some off-limits foods such as ice cream, cheese, and other rich desserts would not be allowed in the house. They had to be consumed in another location. Debra and her husband also took the teenagers to the health-food store to purchase healthier snacks. It was important to give the children some say in what they ate. Finally, the entire family came to two of my lectures. After that, Debra's children chose a healthy diet for themselves as well.

It may not work out the same way for you. But the main point to bring home is compromise and patience.

What if I Don't Go All the Way?

The nutrient formula (H = N/C) allows you to approximate the relative disease-fighting power of your diet. If you are like most Americans, whose diets are only 5 to 6 percent nutrient-dense foods, any step you take in the right direction will lessen the risks to your health.

If you improve your diet now, and begin consuming even 60 percent of your calories from nutrient-dense plant foods (that's ten times as much vegetation as the average American consumes now), it is reasonable to expect a 60 percent decrease in your risk of cancer or heart attack.

Falling off the plan for one meal should give you more incentive to continue the rest of the week without a setback. Jump right back so that you eat healthy for the rest of the week so as to make the one meal off the diet almost meaningless. In other words, follow the 90 percent rule. The 90 percent rule allows you some leeway for imperfection and special occasions or to have a treat once in a while. You can still retain the benefits and your healthy slim body if you follow that less-than-perfect "special occasion meal" with twenty healthy meals.

Focus on Your Actions, the Results Will Follow

You have now received a considerable education in human nutrition by reading this book. In my experience, knowledge about this subject provides the most effective and powerful impetus for change. Superior health and optimal weight are no longer a matter of chance, but a matter of choice. Try not to focus too much on the weight; focus on what you are doing. The weight will drop naturally as a result of eating intelligently, exercising, and adopting a healthy lifestyle. Neither you nor I am totally in control of the amount of weight that you lose or the speed at which you lose it. Your body will set the pace and gravitate toward the ideal weight for you when you eat healthfully. Don't worry if a few days go by without your losing weight; your body will lose at the rate it chooses is best. Weigh yourself as much or as little as you like, but most people find once weekly is sufficient to keep track of their results.

Most people lose weight and then stop losing when they have reached their ideal weight. You are not the judge of your ideal weight; your body is. As almost everyone is overweight, many people think they are too thin when they have reached their best weight. I have many patients who, after following my plan to reverse diabetes or heart disease, report, "Everyone tells me I look too thin now." I then measure their periumbilical fat and check their percentage of body fat, and usually show them that they are still not thin enough.

Stay in Control by Setting a Goal

Be realistic and flexible; give your taste buds time to adjust to the new food choices. Changing your behavior is the key to success. Moderation, however, does not mean it's okay to poison ourselves, abuse our body, and then feel guilty. Moderation means recovering quickly when you have slipped up. Some of us need to plan cheats, once a week or twice a month. Keep to those planned times. A cheat every once in a while is okay if it is moderate and as long as you go right back to the program immediately and then don't do it again for at least one week.

Many health authorities and diet advisers recommend only small changes; they are afraid that if the change is too radical, dieters will give the whole thing up and gain nothing. I strongly disagree. My work over the past twenty years has shown that those who have jumped in with full effort the first six weeks have been the individuals most likely to stick with the plan and achieve results, month after month. Those who try to get into it gradually are the ones most likely to revert back to their former way of eating. Under the gradual approach, they "yo-yo" back and forth between their old bad behaviors and good ones. Change is hard. Why not do more and glean the results you have always been after quickly and permanently?

The Drug of Choice for Most Americans—Food!

Most overweight individuals are addicted to food. This means almost all Americans are food addicts. *Addicted* means that you feel ill or uncomfortable should you not continue your usual habits. Unlike tobacco and drug addiction, however, food addiction is socially acceptable.

Most people thrust into an environment with an unlimited supply of calorie-rich, nutrient-poor food will become compulsive overeaters. That is, the craving for food and the preoccupation with eating, and the resultant loss of control over food intake, are the natural consequences of nutrient paucity. The resulting stress on our system can be toxic.

Obviously, there are complicated emotional and psychological factors that make it more difficult for some to achieve success at overcoming food addiction. Additionally, some physical changes may initially discourage you. Stopping caffeine, reducing sodium, and dropping saturated fat from your diet while increasing fiber and nutrients may result in increased gas, headaches, fatigue, and other withdrawal symptoms. These symptoms are temporary and rarely last longer than one week. Eventually the

308 Joel Fuhrman, M.D.

high volume of food and high nutrient content will help prevent long-term food cravings.

The large quantity of food permitted and encouraged on this program makes you less stressed about overeating. Food cravings and addictive symptoms end for almost everyone because this diet satisfies a person's desire to eat more food.

Halting stimulating behavior such as overeating unmasks the fatigue that was always there. The power reserve in a battery is proportional to its use. The less we use it, the more life it has and the stronger it remains. Likewise, when there is continual stress on your body from stimulating foods and caffeine, it gives the false sensation that we have energy, when actually we are using up our nerve energy faster. This ages us. The fatigue is hidden by the stimulating (aging-inducing) effects of sugar, caffeine, and toxic protein load. Now that you are eating in a health-supporting manner, you may be in better touch with the sleep your body needs, and sleep better as a result.

Some cravings and food behaviors have emotional overtones from childhood or compensate for stress and emotional dysfunction. Some food-addicted people eat compulsively in spite of their awareness of the consequences. These people need a more intensive program than a book can provide. Similar to a twelve-week drug-rehabilitation program, an intensive food recovery program should include counseling. Food reeducation can work even for the most difficult cases. You no longer have an excuse to fail; all you need is the commitment.

This program is not for everybody, because added to the desire to lose weight must be the willingness to make a commitment to achieve wellness. Once that commitment is made, however, there need not be any failures; with proper support and this program, everyone can succeed.

Go for it.

9

Sculpting Our Future
in the Kitchen

MENU PLANS AND RECIPES

Case Study:
Anthony lost 160 pounds, lowered his blood pressure,
and no longer experiences migraines.

I am 6 feet 4 inches tall and at thirty-three years old weighed 360 pounds. I was on medication for high blood pressure, experienced frequent migraines, had a 54-inch waist, and was having difficulty getting a twenty-year life insurance policy. I was a longtime vegetarian who thought I ate well!

I had been struggling with my weight since I was thirteen years old. Through the years, I'd tried all sorts of diets and weight-loss methods. Some things worked for a little while, but the weight never stayed off for very long. With the upcoming birth of my second son, I decided to get serious about becoming healthy once again. I had become very frustrated by all the weight-loss information

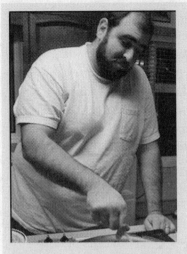 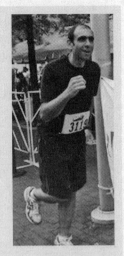

and diet plans available and was not sure what to do, but I knew I had to do something. To get started, I made a New Year's resolution to give up soda and sweets and set a goal to lose fifty pounds by the end of the year.

A few months later, without having lost a single pound, I was frustrated once again. In another attempt to find some useful weight-loss information, I came across Dr. Fuhrman's book *Eat to Live*. The information in the book made a lot of sense to me, and I began making changes in my diet immediately.

I gradually added more and more vegetables to my lunch and dinner meals. By the time my son was born, two months after purchasing *Eat to Live*, I had lost thirty pounds. I continued making gradual changes in my diet for the next several months until I reached a point where about 90 percent of my diet was from foods such as vegetables, fruits, beans, nuts, and seeds. By the end of that year, I had lost a total of ninety pounds, was off blood pressure medication, no longer experienced migraines, and had blown away my goal of losing fifty pounds for the year. I was feeling absolutely great!

With all of my newfound energy, I decided that I wanted to start exercising, so I began running. I gradually increased the amount of running I was doing, continued eating right, and ran my first 5K. At that point I was hooked on living a healthy lifestyle that included eating right and exercising regularly. I continued following Dr. Fuhrman's recommended style of eating and also continued increasing the amount of running I was doing. I ran the Philadelphia Half Marathon in 1 hour 48 minutes 21 seconds! This desire to exercise was amazing to me. I was never into sports or exercise, and the fact that it was so easy for me now was incredible.

Even with this increase in exercise, I continued to lose almost exactly eight pounds a month for about eighteen months, until my weight loss stopped just as suddenly as it began. At this point I weighed 197 pounds, was able to get a life insurance policy, and was in the best shape of my life. Now, more than eighteen months after my body weight leveled off, I still weigh right around 200 pounds, bringing my total weight loss to 160 pounds! I enjoy running regularly and participate in races of various distances throughout the year.

I am proud to be a positive role model for my sons, Evan and Henry. Being able to keep up with them today and knowing that I will continue to be an active part of their lives for years to come make me realize that becoming healthy is the most important thing I have done for myself and my family.

I eat a quick and easy-to-prepare diet, and I eat simply. Most days I eat fruit and nuts for breakfast and something quick for lunch, such as a few fruits and a salad with a healthy serving of broccoli (frozen is fine), peas (frozen is fine), or beans on top and a light dressing. I eat healthfully with little work or effort. Likewise, I have tried to make these menus simple. However, you can modify them significantly and use your own ideas and recipes as long as you obey the guidelines outlined in the previous chapter. The foods or recipes can be switched around and eaten in different combinations or at different meals.

Fourteen days of menu plans and delicious recipes follow. Keep in mind that in the real world you would not necessarily make all these different dishes and recipes each week. Most of us make a soup or a main dish and use the leftovers for lunch or even dinner the next day. Remember, you must rethink what you consider a normal portion. Your former side dishes (such as salads, soups, and vegetables) now become the main dishes, and so the portion sizes of these lower-calorie foods are much larger. It is almost impossible to eat too much food, only too much of the wrong food. Make your life simple. Enjoy food, but don't have your life revolve around a menu plan. This diet is delicious; it involves no sacrifice, only different choices.

The first week of sample menus that follow is vegetarian and is designed for aggressive weight loss and for those who have had difficulty losing weight in the past. This kind of vegetarian diet is also appropriate for those looking to reverse heart disease or diabetes. You cannot expect to significantly reverse atherosclerosis (blockages in your arteries), diabetes, or high blood pressure unless you restore yourself to a normal weight. It is the combination of the healthy, nutrient-dense diet and the fat leaving your body that brings about predictable improvement in many health conditions.

The second week of sample menus is slightly less aggressive. The menus include some animal products (less than twelve ounces per week) and a small amount of oil (no more than one teaspoon per day). A small amount of animal products can be added to any vegetable or bean dish for flavor, if desired, as long you keep it below twelve ounces per week. Use white meat, fish, eggs, or low-fat dairy. Avoid processed, cured, or barbecued meats and full-fat dairy. You can make the nonvegetarian menus stricter and more effective by excluding all oil and limiting the portion size of the whole grains or starchy vegetables.

Remember, you can eat as much as you want of raw and cooked nonstarchy vegetables and fresh and unsweetened fruits. Try to include a serving of beans in your diet each day, as well as one ounce (about one-quarter cup) of raw nuts and seeds. Limit yourself to one serving per day of whole grains or starchy vegetables. Feel free to experiment. Substitute and add the healthy foods and seasonings that you enjoy. Since you are giving up lots of unhealthy foods, treat yourself to lots of delicious and exotic fruits. Try different fresh herbs and spices to season your food. They are salt-free and very high in antioxidants and phytonutrients.

Weekly Shopping List

Always keep a good assortment of healthy food in the house. A key to success is having the right kind of food available to prevent being tempted by the wrong kind of food. I suggest the following items.

Vegetables to be eaten raw—carrots, celery, peppers, tomatoes, cucumbers, mushrooms, lettuce and other salad greens, snow peas, sugar snap peas, and tomatoes.

Vegetables for cooking (fresh or frozen)—broccoli, cauliflower, eggplant, mushrooms, tomatoes, cabbage, string beans, kale, Swiss chard, mustard greens, spinach, Brussels sprouts, asparagus, onions, and garlic.

Fruits (fresh or frozen)—strawberries, blueberries, raspberries, kiwifruit, apples, oranges, pineapple, melons, lemons, limes, grapes, pears, bananas, mangoes, plums, peaches, and cherries.

Raw nuts and seeds—walnuts, almonds, cashews, pistachios, sunflower seeds, pumpkin seeds, unhulled sesame seeds, hemp seeds, flaxseeds, and chia seeds.

Ingredients for homemade soups—carrots, celery, garlic, onions, zucchini, fresh and dried herbs, no-salt seasoning, leeks, turnips, dried beans, lentils, and split peas.

Other staples—flavored and balsamic vinegars, lemons (juice is great in a salad, soup, or vegetable dish), tomato sauce (no salt added), salsa (no salt added), avocados, tofu, edamame (green soybeans), and old-fashioned rolled oats.

Fresh or dried herbs and seasonings—basil, oregano, dill, parsley, cilantro, chives, rosemary, thyme, ginger, garlic cloves or garlic powder, onion powder, mint, chili powder, cumin, Cajun seasoning, pepper, curry powder, cinnamon, Mrs. Dash, and Dr. Fuhrman's VegiZest or MatoZest.

The following menus and recipes are examples of diets and dishes rich in nutrients and fiber, consistent with the basic principles of healthful eating. I have included my favorite recipes and those that have become the most popular with my readers and patients. These recipes are among the highest rated at my Member Center at DrFuhrman.com.

7 Days of Vegetarian Meal Plans
(For Aggressive Weight Loss)

*Recipes follow

Day One

BREAKFAST
Strawberries, orange, and cantaloupe sprinkled
    with ground flaxseeds or hemp seeds

LUNCH
Mixed green salad topped with beans and
    balsamic or flavored vinegar
Portobello–Red Pepper Pita*

DINNER
Mixed greens and watercress salad with red
    peppers and Tofu Ranch Dressing*
Golden Austrian Cauliflower Cream Soup*
Strawberries sprinkled with cocoa powder

Day Two

BREAKFAST
Quick Banana Breakfast to Go*

LUNCH
Raw vegetables (carrots, red bell peppers, and
    celery)
Steamed Broccoli with Sesame Ginger Sauce* or
    Red Lentil Sauce*
Melon or other fresh fruit

DINNER

Salad with lemon juice and shredded pear
Chard and Vegetable Medley*
Jenna's Peach Freeze*

Day Three

BREAKFAST

Eat Your Greens Fruit Smoothie*

LUNCH

Black Bean Mango Salad*
Pineapple or other fresh fruit

DINNER

Romaine and arugula salad with Apple Pie
    Dressing*
Dr. Fuhrman's Famous Anti-Cancer Soup*

Day Four

BREAKFAST

Dried apricots soaked in soy, hemp, or almond
    milk

LUNCH

Mixed green salad topped with white beans and
    walnuts and Dijon Date Dressing*
Fresh or frozen berries

DINNER

Raw vegetables (string beans, carrots, broccoli,
    and peppers)

Simple Guacamole*
Lisa's Lovely Lentil Stew*
Collards and Carrots with Raisins*

Day Five

BREAKFAST
Blue Apple-Nut Oatmeal*

LUNCH
Edamame with no-salt seasoning
Bean Enchiladas*
Papaya with lime or other fresh fruit

DINNER
Romaine and napa cabbage salad with lemon or
    flavored vinegar
Thai Vegetable Curry*
Cantaloupe Slush*

Day Six

BREAKFAST
Creamy Fruit and Berry Smoothie*

LUNCH
Raw vegetables (carrots, celery, snow peas, and
    mushrooms) with salsa
Simple Bean Burgers* with lettuce and tomato
Kiwifruit or other fruit

DINNER
Mixed greens and arugula salad with assorted
    vegetables and Creamy Blueberry Dressing*

Eggplant Roll-ups*
Steamed asparagus

Day Seven

BREAKFAST

Mixed tropical fruit (pineapple, mango, and
banana) sprinkled with flaxseeds and
unsweetened coconut

LUNCH

Raw vegetables (red peppers, zucchini, and
sugar snap peas)
Black Bean Hummus*
Healthy tortilla or pita crisps (Cut whole grain
tortillas or pitas into small triangles and
place in oven at low temperature until
crisp.)
Apple or pear

DINNER

Easy Three-Bean Vegetable Chili*
Great Greens*
Banana Walnut Ice Cream*

7 Days of Nonvegetarian Meal Plans

(Less Strict for Moderate Weight Loss)

Day One

BREAKFAST

Quick Banana Breakfast to Go*

LUNCH

Raw vegetables (carrots, broccoli, and
cucumbers) with Healthy Thousand Island
Dressing*

Black Bean Lettuce Bundles*

Watermelon or other fresh fruit

DINNER

Asian Vegetable Stir-fry*

Strawberries or other fresh fruit with Almond
Chocolate Dip*

Day Two

BREAKFAST

Fruit and nut bowl (assorted fresh fruit
sprinkled with nuts and/or seeds)

LUNCH

Turkey (2 ounces) with mixed greens, broccoli
sprouts, tomato, and mustard on sprouted
grain bread (vegan option: substitute Herbed
White Bean Hummus* for turkey)

Grapes or other fresh fruit

DINNER

Romaine and watercress salad with Balsamic
Vinaigrette*

Tomato Bisque*

Yummy Banana Oat Bars*

Day Three

BREAKFAST

Chocolate Smoothie*

LUNCH

Vegetable Bean Burrito*
Sliced avocado
Orange or other fresh fruit

DINNER

Romaine salad with Caesar Salad Dressing* or
    other nonfat, low-sodium dressing
No-Meat Balls* with low-sodium or no-salt-
    added pasta sauce
Baked spaghetti squash
Spinach and Brussels Sprouts Marinara*

Day Four

BREAKFAST

Vegetable Omelet* topped with salsa

LUNCH

Asparagus Shiitake Salad with Creamy Sesame
    Dressing*
Mixed berries

DINNER

Raw vegetables with Herbed White Bean
    Hummus*
High Cruciferous Vegetable Stew*

Day Five

BREAKFAST

Blue Apple-Nut Oatmeal*

LUNCH

Pita Stuffed with Greens and Russian Fig
 Dressing*
Pineapple or other fresh fruit

DINNER

Mixed greens and arugula salad with tomatoes
 and Tofu Ranch Dressing*
No-Pasta Vegetable Lasagna*
Cara's Apple Strudel*

Day Six

BREAKFAST

Banana-Cashew Lettuce Wrap*

LUNCH

Walnut-Pear Green Salad*
Easy Vegetable Pizza*

DINNER

Southern-Style Mixed Greens*
Black Forest Cream of Mushroom Soup*

Day Seven

BREAKFAST

Blended Mango Salad*

LUNCH

Mixed greens and watercress salad with
assorted vegetables, topped with white beans
and sunflower seeds, choice of Eat to Live
dressing or flavored vinegar

Cantaloupe or other fresh fruit

DINNER

Broiled fish fillets topped with Mango Salsa*

Kale with Cashew Cream Sauce*

Brown and wild rice with water-sautéed onions

Chocolate Cherry Ice Cream*

The Eat to Live Recipes

Smoothies and Blended Salads

Breakfast

Dips, Dressings, and Sauces

Salads

Soups and Stews

Main Dishes

Desserts

Cook to Live

Soups and Stews

Soups and stews are critical components of this eating style. When vegetables are simmered in a soup, all the nutrients are retained in the liquid. Many of my soup recipes use fresh vegetable juices, especially carrot juice. These juices provide a very tasty anti-oxidant-rich base. If you don't have a juicer, consider purchasing one. If you are short on time, bottled carrot juice and other vegetable juices can be purchased at most health-food stores.

To create "cream" soups, blend in raw cashews or cashew butter. This provides a creamy texture and rich flavor.

A big advantage of homemade soups is that they make wonderful leftovers. Soups generally keep well for up to four days in the refrigerator but should be frozen if longer storage is desired.

Should you occasionally choose to use a prepared soup, keep in mind that your overall daily sodium intake ideally should remain under 1,000 mg. Natural whole foods provide about 400 to 700 mg of sodium per day, which allows for a leeway of about 300 mg. Be sure to read labels. You will be amazed at how much sodium canned soups and other processed foods contain. Try to select no-salt-added options.

Salad Dressings and Dips

Salad dressings usually start with oil and vinegar: the oil provides the fat, and the vinegar provides the acidity. My salad dressings use whole foods such as raw almonds and cashews, other raw nuts and seeds, avocado, and tahini as the fat sources. Use a food processor or high-powered blender to blend nuts or seeds with other healthy ingredients to create smooth, creamy dressings.

Smoothies

Delicious smoothies are made by blending a mixture of fruits and raw leafy greens. Blending raw vegetables with fruits is an efficient way to increase your nutrient absorption. The cell walls of the foods are efficiently crushed, making it easier for your body to absorb the beneficial phytochemicals contained within. A powerful blender such as a Vita-Mix is very helpful for making smoothies and fruit sorbets.

Cooking Beans

It is advisable to soak most dried beans or legumes overnight before cooking.

Replace the soaking water with two to three cups of fresh water for each cup of beans when cooking them. Most beans require about one and a half to two hours of cooking to become soft. Lentils and split peas require only one hour and need not be soaked prior to cooking.

Make sure beans are thoroughly cooked, as they are more difficult to digest when undercooked. Keep in mind that it is important to chew them thoroughly. As you get in the habit of eating beans regularly, you will digest them better.

Water Sautéing

A basic cooking technique used in some of our recipes is water sautéing. This is used instead of cooking with oil. Water sautéing is simple and good for stir-fries, sauces, and many other dishes. To water sauté, heat a skillet on high heat until water sputters when dropped in the pan. Use small amounts (two to three tablespoons) of water in the hot skillet, wok, or pan, covering the pan occasionally and adding more water as necessary until the vegetables are tender. If stir-frying a vegetable dish, other alternatives to oil include no-salt vegetable broth, coconut water, wine, or fruit juice.

The Eat to Live Recipes

Smoothies and Blended Salads

BLENDED MANGO SALAD

Serves 2

> 1 ripe mango, chilled
> 1 cup chopped spinach
> 4 cups chopped romaine lettuce
> ¼ cup unsweetened soy, hemp, or almond milk

Peel and chop the mango and place in a food processor or high-powered blender. Add the spinach and half the lettuce. Blend until well combined. Add the milk and remaining lettuce. Blend until creamy.

CHOCOLATE SMOOTHIE

SERVES 2

> 5 ounces baby spinach
> 2 cups frozen blueberries
> ½ cup unsweetened soy, hemp, or almond milk
> 1 banana
> 2–4 dates, pitted
> 2 tablespoons natural cocoa powder
> 1 tablespoon ground flaxseeds

Blend all the ingredients in a high-powered blender until smooth and creamy.

CREAMY FRUIT AND BERRY SMOOTHIE

SERVES 2

> 1 cup pomegranate juice
> ½ cup unsweetened soy, hemp, or almond milk
> ½ cup frozen strawberries
> ½ cup frozen blueberries
> ½ cup frozen peaches
> 1 banana
> 2 tablespoons ground flaxseeds

Blend all the ingredients in a high-powered blender until smooth and creamy.

EAT YOUR GREENS FRUIT SMOOTHIE

SERVES 2

> 5 ounces baby spinach
> 1 banana
> 1 cup frozen blueberries
> ½ cup unsweetened soy, hemp, or almond milk
> ½ cup pomegranate juice or other unsweetened fruit juice
> 1 tablespoon ground flaxseeds

Blend all the ingredients in a high-powered blender until smooth and creamy.

Breakfast

BANANA-CASHEW LETTUCE WRAP

SERVES 2

> ¼ cup raw cashew butter
> 12 romaine lettuce leaves
> 2 bananas, thinly sliced

Spread about 1 teaspoon cashew butter on each lettuce leaf. Lay a few banana slices on the butter and roll up like a burrito.

Note: This makes a delicious, healthy breakfast or snack.

BLUE APPLE-NUT OATMEAL

SERVES 2

> 1⅔ cups water
> ¼ teaspoon cinnamon

¼ *cup old-fashioned rolled oats*
2 *tablespoons dried currants*
1 *cup fresh or frozen blueberries*
1 *banana, sliced*
1 *apple, peeled, cored, and chopped or grated*
2 *tablespoons chopped walnuts*

In a saucepan, combine the water, cinnamon, oats, and currants. Simmer until the oatmeal is creamy. Add the blueberries and banana. Cook for 5 minutes, or until hot, stirring constantly. Mix in the apples and nuts.

QUICK BANANA BREAKFAST TO GO

Serves 2

2 *cups fresh or frozen blueberries*
2 *bananas, sliced*
½ *cup old-fashioned rolled oats*
⅓ *cup pomegranate juice*
2 *tablespoons chopped walnuts*
1 *tablespoon raw sunflower seeds*
2 *tablespoons dried currants (optional)*

Combine all the ingredients in a small microwave-proof bowl. Heat in the microwave for 3 minutes.
Note: For on the go, combine all the ingredients in a resealable container and eat later, either hot or cold.

Dips, Dressings, and Sauces

APPLE PIE DRESSING

SERVES 4

> 2 apples, peeled and cored
> ¼ cup fresh-squeezed orange juice
> cinnamon to taste

Blend all the ingredients in a food processor or high-powered blender until smooth and creamy.

BALSAMIC VINAIGRETTE

SERVES 5

> ½ cup water
> ¼ cup plus 2 tablespoons roasted garlic rice vinegar
> 2 tablespoons olive oil
> ¼ cup balsamic vinegar
> ¼ cup 100% grape fruit spread or raisins
> 4 cloves garlic, pressed
> 1 teaspoon dried oregano
> ½ teaspoon dried basil
> ½ teaspoon onion powder

Blend all the ingredients in a food processor or high-powered blender until smooth and creamy.

BLACK BEAN HUMMUS

Serves 6

> 1½ cups cooked black beans or 1 (15-ounce)
>   can no-salt-added or low-sodium black
>   beans, drained and rinsed
> 2 tablespoons water
> 2 tablespoons fresh lemon juice
> 2 tablespoons Dr. Fuhrman's VegiZest or other
>   no-salt seasoning
> 2 tablespoons raw tahini
> 2 teaspoons Bragg Liquid Aminos or low-
>   sodium soy sauce
> ½ teaspoon ground cumin
> ½ clove garlic, chopped
> dash cayenne pepper, or more to taste
> dash paprika, for garnish

Blend all the ingredients except the paprika in a food processor or high-powered blender until smooth, scraping down the sides as needed. Add more seasoning to taste. Add more water to achieve the desired consistency. Garnish with paprika.

Note: Serve with vegetables such as baby carrots, broccoli florets, zucchini, cucumbers, romaine lettuce leaves, or steamed asparagus spears.

CAESAR SALAD DRESSING/DIP

Serves 4

> 4 cloves garlic
> ⅔ cup unsweetened soy, hemp, or almond milk

⅓ cup raw cashew butter or ⅔ cup raw
   cashews
1 tablespoon plus 1 teaspoon fresh lemon juice
1½ tablespoons nutritional yeast
2 teaspoons Dijon mustard
dash black pepper

Preheat the oven to 350 degrees. Break the garlic cloves apart, leaving on the papery skins. Roast for about 25 minutes, or until mushy. When cool, remove the skins and blend with the remaining ingredients in a food processor or high-powered blender until creamy and smooth.

CREAMY BLUEBERRY DRESSING

SERVES 4

2 cups fresh or frozen (thawed) blueberries
½ cup pomegranate juice
¼ cup raw cashew butter or ½ cup raw
   cashews
3 tablespoons Dr. Fuhrman's Wild Blueberry
   Vinegar or other fruit-flavored vinegar

Blend all the ingredients in a food processor or high-powered blender until smooth and creamy.

DIJON DATE DRESSING/DIP

SERVES 4

1 cup water
⅓ cup raw cashew butter or ⅔ cup raw
   cashews

4 tablespoons Dr. Fuhrman's Riesling Raisin
   Vinegar or balsamic vinegar
2 tablespoons Dr. Fuhrman's VegiZest or other
   no-salt seasoning
2 tablespoons Dijon mustard
4–6 dates, pitted
1–2 cloves garlic, minced

Blend all the ingredients in a food processor or high-powered blender until smooth and creamy.

HEALTHY THOUSAND ISLAND DRESSING

SERVES 4

½ cup raw cashew butter or 1 cup raw cashews
½ cup unsweetened soy, almond, or hemp
   milk
2 tablespoons balsamic vinegar
2 tablespoons fresh lemon juice
1 teaspoon dried dill weed
1 teaspoon onion powder
½ teaspoon garlic powder
3 tablespoons tomato paste
1 rounded tablespoon date sugar or 1–2 dates,
   pitted
¼ cucumber, peeled
¼ cucumber, peeled and finely chopped
¼ cup finely chopped onion

In a food processor or high-powered blender, blend
the cashews, milk, vinegar, lemon juice, dill, onion
powder, garlic powder, tomato paste, date sugar,

and peeled cucumber until smooth. Transfer to a small bowl and fold in the finely chopped cucumber and onion.

HERBED WHITE BEAN HUMMUS

SERVES 2

>   2 cups cooked or canned no-salt-added or low-sodium white beans, drained and rinsed
>   1 tablespoon fresh lemon juice
>   2 tablespoons unhulled sesame seeds
>   2 tablespoons red wine vinegar
>   ½ teaspoon Dijon mustard
>   2 tablespoons water
>   ¼ cup chopped fresh basil
>   2 tablespoons chopped fresh thyme

Blend the beans, lemon juice, sesame seeds, vinegar, mustard, and water in a high-powered blender or food processor until smooth. Add the basil and thyme and pulse very briefly. Do not overprocess; the herbs should be visible in small pieces.

RED LENTIL SAUCE

SERVES 4

>   ½ cup dried red lentils
>   1 medium onion, chopped
>   1 clove garlic, chopped
>   1½ cups carrot juice
>   1 tablespoon Dr. Fuhrman's VegiZest or other no-salt seasoning

1 teaspoon ground cumin
½ teaspoon balsamic vinegar

Place the lentils, onion, garlic, and carrot juice in a saucepan. Bring to a boil, cover, and simmer for 20 to 30 minutes, until the lentils are soft and pale. Add more carrot juice if needed. Blend the cooked lentil mixture, VegiZest, cumin, and vinegar in a food processor or high-powered blender to a smooth puree. Add more carrot juice if it is too thick.

Note: Serve with steamed broccoli, cauliflower, or other vegetables.

MANGO SALSA

SERVES 4

1 ripe mango, peeled, pitted, and cut into small
   pieces
3 green onions, chopped
2 tablespoons chopped fresh cilantro
1 tablespoon fresh lemon juice
2 teaspoons seeded and chopped jalapeño

Combine all the ingredients in a small bowl.

SESAME GINGER SAUCE

SERVES 4

⅔ cup water
½ cup raw tahini
2 tablespoons fresh lemon juice
1 teaspoon white miso

1 tablespoon finely grated fresh ginger
2 dates, pitted
1 clove garlic, pressed
dash crushed red pepper flakes

Blend all the ingredients in a food processor or high-powered blender. Add more water if needed to achieve the desired consistency.

Note: Serve with steamed or water-sautéed vegetables. This sauce goes well with bok choy, asparagus, or kale.

SIMPLE GUACAMOLE

SERVES 4

2 ripe avocados, peeled and pitted
½ cup finely chopped onion
¼ cup minced fresh cilantro
2 tablespoons fresh lime juice
¼ teaspoon ground cumin
¼ teaspoon freshly ground black pepper

Using a fork, mash the avocados in a small bowl. Add the remaining ingredients and stir well. Cover and chill.

TOFU RANCH DRESSING/DIP

SERVES 4

6 ounces silken tofu
3 dates, pitted
1 clove garlic, peeled
¼ cup finely chopped green onion

3 tablespoons water
2 tablespoons fresh lemon juice
1½ tablespoons dried Italian seasoning
1 tablespoon chopped fresh parsley
1 tablespoon chopped fresh dill
1 teaspoon Bragg Liquid Aminos or low-
   sodium soy sauce
dash cayenne pepper (optional)

Blend all the ingredients in a high-powered blender or food processor until smooth and creamy.

Note: Use as a dressing, dip, spread, or mayonnaise substitute in your favorite recipes. Store in the refrigerator in an airtight container for up to 5 days.

Salads

ASPARAGUS SHIITAKE SALAD
WITH CREAMY SESAME DRESSING

SERVES 4

For the Creamy Sesame Dressing:
   ⅔ cup plus 2 tablespoons unhulled sesame seeds
   1 cup unsweetened soy, hemp, or almond milk
   2 tablespoons Dr. Fuhrman's Riesling Raisin
      Vinegar or rice vinegar
   1 tablespoon raw cashew butter or 2 table-
      spoons raw cashews
   1 teaspoon toasted sesame oil
   7 dates, pitted, or to taste, soaked in water for
      30 minutes (soaking liquid reserved)
   ½ clove garlic, chopped

For the salad:

   2 *medium beets, peeled and sliced ½ inch thick*
   ½ cup water
   8 *ounces shiitake mushrooms, sliced*
   1 *pound asparagus, cut diagonally into 2-inch*
      pieces
   1 *tablespoon Dr. Fuhrman's VegiZest or other*
      no-salt seasoning
   1 *teaspoon garlic powder*
   1 *medium red bell pepper, seeded and thinly*
      sliced
   ½ cup sliced water chestnuts
   4 *cups watercress*
   2 *cups bean sprouts*

To make the dressing, lightly toast 2 tablespoons of the sesame seeds in a pan over medium heat for 5 minutes, shaking the pan frequently. Set aside.

In a food processor or high-powered blender, blend the remaining ⅔ cup sesame seeds along with other dressing ingredients except the soaking liquid, until smooth and creamy. Stir in the sesame seeds. Use the soaking liquid to thin the dressing as needed.

To make the salad, preheat the oven to 400 degrees. Place the beets and water in a baking pan. Cover and roast for 20 minutes. Continue roasting, uncovered, until tender. If needed, add more water to keep the beets from drying out. Set aside.

Meanwhile, water sauté the mushrooms over high heat for about 5 minutes, using only enough water to keep them from scorching. When the mushrooms are tender and juicy, add the asparagus and water sauté until slightly tender but still crisp, about 5 minutes. Toss with the VegiZest and garlic powder. Remove from the heat and toss with the bell pepper and water chestnuts.

Place the watercress on a plate and pile the vegetable mixture on top. Drizzle the dressing over all, topping with the bean sprouts. Arrange the roasted beets around the edge.

BLACK BEAN MANGO SALAD

SERVES 3

> 1 mango, peeled, pitted, and cubed
> 2 tablespoons chopped fresh cilantro
> 4 green onions, thinly sliced
> 1 medium red bell pepper, seeded and
>   chopped
> ½ cup frozen corn, thawed, or fresh corn
>   off the cob
> 3 cups cooked black beans or 2 (15-ounce)
>   cans no- or low-salt black beans, drained
>   and rinsed
> 3 tablespoons fresh lime juice
> 1 teaspoon minced fresh garlic
> 1 teaspoon dried oregano
> 1 teaspoon ground cumin
> dash chili powder
> 9 cups chopped romaine lettuce

If using fresh corn, water sauté for 5 minutes or until tender. Mix all the ingredients except the let-

tuce in a bowl. Let stand for at least 15 minutes.
Serve on top of the lettuce.

Note: The vegetable mixture without the mango can be
made a day ahead and refrigerated. Add the mango and a
splash of lime juice just before serving.

SOUTHERN-STYLE MIXED GREENS

SERVES 2

> 1 cup water
> 1 clove garlic, minced
> dash black pepper
> 1½ cups cooked black-eyed peas or 1
>   (15-ounce) can no-salt-added or low-
>   sodium black-eyed peas, drained and rinsed
> 1 cup seeded and chopped yellow bell pepper
> 1 cup chopped fresh tomato
> ⅓ cup chopped fresh parsley
> ¼ cup chopped red onion
> 2 tablespoons balsamic or fig vinegar
> 10 ounces (about 7 cups) mixed salad greens

Combine the water, garlic, and black pepper in a
large saucepan; bring to a boil. Add the black-eyed
peas; cover and simmer over low heat for 10 minutes. Drain.

In a bowl, combine the black-eyed peas, bell
pepper, tomato, parsley, onion, and vinegar. Cover
and chill for 3 hours or overnight. Serve over the
salad greens.

Note: If you can't find no- or low-salt black-eyed peas, use
no- or low-salt small white beans instead.

WALNUT-PEAR GREEN SALAD

SERVES 2

> *8 ounces (about 5 cups) baby greens*
> *2 ounces (about 2 cups) arugula or watercress*
> *1 pear, peeled, cored, and grated*
> *¼ cup dried currants*
> *¼ cup walnuts, chopped*
> *2 tablespoons Dr. Fuhrman's D'Anjou Pear
>   Vinegar or rice vinegar*
> *2 teaspoons olive oil*
> *2 pears, peeled, cored, and sliced*
> *¼ cup walnut halves*

Combine the baby greens, arugula, grated pear, currants, and walnuts in a bowl. Toss with the vinegar and olive oil. Top with the sliced pears and walnut halves.

Note: Use watercress as often as possible in salads for nutrient density.

Soups and Stews

BLACK FOREST CREAM OF
MUSHROOM SOUP

SERVES 6

> *2 tablespoons water*
> *2 pounds mixed fresh mushrooms (button,
>   shiitake, cremini), sliced ¼ inch thick*
> *2 cloves garlic, minced or pressed*
> *2 teaspoons herbes de Provence*

5 cups carrot juice

3 cups unsweetened soy, hemp, or almond
  milk, divided

2 carrots, coarsely chopped

2 medium onions, chopped

¾ cup fresh or frozen corn kernels

1 cup chopped celery

3 leeks, cut into ½-inch-thick rounds

¼ cup Dr. Fuhrman's VegiZest or other no-salt
  seasoning

¼ cup raw cashews

1 tablespoon fresh lemon juice

1 tablespoon chopped fresh thyme

2 teaspoons chopped fresh rosemary

2 (15-ounce) cans no-salt-added or low-
  sodium white beans (northern, navy,
  cannellini), drained and rinsed

5 ounces baby spinach

¼ cup chopped fresh parsley, for garnish
  (optional)

Heat the water in a large sauté pan. Sauté the mushrooms, garlic, and herbes de Provence for about
5 minutes, or until tender, adding more water if
necessary to prevent from sticking. Set aside.

In a large soup pot, bring the carrot juice, 2½ cups
of the milk, the carrots, onion, corn, celery, leeks,
and VegiZest to a boil. Reduce the heat and simmer
until the vegetables are tender, about 30 minutes.

In a food processor or high-powered blender,
puree the cashews and remaining ½ cup milk. Add
half of the soup liquid and vegetables, the lemon

juice, thyme, and rosemary. Blend until smooth and creamy.

Return the pureed soup mixture to the pot. Add the beans, spinach, and sautéed mushrooms. Heat until the spinach is wilted. Garnish with the parsley, if desired.

DR. FUHRMAN'S FAMOUS ANTI-CANCER SOUP

SERVES 10

½ cup dried split peas
½ cup dried beans (can use any variety)
4 cups water
4 medium onions chopped
6–8 medium zucchini, cut into 1-inch pieces
3 leek stalks, coarsely chopped
2 bunches kale, collard greens, or other greens, tough stems and center ribs removed and leaves chopped
5 pounds carrots, juiced (5–6 cups juice; see note)
2 bunches celery, juiced (2 cups juice; see note)
2 tablespoons Dr. Fuhrman's VegiZest or Mrs. Dash
1 cup raw cashews
8 ounces fresh mushrooms (shiitake, cremini, and/or oyster), chopped

Place the split peas, beans, and water in a very large pot over low heat. Bring to a boil and simmer for 30 minutes. Add the onions, zucchini, leeks, and kale to the pot. Add the carrot juice, celery juice, and VegiZest. Simmer until the onions, zucchini, and leeks are soft, about 40 minutes.

Remove 2 cups of the soup liquid, being careful to leave the beans and at least half of the kale in the pot. Using a high-powered blender or food processor, blend the soup liquid with the cashews. Return the creamy mixture to the pot. Add the mushrooms and simmer for 30 minutes, or until the beans are soft.

Note: Freshly juiced organic carrots and celery will maximize the flavor of this soup.

GOLDEN AUSTRIAN CAULIFLOWER CREAM SOUP

SERVES 4

> 1 *head cauliflower, cut into pieces*
> 3 *carrots, coarsely chopped*
> 1 *cup coarsely chopped celery*
> 2 *leeks, coarsely chopped*
> 2 *cloves garlic, minced*
> 2 *tablespoons Dr. Fuhrman's VegiZest or other no-salt seasoning*
> 2 *cups carrot juice*
> 4 *cups water*
> ½ *teaspoon nutmeg*
> 1 *cup raw cashews*
> 5 *cups chopped kale leaves or baby spinach*

Place all the ingredients except the cashews and kale in a pot. Cover and simmer for 15 minutes or until the vegetables are just tender. Steam the kale until tender. (If you are using spinach there is no need to steam it. It will wilt in the hot soup.)

In a food processor or high-powered blender, blend two-thirds of the soup liquid and vegetables with the cashews until smooth and creamy. Return to the pot and stir in the steamed kale (or raw spinach).

HIGH CRUCIFEROUS VEGETABLE STEW

SERVES 10

> 4 cups water
> 2½ cups carrot juice
> ½ cup dried split peas
> ½ cup dried lentils (red lentils make the prettiest soup)
> ½ cup dried adzuki beans, soaked overnight, or no- or low-salt canned adzuki beans, drained and rinsed
> 1 bunch kale, tough stems and center ribs removed and leaves coarsely chopped
> 1 bunch collard greens, tough stems and center ribs removed and leaves coarsely chopped
> 1 head broccoli, cut into florets
> 8 ounces fresh or frozen Brussels sprouts, cut in half if large
> 8 ounces shiitake mushrooms, cut in half
> 10 ounces celery stalks, cut into 1-inch pieces
> 3 leeks, coarsely chopped
> 3 carrots, cut into 1-inch pieces
> 3 parsnips, cut into 1-inch pieces

3 *medium onions, chopped*

4 *medium zucchini, cubed*

4 *cloves garlic, chopped, or 2 teaspoons garlic powder*

1 *(28-ounce) can chopped tomatoes, no-salt-added or low-sodium*

¼ *cup Dr. Fuhrman's VegiZest or other no-salt seasoning*

2 *tablespoons Mrs. Dash*

¼ *cup chopped fresh parsley*

1 *cup broccoli sprouts (optional)*

Place all the ingredients except the parsley and sprouts in a large soup pot. Cover and bring to a simmer, cooking until the adzuki beans are tender, about 1½ hours. (If using canned adzuki beans, simmer until the vegetables, lentils, and split peas are tender and the flavors blend, about 1 hour.) In a food processor or high-powered blender, blend one-quarter of the soup until smooth. Return to the soup pot and stir in the parsley and broccoli sprouts (if using).

LISA'S LOVELY LENTIL STEW

SERVES 4

2 *cups dried lentils*

6 *cups water*

½ *medium onion, finely chopped*

⅛ *teaspoon black pepper*

1 *teaspoon dried basil*

3 *large, ripe tomatoes, chopped*

1 *celery stalk, finely chopped*

Place the lentils, water, onion, pepper, and basil in a pot and simmer for 30 minutes. Add the tomato and celery and simmer for an additional 15 minutes, or until the lentils are tender.

TOMATO BISQUE

SERVES 6

> 3 cups carrot juice
> 1½ pounds tomatoes, chopped, or 1
>   (28-ounce) can whole tomatoes, no-salt-
>   added or low-sodium (San Marzano variety
>   is best; lower acid and sweeter.)
> ¼ cup sun-dried tomatoes, chopped
> 2 celery stalks, chopped
> 1 small onion, chopped
> 1 leek, chopped
> 1 large shallot, chopped
> 3 cloves garlic, chopped
> 1 small bay leaf
> pinch saffron (optional)
> 1 teaspoon dried thyme, crumbled
> 2 tablespoons Dr. Fuhrman's MatoZest or
>   other no-salt seasoning
> ½ cup raw cashews
> ¼ cup chopped fresh basil
> 5 ounces baby spinach

In a large saucepan, combine all the ingredients except the cashews, basil, and spinach. Simmer for 30 minutes. Discard the bay leaf. Remove 2 cups of the vegetables with a slotted spoon and set aside.

Puree the remaining soup and cashews in a food processor or high-powered blender until smooth. Return the reserved vegetables to the pot. Stir in the basil and spinach and let the spinach wilt.

Main Dishes

ASIAN VEGETABLE STIR FRY

SERVES 4

> 14 ounces extra-firm tofu, cubed
> 1 teaspoon Bragg Liquid Aminos or low-sodium soy sauce
> ¼ teaspoon crushed red pepper flakes
> ½ cup brown rice and/or wild rice
> 2 tablespoons Spike salt-free seasoning or other no-salt seasoning
> ¼ cup unhulled sesame seeds

For the sauce:

> ¼ cup plus 2 tablespoons 100% apricot fruit spread
> ¼ cup unsalted natural peanut butter or raw cashew butter
> 2 tablespoons fresh chopped ginger
> 4 cloves garlic, chopped
> 4 teaspoons Dr. Fuhrman's VegiZest or other no-salt seasoning
> ⅓ cup water
> ¼ cup Dr. Fuhrman's Black Fig Vinegar or balsamic vinegar
> 1 teaspoon arrowroot powder
> ¼ teaspoon crushed red pepper flakes

For the vegetables:

> 2 tablespoons water
> 1 medium onion, cut into wedges and separated into 1-inch strips
> 4 cups small broccoli florets
> 2 carrots, cut diagonally into ⅓-inch pieces
> 4 medium red bell peppers, seeded and cut into 1-inch squares
> 1 cup sugar snap peas or snow peas, strings removed
> 2 cups bok choy, cut into bite-size pieces
> 3 cups fresh mushrooms (shiitake, porcini, and/or cremini), stems removed, sliced
> 1 pound fresh spinach
> ½ cup raw cashews, coarsely chopped
> 1¼ pounds romaine lettuce, shredded

Marinate the tofu for 30 minutes in the liquid aminos, red pepper flakes, and Spike. While the tofu marinates, cook the rice according to the package directions. Set aside.

Preheat the oven to 350 degrees. Toss the marinated tofu with the sesame seeds. Bake the sesame-coated tofu in a nonstick baking pan for 30 to 40 minutes, until golden.

To make the sauce, place all the ingredients in a food processor or high-powered blender and blend until smooth. Transfer to a small bowl and set aside.

Heat water in a large pan and water sauté the onion, broccoli, carrots, bell peppers, and peas for 5 minutes, adding more water as necessary to keep vegetables from scorching. Add the bok choy and mushrooms, cover, and simmer until the vegetables are just tender. Remove the cover and cook off most of the water. Add the spinach and toss until wilted.

Add the sauce and stir until all the vegetables are glazed and the sauce is hot and bubbly, about 1 minute. Mix in the cashews and baked tofu. Serve the stir fry over the shredded lettuce along with ¼ cup rice per person.

Note: This recipe looks harder than it is. It is well worth the time it takes to make it and is great for company.

Variation: Stir-fry beans or small pieces of chicken breast or shrimp with the vegetables.

BEAN ENCHILADAS

SERVES 4

1 medium green bell pepper, seeded and chopped
½ cup sliced onion
1 (8-ounce) can tomato sauce, divided,
   no-salt-added or low-sodium
2 cups cooked or canned no-salt-added or low-
   sodium pinto or black beans, drained and
   rinsed
1 cup frozen corn, thawed, or fresh corn off
   the cob
1 tablespoon chopped fresh cilantro
1 tablespoon chili powder
1 teaspoon ground cumin
1 teaspoon onion powder
⅛ teaspoon cayenne pepper (optional)
6–8 corn tortillas

Sauté the bell pepper and onion in 2 tablespoons of the tomato sauce until tender. Stir in the remaining tomato sauce, beans, corn, cilantro, chili powder, cumin, onion powder, and cayenne (if using); simmer for 5 minutes. Spoon about ¼ cup of the bean mixture on each tortilla and roll up. Serve as is or bake for 15 minutes in a 375-degree oven.

BLACK BEAN LETTUCE BUNDLES

SERVES 4

> 2 cups cooked or canned no-salt-added or low-sodium black beans, drained and rinsed
> ½ large, ripe avocado, peeled, pitted, and mashed
> ½ medium green bell pepper, seeded and chopped
> 3 green onions, chopped
> ⅓ cup chopped fresh cilantro
> ⅓ cup mild no-salt-added or low-sodium salsa
> 2 tablespoons fresh lime juice
> 1 clove garlic, minced
> 1 teaspoon ground cumin
> 8 large romaine lettuce leaves

In a bowl, mash the beans and avocado together with a fork until well blended and only slightly chunky. Add all the remaining ingredients except the lettuce and mix.

Place approximately ¼ cup of the mixture in the center of each lettuce leaf and roll up like a burrito.

CHARD AND VEGETABLE MEDLEY

SERVES 4

½ cup water, divided, plus more as needed
4 cloves garlic, minced or pressed
1 medium onion, coarsely chopped
2 tablespoons Dr. Fuhrman's VegiZest or other
   no-salt seasoning
1 teaspoon Spike salt-free seasoning
4 small yellow squash, cut into ½-inch-thick
   slices
2 bunches red or green Swiss chard, tough
   stems removed and leaves coarsely chopped
1 large red bell pepper, seeded and cut into
   ½-inch pieces
1 cup cherry tomatoes cut in half
2 tablespoons balsamic vinegar

Place ¼ cup of the water, the garlic, onion, Vegi-Zest, Spike seasoning, and yellow squash in a large soup pot. Simmer until the onion is soft, about 3 minutes, adding more water if necessary. Add the Swiss chard, bell pepper, tomatoes, and remaining ¼ cup water. Cover and simmer for about 12 minutes, until the vegetables are tender. Remove the vegetables with a slotted spoon. Add the balsamic vinegar to the pot and reduce over high heat until syrupy. Pour over the vegetables.

COLLARDS AND CARROTS WITH RAISINS

SERVES 4

> 4 bunches collard greens, tough stems and cen-
> ter ribs removed and leaves chopped
> 4 carrots, grated
> 1 medium cucumber
> ¼ cup raisins
> ¼ cup raw almond butter
> 2 teaspoons Dr. Fuhrman's Riesling Raisin
> Vinegar or balsamic vinegar
> 1 teaspoon nutritional yeast
> black pepper to taste

Steam the collard greens for 15 minutes. Add the grated carrot and steam for another 5 minutes. Remove from pan and place in a bowl. Blend the remaining ingredients in a food processor or high-powered blender until smooth. Add the sauce to the collards and carrots and toss.

EASY THREE-BEAN VEGETABLE CHILI

SERVES 6

> 1 pound firm tofu, frozen, then defrosted
> 5 teaspoons chili powder, or more to taste
> 1 teaspoon ground cumin
> 10 ounces frozen onions
> 3 cups frozen broccoli, thawed and finely
> chopped
> 3 cups frozen cauliflower, thawed and finely
> chopped

3 cloves garlic, chopped
1 can (15-ounce) pinto beans, no-salt-added or
   low-sodium, rinsed and drained
1 can (15-ounce) black beans, no-salt-added or
   low-sodium, rinsed and drained
1 can (15-ounce) red beans, no-salt-added or
   low-sodium, rinsed and drained
1 (28-ounce) can diced tomatoes,
   no-salt-added
1 (4-ounce) can chopped mild green chilies,
   drained
2½ cups fresh or frozen corn kernels
2 large zucchini, finely chopped

Squeeze the excess water out of thawed tofu and crumble. Place the crumbled tofu, chili powder, and cumin in a soup pot and quickly brown. Add the remaining ingredients and simmer, covered, for 2 hours.

EASY VEGETABLE PIZZA

SERVES 4

4 large whole wheat pitas
2 cups no-salt-added or low-sodium pasta
   sauce
½ cup chopped shiitake mushrooms
½ cup chopped red onion
10 ounces frozen broccoli florets, thawed and
   finely chopped
1 cup shredded nondairy mozzarella-type
   cheese

Preheat the oven to 200 degrees. Place pitas on two baking sheets and warm for 15 minutes. Remove from oven and spoon on the pasta sauce. Sprinkle evenly with the mushrooms, onion, broccoli, and cheese. Bake for 30 minutes.

EGGPLANT ROLL-UPS

SERVES 6

> 2 large eggplants, peeled and sliced lengthwise
>   ½ inch thick
> 2–3 tablespoons water
> 2 medium red bell peppers, seeded and coarsely
>   chopped
> 1 medium onion, coarsely chopped
> 1 cup chopped carrot
> ½ cup chopped celery
> 4 cloves garlic, chopped
> 8 ounces baby spinach
> 1 tablespoon Dr. Fuhrman's VegiZest or other
>   no-salt seasoning
> 2 cups no-salt-added or low-sodium pasta
>   sauce, divided
> 6 ounces nondairy mozzarella-type cheese,
>   shredded

Preheat the oven to 350 degrees. Lightly oil a non-stick baking pan. Arrange the eggplant in a single layer in the pan. Bake for about 20 minutes, or until flexible enough to roll up easily. Set aside.

Heat 2 tablespoons water in a large pan, add the bell pepper, onion, carrot, celery, and garlic; sauté until just tender, adding more water if needed. Add the spinach and VegiZest. Transfer to a mixing bowl. Mix in 2 to 3 tablespoons of the pasta sauce and all of the shredded cheese.

Spread about ¼ cup of the pasta sauce in a baking pan. Put some of the vegetable mixture on each eggplant slice, roll up, and place in the pan. Pour the remaining sauce over the eggplant rolls. Bake for 20 to 30 minutes, until heated through.

GREAT GREENS

SERVES 5

> 1 large bunch kale, tough stems and center ribs removed and leaves chopped
> 1 bunch Swiss chard, tough stems removed and leaves chopped, or 5 ounces spinach
> 1 tablespoon Dr. Fuhrman's Spicy Pecan Vinegar or other flavored vinegar
> ½ tablespoon Dr. Fuhrman's VegiZest or other no-salt seasoning
> 1 clove garlic, minced
> 1 teaspoon dried dill
> 1 teaspoon dried basil
> black pepper to taste

Steam the kale for 10 minutes. Add the Swiss chard and steam for another 10 minutes or until tender. Transfer to a bowl. Combine the remaining ingredients and add to the greens. If desired, add 2 to 3 tablespoons of the steaming water to adjust the consistency.

KALE WITH CASHEW CREAM SAUCE

SERVES 4

> 2 large bunches kale, tough stems and center
>   ribs removed
> 1 cup raw cashews
> 1 cup hemp, soy, or almond milk
> ¼ cup onion flakes
> 1 tablespoon Dr. Fuhrman's VegiZest or other
>   no-salt seasoning (optional)

Steam the kale for 15 minutes or until tender. Meanwhile, blend the cashews, milk, onion flakes, and VegiZest in a food processor or high-powered blender until smooth and creamy. When the kale is done, press it with paper towels to remove any excess water, chop, and mix with the sauce.

NO-MEAT BALLS

SERVES 6 (makes 18 balls)

> 1–2 tablespoons water or no-salt-added or
>   low-sodium vegetable broth
> ½ cup diced onion
> 3 cloves garlic, roasted (see page 000) and
>   mashed
> ¼ cup diced celery
> 2 tablespoons minced fresh parsley
> ¼ teaspoon dried sage
> 1 teaspoon dried basil
> 1 teaspoon dried oregano

1½ cups cooked lentils or 1 (15-ounce) can
   lentils, no-salt-added or low-sodium,
   drained and rinsed
¼ cup cooked brown rice
2–3 tablespoons tomato paste
1 tablespoon arrowroot powder or whole
   wheat flour
2 tablespoons Dr. Fuhrman's MatoZest or
   other no-salt seasoning
2 tablespoons nutritional yeast
freshly ground black pepper to taste
2 tablespoons vital wheat gluten flour, for a
   chewier consistency (optional)

Preheat the oven to 350 degrees. In a sauté pan, heat
1 tablespoon water. Add the onion and garlic and
sauté for 5 minutes. Add the celery, parsley, sage,
basil, and oregano. Sauté for another 5 minutes,
adding more water as needed to prevent sticking.

In a large bowl, combine the sautéed vegetables
with the remaining ingredients and mix well. Mash
lightly with a potato masher. With wet hands, form
2 tablespoons of the lentil mixture into a smooth
ball. Repeat. Place the balls on a very lightly oiled
baking sheet and bake for 30 minutes.

Note: Serve with your favorite no- or low-salt marinara
sauce.

NO-PASTA VEGETABLE LASAGNA

SERVES 8

For the lasagna "noodles":
   2 large eggplants, sliced lengthwise ¼ inch thick
   3 small zucchini, sliced lengthwise as thinly as
      possible
   3 small yellow squash, sliced lengthwise as
      thinly as possible
For the tofu "ricotta":
   16 ounces silken tofu
   1 small onion, cut into quarters
   4 cloves garlic, cut in half
   ½ cup fresh basil leaves
   1¼ pounds firm tofu, squeezed dry and
      crumbled
   ¼ cup Dr. Fuhrman's VegiZest or other no-salt
      seasoning
   2 tablespoons dried Italian seasoning
   1 cup grated nondairy mozzarella cheese
For the vegetables:
   2 heads broccoli, coarsely chopped
   4 cups sliced mixed fresh mushrooms (shiitake,
      cremini, oyster)
   4 medium bell peppers (red, yellow, and/or
      orange), seeded and chopped
   7 ounces baby spinach
   3 cups no- or low-salt pasta sauce, divided
   shredded fresh basil, for garnish

To make the lasagna noodles, preheat the oven to
350 degrees. Wipe a baking pan with a small amount

of olive oil. Place the eggplant, zucchini, and yellow squash in the pan and bake for 10 minutes, or until flexible but not completely cooked. Work in batches if necessary. Set aside.

While the "noodles" are baking, make the tofu "ricotta." Puree the silken tofu, onion, and garlic in a food processor or high-powered blender. Add the basil leaves and pulse to coarsely chop. Transfer to a medium bowl and mix in the crumbled firm tofu. Add the VegiZest, Italian seasoning, and grated cheese. Set aside.

To prepare the vegetables, sauté broccoli, mushrooms, bell peppers, and spinach, without water, over low heat for 5 minutes, just until tender.

To assemble the lasagna, spread a thin layer of pasta sauce on the bottom of a baking dish. Layer eggplant slices, sautéed vegetables, yellow squash slices, zucchini slices, and tofu "ricotta," then spread with pasta sauce. Repeat the layer, ending with the tofu "ricotta." Spread the remaining pasta sauce on top and bake at 350 degrees, uncovered, for 1 hour, or until hot and bubbly. Garnish with the shredded basil.

PITA STUFFED WITH GREENS AND RUSSIAN FIG DRESSING

SERVES 1

> several leaves kale, Swiss chard, or mustard
>   greens, tough stems removed
> 1 teaspoon fresh lemon juice
> dash garlic powder

3 tablespoons no-salt-added or low-sodium
    pasta sauce
1 tablespoon raw almond butter
1 tablespoon Dr. Fuhrman's Black Fig Vinegar
1 whole grain pita
2 thin slices red onion
Sliced tomato

Steam the greens until tender, about 15 minutes. Sprinkle with the lemon juice and garlic powder. Let cool.

Blend the pasta sauce, almond butter, and vinegar in a food processor or high-powered blender until smooth. Stuff the pita with the greens, red onion, and tomato. Top with the dressing.

PORTOBELLO–RED PEPPER PITA

SERVES 4

4 large portobello mushrooms, stems removed
½ large red onion, thinly sliced
4 whole wheat pitas
2 cups arugula leaves
2 medium roasted red peppers from a jar,
    seeded and cut into ½-inch-thick slices

For the tahini spread:
¾ cup raw tahini
½ cup water
1 tablespoon fresh lemon juice
1 medjool date or 2 deglet noor dates, pitted
    and chopped
1 clove garlic, chopped

1 tablespoon Dr. Fuhrman's VegiZest or other
   no-salt seasoning
1 teaspoon Bragg Liquid Aminos or low-
   sodium soy sauce

Preheat the oven to 375 degrees. Arrange the mushrooms and onion on a baking sheet and roast until
tender, 15 to 20 minutes.

Meanwhile, make the tahini spread by blending
all the ingredients together in a food processor or
high-powered blender until creamy.

When the mushrooms and onion are done, split
the pitas in half horizontally and warm slightly.
Spread generous amount of the tahini spread on the
top half of each pita. Place ½ cup arugula, 1 mushroom cap (pat dry with paper towels to absorb any
excess liquid), and one-quarter of the onion and
roasted red pepper on the bottom half of each pita.
Assemble the sandwiches.

SIMPLE BEAN BURGERS

SERVES 6

¼ cup raw sunflower seeds
2 cups cooked or canned red or pink beans,
   no-salt-added or low-sodium, drained and
   rinsed
½ cup minced onion
2 tablespoons low-sodium ketchup
1 tablespoon wheat germ or old-fashioned
   rolled oats
½ teaspoon chili powder

Preheat the oven to 350 degrees. Lightly oil a baking sheet with a little olive oil on a paper towel.

Chop the sunflower seeds in a food processor or with a hand chopper. Mash the beans in the food processor or with a potato masher and mix with the sunflower seeds. Mix in the remaining ingredients and form into six patties. Place the patties on the baking sheet and bake for 25 minutes. Remove from the oven and let cool slightly, until you can pick up each patty and compress it firmly in your hands to re-form the burger. Return the patties to the baking sheet, bottom side up, and bake for another 10 minutes.

SPINACH AND BRUSSELS SPROUTS MARINARA

SERVES 4

> 1 pound Brussels sprouts
> 14 ounces baby spinach
> ¼ cup water
> 4 cloves garlic, minced
> 1 small onion, chopped
> 1 (14.5-ounce) can no- or low-salt chopped tomatoes
> 1 tablespoon Dr. Fuhrman's VegiZest or other no-salt seasoning

Steam the Brussels sprouts and spinach for 8 minutes, or until the Brussels sprouts are almost tender. Meanwhile, heat the water in a large pot and water sauté the garlic and onion until the onion is tender, about 5 minutes. Add the Brussels sprouts and spinach, chopped tomatoes, and VegiZest. Simmer for 10 minutes.

THAI VEGETABLE CURRY

SERVES 8

4 cloves garlic, finely chopped

2 tablespoons finely chopped fresh ginger

2 tablespoons chopped fresh mint

2 tablespoons chopped fresh basil

2 tablespoons chopped fresh cilantro

2 cups carrot juice

1 medium red bell pepper, seeded and thinly sliced

1 large eggplant, peeled if desired and cut into 1-inch cubes

2 cups green beans cut into 2-inch pieces

3 cups sliced shiitake mushrooms

1 (8-ounce) can bamboo shoots, drained

2 tablespoons Dr. Fuhrman's VegiZest or other no-salt seasoning

½ teaspoon curry powder

2 cups watercress leaves, divided

3 tablespoons unsalted natural chunky peanut butter

2 pounds firm tofu, cut into ¼-inch-thick slices

½ cup light coconut milk

½ cup raw cashews, chopped

chopped fresh mint, basil, or cilantro leaves, for garnish (optional)

Place the garlic, ginger, mint, basil, cilantro, carrot juice, bell pepper, eggplant, green beans, mushrooms, bamboo shoots, VegiZest, curry powder, and 1 cup of the watercress in a wok or large skillet. Bring to a boil, cover, and simmer, stirring occasionally, until all the vegetables are tender. Mix in the peanut butter. Add the tofu, bring to a simmer, and toss until hot. Add the coconut milk and heat through. Top with the remaining 1 cup watercress and the cashews. Garnish with mint, basil, or cilantro leaves, if desired.

Note: This can be served over brown rice or quinoa. Frozen vegetables may be used instead of fresh.

VEGETABLE BEAN BURRITO

Serves 6

> 2–3 tablespoons water
> 1 head broccoli florets, chopped
> ½ head cauliflower florets, chopped
> 2 carrots, chopped
> 2 medium red bell peppers, seeded and chopped
> 1 medium zucchini, chopped
> 1 medium onion, chopped
> 4 cloves garlic, chopped
> 1½ tablespoons Dr. Fuhrman's VegiZest or other no-salt seasoning
> 1 teaspoon dried basil
> 1 teaspoon dried oregano
> 1 teaspoon dried parsley
> 1 cup raw cashews

½ cup unsweetened soy, hemp, or almond milk

1½ cups cooked pinto beans or 1 (15-ounce) can no-salt-added or low-sodium pinto beans, drained and rinsed

6 whole wheat tortillas or large romaine lettuce leaves

Place 2 tablespoons water, the broccoli, cauliflower, carrot, bell pepper, zucchini, onion, garlic, VegiZest, basil, oregano, and parsley in a large covered pot. Sauté for 15 minutes, or until tender, adding more water if needed. In the meantime, place cashews and milk in a food processor or high-powered blender and blend until smooth. Add the cashew mixture and beans to the vegetables and mix thoroughly. Spread the mixture on the tortillas and roll up to form burritos.

VEGETABLE OMELET

SERVES 2

1 medium onion, diced

1 medium green or red bell pepper, seeded and diced

1½ cups chopped shiitake mushrooms

1 cup diced fresh tomato

¼ teaspoon dried basil

4 eggs, beaten

black pepper to taste (optional)

Lightly wipe a skillet with olive oil. Sauté the onion, bell pepper, mushrooms, and tomato over medium heat for 10 minutes, or until tender. Add the basil and eggs and cook over medium-high heat until done, about 8 minutes, turning over with a spatula halfway through cooking. Sprinkle with black pepper, if desired.

Desserts

ALMOND CHOCOLATE DIP

SERVES 10

> 1⅓ cups raw almonds or ⅔ cup raw
>   almond butter
> 1 cup unsweetened soy, hemp, or almond
>   milk
> 1 teaspoon vanilla extract
> 1 tablespoon natural cocoa powder
> ⅔ cup dates, pitted

Blend all the ingredients in a high-powered blender until smooth and creamy, adding more milk if necessary.

Note: Use as a dipping sauce for fresh strawberries and fruit slices.

BANANA WALNUT ICE CREAM

SERVES 2

> 2 ripe bananas, frozen (see note)
> ⅓ cup vanilla soy, hemp, or almond milk
> 2 tablespoons chopped walnuts

Blend all the ingredients in a high-powered blender until smooth and creamy.

Note: Freeze ripe bananas at least 24 hours in advance. To freeze, peel, cut into thirds, and wrap tightly in plastic wrap.

CANTALOUPE SLUSH

Serves 3

> 1 cantaloupe, rind removed, seeded, and cut into pieces
> 2 cups ice
> 6–8 medjool dates, pitted

Blend all the ingredients in a high-powered blender until smooth.

Variation: Use peaches or nectarines instead of cantaloupe.

CARA'S APPLE STRUDEL

Serves 4

> ¼ cup apple juice
> ¾ teaspoon vanilla extract
> 1 teaspoon cinnamon
> 1 egg white
> ¼ cup vanilla soy, hemp, or almond milk
> 3 apples, peeled, cored, and chopped
> ¼ cup raisins, chopped
> ½ cup old-fashioned rolled oats or oatmeal flakes

Preheat the oven to 350 degrees. In a bowl, mix the apple juice, vanilla, cinnamon, egg white, and milk until combined. Stir in the apple, raisins, and oats. Pour into an 8-by-8-inch baking dish. Bake, uncovered, for 1 hour.

CHOCOLATE CHERRY ICE CREAM

SERVES 2

> ½ cup vanilla soy, hemp, or almond milk
> 1 tablespoon natural cocoa powder
> 4 dates, pitted
> 1½ cups dark sweet frozen cherries

Blend all the ingredients in a high-powered blender until smooth and creamy. If using a regular blender, add only half the cherries and blend until smooth, then add the remaining cherries and continue to blend.

Variation: Use berries or banana instead of cherries. Freeze ripe bananas at least 24 hours in advance. To freeze, peel, cut into thirds, and wrap tightly in plastic wrap.

JENNA'S PEACH FREEZE

SERVES 2

> 1 ripe banana, frozen (see note)
> 3 peaches or nectarines, peeled and pitted
> 2 medjool dates or 4 deglet noor dates, pitted
> ¼ cup vanilla soy, hemp, or almond milk
> 1 teaspoon vanilla extract
> ⅛ teaspoon cinnamon

Blend all the ingredients in a high-powered blender until smooth and creamy.

Note: Freeze ripe bananas at least 24 hours in advance. To freeze, peel, cut into thirds, and wrap tightly in plastic wrap.

YUMMY BANANA-OAT BARS

SERVES 8

> 2 cups quick-cooking rolled oats (not instant)
> ½ cup shredded coconut
> ½ cup raisins or chopped dates
> ¼ cup chopped walnuts
> 2 large, ripe bananas, mashed
> ¼ cup unsweetened applesauce (optional; see note)
> 1 tablespoon date sugar (optional; see note)

Preheat the oven to 350 degrees. Mix all the ingredients in a large bowl until well combined. Press into a 9-by-9-inch baking pan and bake for 30 minutes. Cool on a wire rack. When cool, cut into squares or bars.

Note: Add the applesauce and date sugar for sweeter, moister bars.

Frequently Asked Questions

You now have the knowledge that you need to eat to live. Much of this information may be new and contradictory to what you have learned in the past. The questions and answers that follow are intended to solidify and reinforce what I have covered and help you clear up any uncertainties.

Should I take vitamins and other nutritional supplements?

I often recommend that people take sensibly designed, high-quality vitamin and mineral supplements to ensure that they get enough vitamin D, vitamin B_{12}, zinc, and iodine. It is also a good idea to take supplemental omega-3 fatty acids or DHA. Very few individuals eat perfectly, and some of us require more of certain nutrients than others, so it makes sense to be sure to ingest adequate amounts of all of these important substances.

Deficiency of vitamin D, the sunshine vitamin, is very common. Many of us avoid sun exposure, wear sunscreen daily, or spend most of our time indoors. Recent studies indicate that average serum vitamin D levels of Americans have dropped in the past decade. This drop was associated with an overall increase in vitamin D insufficiency in nearly three out of four adolescent and adult Americans.[1]

Avoiding the sun may protect against skin damage, but a vitamin D deficiency can contribute to the progression of osteoporosis. It has also been associated with higher rates of certain cancers and autoimmune diseases.[2] A 2009 meta-analysis of nineteen studies established a strong inverse relationship between circulating vitamin D levels and breast cancer: women in the highest vitamin D range reduced their risk of breast cancer by 45 percent.[3] Another 2009 review of twenty-five studies found that sufficient vitamin D levels were consistently associated with reduced risk of colorectal cancer.[4]

Vitamin B_{12} helps make red blood cells and keeps your nervous system working properly. It is found mainly in foods of animal origin. Although individuals whose diets are low in animal products dramatically reduce their risk of developing certain diseases and increase life expectancy, they need a supplemental source of vitamin B_{12}. Some people are unable to absorb the vitamin B_{12} found naturally in food (particularly those in the over-fifty age group),[5] and so a supplement is often necessary to optimize immune function, especially in older people.

I instruct my patients to avoid salt, which is iodinated. Since salt is the primary source of iodine in most people's diets, a multivitamin can ensure adequate iodine intake for those who avoid salt.

It is also a good idea to take some extra DHA (the omega-3 fatty acid docosahexaenoic acid). This essential fatty acid is known for its importance in healthy brain function and cardioprotection. It is naturally converted from the omega-3 fats found in certain green vegetables, walnuts, flaxseeds, chia seeds, and hemp seeds. Studies show that people have varying abilities to make this conversion. Many cannot derive enough of these essential fatty acids from natural food sources, and men generally convert less than women, especially as they age.

The main problem with taking typical supplements is that they may expose you to extra nutrients you do not need. More is not always better. While most people can certainly benefit from a sensibly designed multivitamin plus additional vitamin D and omega-3 fatty acids, it is important to make the right choices. Excessive quantities of some vitamins and minerals can be toxic or have long-term negative health effects.

Avoid taking supplements that contain these ingredients: vitamin A, high-dose (200 IU or greater) isolated vitamin E, folic acid, beta-carotene, and copper. Ingesting vitamin A or beta-carotene from supplements instead of food may interfere with the absorption of other crucially important carotenoids, such as lutein and lycopene, thus potentially increasing your cancer risk.[6]

Folic acid is the synthetic form of folate added to food or used as an ingredient in vitamin supplements. Folate is found naturally in fruits, vegetables, grains, and other foods. Too much folate obtained naturally from food is not a concern. It comes naturally packaged in balance with other micronutrients, and the body regulates its absorption.[7] Everyone, including pregnant women, should be getting adequate amounts of folate from natural plant sources. Recently, there have been some troubling studies connecting folic acid supplementation and cancer. More and more evidence suggests that folic acid supplementation may significantly increase the risk of cancer.[8]

Remember, dietary supplements are *supplements*, not substitutes for a healthy diet. Supplements alone cannot offer optimal protection against disease, and you cannot make an unhealthy diet into a healthy one by consuming supplements.

Could restricting my intake of animal products or eating a strict vegetarian diet cause me to develop vitamin deficiencies?

A strict vegetarian diet is deficient in meeting the vitamin B_{12} needs of some individuals. If you choose to follow a complete vegetarian (vegan) diet, it is imperative that you consume a multivitamin or other source of B_{12}, such as fortified soy milk. My vegetarian menu plans and dietary suggestions are otherwise rich in calcium and contain sufficient iron from green vegetables and beans. They contain adequate protein and are extremely nutrient-dense.

My observations suggest that vegetarians would be foolish not to play it safe, either by taking a B_{12} supplement or a multivitamin or by consuming foods that have been fortified with vitamin B_{12}. Another option for those who loathe taking vitamins is to have their blood checked periodically. Checking your B_{12} level alone is not sufficient. Your methylmalonic acid (MMA) must be checked to accurately gauge if the level of B_{12} in your body is enough for you.

What about supplements or herbs to help me lose weight?

Don't be conned by diet pills, magic in a bottle, or fat absorbers. Anything really effective is not safe, and those that are safe are not effective. To deal with the real problem, you must make real changes. Here is some data on four of the most popular remedies.

Acai berries: While all berries are anti-inflammatory and high in antioxidants, the overhyped Brazilian acai (pronounced a-sigh-EE) berries offer no additional magical health or weight-loss benefits. There is no evidence to suggest that acai products will help you shed pounds, flatten your tummy, cleanse your colon, enhance your sexual desire, cure baldness, or perform any of the other commonly advertised functions. The expensive acai berry comes as a juice, pulp, powder, and capsule and is a triumph of marketing over science. In fact, companies selling acai fruits are under investigation after numerous consumer complaints.

Garcinia cambogia (hydroxycitric acid): In spite of an interesting theory and some intriguing animal studies, the human studies are unimpressive. In the best study to date, 135 patients were double-blinded to receive either 1,500 mg per day of hydroxycitric acid or a placebo. They were all placed on a high-fiber, low-calorie diet. After twelve weeks, the placebo group had lost more weight.[9] Conclusion: garcinia cambogia doesn't work.

Chitosan: This form of chitin, derived from the shells of crustaceans, supposedly traps fat in the intestine and is frequently advertised as Fat Absorb. A review of the data available seems to indicate that you would have to consume an entire bottle every day to have much of a reduction in fat absorption. The amount of fat absorbed is minuscule, and clinical data shows that Chitosan does not promote weight loss.[10] Conclusion: Chitosan doesn't work.

Ephedra alkaloids (ma huang): Although this natural stimulant has a small effect on reducing appetite, the FDA has issued a warning regarding serious and potentially lethal side effects associated with the use of products containing ephedra, including arrhythmias, heart attacks, strokes, psychosis, abnormal liver function, seizures, rapid heart rate, anxiety, and stomach pain.[11] Ephedra is so dangerous that it has been linked with fatalities—even a low dose has detrimental health effects. Conclusion: it's not worth the risk.

What about drugs for weight loss?

Remember: for anything to be effective, you have to be on it forever. Even if the drugs were remarkably effective, you would have to be prepared to stay on them forever; the minute you stopped, the benefits would slowly be lost. In the long run, it is still your diet that determines your health and your weight. The amphetamine-related appetite suppressants have received much press, and they were quite popular until their dangers became better known. They were never approved for long-term use, so it wasn't very wise for people to use them.

The two FDA-approved drugs for weight reduction are Meridia (sibutramine) and Xenical (orlistat). Meridia can cause headaches, insomnia, constipation, dry mouth, and hypertension and is only slightly helpful. Xenical, the fat inhibitor, can cause abdominal pain and diarrhea, and it reduces absorption of the fat-soluble vitamins, such as D, E, and K. It may help those who consume an unhealthful, fatty diet, but even then it is hardly worth the side effects. Overall, drugs are drugs—they are a poor substitute for healthy living.[12]

Can't I eat chocolate, ice cream, or other junk food ever again?

You can eat anything you desire, on occasion, but just don't make a habit of it. Try to be very strict the first three months in order to document how much weight you can expect to lose when you eat sensibly. We are all tempted by these treats. It is easier to resist if you get them out of your house completely. All cheating should be done outside your home. If possible, associate with friends who will support you in recovering your health—or may join you in trying to be healthy.

Once you regain your health and feel great, you are less likely to crave these foods or be so tempted. Then, when you do deviate from a healthful diet, it is likely you will feel poorly, have a persistent dry mouth, and not sleep well. If you go off your diet and eat junk food on occasion, mark it on your calendar and consider it a special occasion that you won't repeat too often.

Nobody is perfect; however, do not let your weight yo-yo. You must adhere to the plan strictly enough so that you never put back on whatever weight you take off.

Is exercise essential for success in weight loss, and what type of exercise is best?

Exercise is important, but if your ability to be active and exercise is limited, do not despair. My more aggressive menu plans will still enable you to lose weight.

Obviously, those unable to exercise require a stricter diet. Some people have health conditions that preclude them from exercising much. However, you should still try to devise an exercise prescription to fit your capabilities. Almost everyone can do something; even those who cannot walk can do arm exercises with light weights and use an arm cycle.

Exercise will facilitate your weight loss and make you healthier. Vigorous exercise has a powerful effect on promoting longevity. If you have the will to adopt this plan and take good care of yourself, you will find the will to exercise. "No time to exercise" is not an excuse. If you have time to brush your teeth, take a shower, or go to the bathroom, you can make some time to exercise. Take frequent five-minute exercise breaks—walk stairs or stand up then sit down slowly in your chair twenty times. Even people with no time to exercise or join a health club can go up and down stairs in their home or place of work. Try doing as many flights as you can two or three times a day. Walking twenty or more flights a day is an effective way to achieve your goal. Most of my patients have a health club in their house—that is, a stairway leading to the upstairs floor and one going down to the basement as well. I ask them to walk up and down the two flights ten times in the morning before they shower and ten times at night. It takes only five minutes, but it really works.

I encourage patients to join a real health club and use a variety of equipment to utilize many body parts for maximum results. The more muscle groups that are exercised, the more metabolically active players you have on your team to help you meet your goals. It is definitely helpful to have access to an assortment of exercise equipment, such as elliptical machines, treadmills, steppers, recumbent bicycles, and numerous resistance machines. When you tire of one machine, you can move on to a new one.

Are there other strategies for success in the weight-loss arena?

This is not a book on stress management, social support, or stimulus control. Entire books have been written on these subjects. Clearly, it is difficult to eat healthfully in our crazy world, where it seems that everyone else is on a mission to commit suicide with food. That said, some of the following suggestions have proven helpful for people trying to lose weight.

Social support: Include family and friends in your plan. Ask others to read this book—not with the purpose of recruiting them to this way of eating, but so they will help you and understand why you are eating this way. If they are truly your friends, they will support you in your desire to improve your health and will try to have the right food choices available when you are around. Maybe they will even join you on your quest. It is extremely helpful to find at least one friend to join you or support you on your road back to superior health.

Stimulus control: Implement strategies to prevent temptation and exposure to sedentary activities or social eating. The most important stimulus-control technique is structuring your environment. This means removing temptation from your home and stocking your cupboards and refrigerator with the proper foods. Eat only at the kitchen table, not while watching television. When you finish dinner, clean up and leave the kitchen area, then brush and floss your teeth, so you are not tempted to return and snack again. Lay out your exercise clothes for the morning so you are reminded to begin your day with your exercise program.

When going out to social situations, eat first or bring your own food if you cannot arrange in advance to have food that meets your needs. Volunteer to bring food for the other guests, too; then you have something you can eat without distress. Try not to make food the center of your life. Keep active with interests that keep you from thinking about eating.

Positive visualization and other relaxation techniques: Progressive muscle relaxation and meditation are designed to reduce tension and provide a distraction for stressful events.[13] For many, stress is a predictor of relapse and unhealthful eating. We need both exercise and sufficient rest and sleep to best deal with the stress in our lives. If you are not sleeping well, you can become overwhelmed more easily by stressful situations. An audiotape or CD to guide you in relaxation can be very helpful in reducing stress and sleeping better.

Self-monitoring: Accept that this diet is a lifetime commitment. The individual most likely to succeed is one who has changed both his habits and his mind-set. Food diaries, weekly weigh-ins, physical activity logs, and goal setting are all effective ways to stay on track. The primary purpose of self-monitoring is to become aware of behaviors and factors that either positively or negatively influence your food and activity choices. Research has consistently demonstrated that self-monitoring is a helpful tool that improves outcome.[14]

I suggest you make a list of goals that losing weight will help you accomplish and post it somewhere in your home where you will see it. Add to it from time to time and check off accomplishments as you achieve them. Make the goals very specific to you, such as the following:

I will be confident about my ability to resist disease.

I will succeed at losing pounds and regaining excellent health.

I will be able to fit into fashionable clothes, including my favorite blue dress.

My cholesterol will improve by at least fifty points.

I will look good in a bathing suit at the pool this summer.

I will have more energy and be able to enjoy bike trips with my children.

My husband/wife/other will find me more attractive.

My job will be less tiring, and I will perform
    better and make more money.

I will save money on health care and will be able
    to save for my retirement.

I will have a better social life and be in a
    position to attract John [or Jane].

My knees and back will stop hurting.

I will gain the respect of my peers.

My allergies, constipation, indigestion,
    headaches, and acne will all resolve.

My fears about a health crisis or death will
    subside.

Additional support from Dr. Fuhrman: I have created a website to provide additional information, tools, and support to help you accomplish your goals. At DrFuhrman.com, you have access to the most current information on health and nutrition, as well as to more inspiring and dramatic stories of sustained weight loss and health recoveries. You can find articles I have written making sense of recent research findings and nutritional medicine—sifting through the myths versus the facts. It's also the best place to find out about my upcoming lectures and events. Every year I organize a weeklong health getaway, which gives you the opportunity to be fully engaged in receiving information critical to your health, enjoy and learn how to make gourmet nutritarian recipes, and develop lifelong friendships with supportive, like-minded people. The getaway offers lectures, cooking demonstrations, exercise classes, and health screenings, along with activities and entertainment, in a beautiful resort setting.

The membership at DrFuhrman.com is specifically designed to ensure your success, whether you need guidance and encouragement or just want to enjoy the information and camaraderie there. Members can turn to the website for ongoing insight, recipes, meal plans, social networking, and even my personal advice. You can read my answers to thousands of questions and ask me your questions, too. In addition, you have the opportunity to connect directly with other members who are just starting out or who have been successful and can pass along helpful tips. Remember, you will reach your goals more quickly when you have the support of others who've already achieved success.

Structured coaching: Some individuals do better when another person tracks their results and provides encouragement. Some people maximize success with a variety of aids, including regular visits to a physician, dietitian, or psychologist. When patients see me each month, we review what they have achieved and what it will take to achieve the goal for the following month. Improvements in blood pressure, weight, lipid levels, liver function, and diabetic parameters are all helpful to keep people focused on achieving their goals. If you are on medication, you will have to visit your physician regularly to adjust the dose and potentially discontinue a medication that you will no longer need as you lose weight. You can also ask your physician to read this book and work with you, supporting you as you earn your way back to total wellness.

In-patient facilities or health retreats: If you do not succeed, or are not able to do so on your own, you are not a failure. Some individuals require a structured environment to get them started on the road to success. For others it is imperative for their health that they succeed at taking weight off relatively quickly. If you are committed to success, there is no reason you should be satisfied with anything less than spectacular results in your health, wellness, and physique. Some individuals may require an initial period of supervision that offers a more disciplined and structured program in which all the food they eat is prepared for them. These people are soon reeducated in proper eating and learn to adjust to the changes they must make. They can taste many different ways to prepare healthy food and learn healthy food preparation.

Is a vegetarian or vegan diet healthier than a diet that contains a small amount of animal products?

I do not know for sure. A preponderance of the evidence suggests that either a near-vegetarian diet or a vegetarian diet is the best. In the massive China-Cornell-Oxford Project, a reduction in cancer rates continued to be observed as participants reduced their animal-food consumption all the way down to one serving per week. Below this level there is not enough data available. Some smaller studies suggest that some fish added to a vegetarian diet provides benefit, which is likely a result of the increased DHA fat from fish.[15] This same benefit most likely could be achieved on a strict vegetarian diet by including ground flaxseeds and nuts that contain omega-3, such as walnuts. If you want to get the benefit from the additional DHA contained in fish yet remain on a strict vegetarian diet, you can take algae-derived DHA.

Whether or not you are a strict vegetarian, your diet must be plant-predominant for optimal health and to maximally reduce your cancer risk. A vegetarian or vegan diet may be healthy or unhealthy, depending on food choices, but a diet similar to the one most Americans consume—i.e., one containing a significant quantity of animal products—cannot be made healthful. For those not willing to give them up, animal products should be limited to twelve ounces or less per week. Otherwise, the risk of disease increases considerably. Many of my patients choose to eat only vegan foods in their home and eat animal products as a treat once a week or so when they are out.

Is a high-nutrient, low-calorie diet the best one for everyone?

I do not recommend the same diet for everyone, but the H = N/C formula never changes. On very rare occasions I come across an individual who requires some modification to this diet. There are some illnesses, such as active inflammatory bowel disease, for which this diet would have to be adjusted because the patient may not tolerate a large amount of raw vegetables and fruits. I do adjust and customize eating plans and nutritional supplements for individuals with unique medical and metabolic needs. If you are one such person, or if you need a healthful way to gain weight, I would hope you would contact me, or another physician with expertise in this area, for more specific advice.

I don't drink six to eight glasses of water daily. Is that bad?

Only those eating an American-style diet, so high in salt and so low in the high-water-content fruits and vegetables, need to drink that much water. On my fiber- and fluid-rich diet, your need for extra water decreases. Three glasses a day is usually sufficient; but if you are exercising or in the heat, then you obviously need to drink more to replenish those liquids lost through perspiration.

How do you modify your recommendations about superior nutrition and disease prevention for children or those not needing to lose weight?

I believe the diet we currently feed our children is the reason we are seeing so many frequent infections and such high levels of allergies, autoimmune disease, and cancer in this country. Unfortunately, what we eat early in life has a more powerful effect on our eventual health (or ill health) than what we eat later in life. I have four children and understand the difficulties of trying to raise healthy children in today's insane world. It seems we are in an environment in which parents are enthusiastically and purposely breeding a nation of sickly and diseased adults.

In my community, parents and neighbors unknowingly attempt to poison their children at every opportunity. They don't merely feed their own children a diet chock-full of sugar and fat, but at every birthday party, athletic event, and social occasion they bring sugar-coated doughnuts, cupcakes, and candy for the entire crowd. I would expect that as parents, we all have the same goal of trying to get our children to eat more nutritious foods: more vegetables, fruits, raw nuts and seeds, and legumes and beans. However, no child will eat healthfully if he or she is allowed to eat unhealthy foods on a regular basis.

The only way to have a child eat healthfully is to clear all unhealthful foods out of the house, so that when the child is hungry, he or she is forced to pick from healthy choices. Children will at least eat healthfully at home if they are presented with only healthy food choices. For more information, consider reading my book *Disease-Proof Your Child*.

The dietary rules in this book are too calorie-restricted and too fat-restricted for a child or thin athlete. However, the principles for healthy eating and longevity do not change. All that has to be done to increase the caloric density and fat density of the diet is to add more wholesome sources of fat and calories, such as raw nuts and seeds, nut butters, and avocados. Starchy vegetables and whole grains can be consumed in larger amounts, and vegetable and grain dishes can be flavored with sauces and dressings made with nuts and seeds.

If you want to gain weight, eating more—or eating differently to bulk up—will add mostly fat to your body. It is exceptionally rare for a person to gain more muscle just from eating more food. Forcing yourself to consume more food than your body wants is not in your best interest. If you want to gain weight, lift weights to add muscle; then the exercise will increase your appetite accordingly. When you eat a healthful diet, nature has you carry only that mass you need; your muscles will enlarge only if additional stress is placed on them. Of course, this book is designed for those who are overweight and desirous of losing weight. Those who are truly excessively thin and need to gain weight may have to modify this eating plan somewhat to meet their individual needs.

Is it dangerous to eat more fruits and vegetables because of the increased consumption of pesticides? Do I have to buy organic?

The effects of ingesting pesticides in the very small amounts present in vegetation are unknown. Bruce Ames, Ph.D., director of the National Institute of Environmental Health Sciences Center at the University of California at Berkeley, who has devoted his career to examining this question, believes these minute amounts pose no risk at all.

He and other scientists support this view because humans and other animals are exposed to small amounts of naturally occurring toxins with every mouthful of organically grown, natural food. The body normally breaks down self-produced metabolic wastes and naturally occurring carcinogens in foods, as well as pesticides, and excretes these harmful substances every minute. Since 99.99 percent of the potential carcinogenic chemicals consumed are naturally present in all food, reducing our exposure to the 0.01 percent that are synthetic will not reduce cancer rates.

These scientists argue that humans ingest thousands of natural chemicals that typically have a greater toxicity and are present at higher doses than the very minute amount of pesticide residues that remain on food. Furthermore, animal studies on the carcinogenic potential of synthetic chemicals are done at doses a thousandfold higher than what is ingested in food. Ames argues that a high percentage of all chemicals, natural or not, are potentially toxic in high doses—"the dose makes the poison"— and that there is no evidence of possible cancer hazards from the tiny chemical residue remaining on produce.

Others believe a slight risk may be present, though that risk may be difficult to prove. There certainly is a justifiable concern that some chemicals have increased toxicity and are potentially harmful at lower doses than are used in rodent experiments. No scientist believes that this means we should reduce our consumption of vegetation, but many (including me) believe it prudent to reduce our exposure to the multiple toxic residues present in our food supply. I certainly advocate avoiding the skins of foods that are reported to have the most pesticide residues. And, of course, all fruits and vegetables should be washed before eating.

If you are concerned about pesticides and chemicals, keep in mind that animal products, such as dairy and beef, contain the most toxic pesticide residues. Because cows and steers eat large amounts of tainted feed, certain pesticides and dangerous chemicals are found in higher concentrations in animal foods. For example, dioxin, which is predominantly found in fatty meats and dairy products, is one of the most potent toxins linked to several cancers in humans, including lymphomas.[16] By basing your diet on unrefined plant foods, you automatically reduce your exposure to the most dangerous chemicals.

According to the Environmental Working Group,[17] these are the "Dirty Dozen" consistently most contaminated fruits and vegetables, ranked from highest to lowest:

1. celery
2. peaches
3. strawberries
4. apples
5. blueberries
6. nectarines
7. bell peppers
8. spinach

9. cherries
10. kale
11. potatoes
12. imported grapes

It would make sense to purchase organically grown versions of these foods.

Onions, sweet corn, asparagus, sweet peas, cabbage, eggplant, broccoli, tomatoes, and sweet potatoes are the vegetables least likely to have pesticides on them. Avocados, pineapples, mangoes, kiwifruit, papayas, watermelon, and grapefruit are the fruits least likely to have pesticide residues on them.

It makes good sense to peel fruits if possible, and not to eat potato skins unless you are able to purchase pesticide-free potatoes. Remove and discard the outermost leaves of lettuce and cabbage if not organically grown; other surfaces that cannot be peeled can be washed with soap and water or a commercial vegetable wash. Washing with plain water removes 25 to 50 percent of the pesticide residue.

Every study done to date on the consumption of food and its relation to cancer has shown that the more fruits and vegetables people eat, the less cancer and heart disease they have. All these studies were done on people eating conventionally grown, not organic, produce. Clearly, the benefit of conventional produce outweighs any hypothetical risk.

My doctor noted that my complexion had turned yellowish and told me to cut back on foods containing carotene, such as mangoes, carrots, and sweet potatoes.

The slight yellow-orange tinge to your skin is not a problem; it is a marker that you are on a healthy diet. On the contrary, any person who does not have some degree of carotenemia in his or her skin is not eating properly, and such an eating pattern places him or her at risk of cancer—including skin cancer. I drink no carrot juice; however, my skin has a slight yellow hue, especially when contrasted with the skin of people eating conventionally. When my patients eat a nutritionally packed diet, their skin changes color slightly as well. Tell your doctor it is he who has the dangerous skin tone. However, I still do not recommend taking vitamin A or high doses of beta-carotene in supplements. Both vitamin A and beta-carotene in supplement form have been linked to increased mortality.[18]

What about the argument about our ancestors being hunter-gatherers who ate lots of meat?

Of course there were primitive populations who ate high-meat diets and there were primitive people who ate plant-predominant diets. Humans were desperate for calories, so they ate whatever they could get their hands on. The two questions we have to look at are these: How long did they live on that diet? What diet for humans gives them the best protection against disease and the greatest chance for longevity in modern times?

Personally, I want to do a lot better than our prehistoric ancestors did. A comprehensive overview and a sensible interpretation of the scientific evidence support the conclusion that we can increase human longevity and prevent disease if we make specific food choices. We still retain our primate physiology—a physiology that depends on high vegetation consumption—which is relevant to explain our ability to thrive on a plant-predominant diet.

Dr. Katharine Milton, at the University of California at Berkeley, is among the few nutritional anthropologists in the world who has worked with and studied cultures and primitive peoples not influenced by modern technology. She has concluded that the diet of both primitive people and wild primates is largely plant-based.[19] The main difference between primitive diets and our own is their consumption of nutrient-dense wild plants and the lack of access to low-nutrient, high-fat foods such as cheese and oil, as well as refined grains.

We have a unique opportunity in human history: we have fresh produce being flown into our food stores from all over the planet. We can take advantage of this abundant variety of fresh vegetation to eat a diet with more phytochemical density and diversity than ever before. We have the opportunity to make decisions about what we eat that were not available to our prehistoric ancestors. Fortunately, we have knowledge that they lacked, and we can use this knowledge to live longer than ever before.

I know you do not recommend butter or margarine, so what do we put on bread and vegetables?

Butter is loaded with a dangerous amount of saturated fat; stick margarines have hydrogenated oils that contain trans fats, which raise LDL, the bad cholesterol. The more solid a margarine is at room temperature, the more trans fat it contains. Adjusting the type of fat consumed, researchers found that butter caused the highest cholesterol level and that varying amounts of margarines and oils had various harmful effects.[20] The best answer is to use nothing, or buy whole grain bread that tastes good without adding a greasy topping. If you love the flavor of butter, sparingly use a tub or liquid margarine that contains no hydrogenated oil. Lots of my patients like no-salt tomato sauce, a tomato-salsa blend, avocado, or stewed mushrooms on bread. Of course, the best way to get out of the habit of eating those greasy toppings is not to eat bread at all.

Are soy products and soybeans a healthy food to eat?

Soy products such as soy burgers, soy milk, and soy cheese are much more popular and available today than in the past. The FDA has approved soy-containing products as heart-healthy and allows health claims for soy protein.

Studies have shown soy's beneficial effects on cholesterol and other cardiovascular risk factors. However, there is no reason not to expect the same results from beans of any type—it's merely that more studies have been done on soy than on other beans.

There are also numerous studies indicating that soybeans are rich in various anti-cancer compounds, such as isoflavones. In spite of popular myths, the scientific literature is clear: the consumption of soybeans, or minimally processed soy products such as tofu and tempeh, is linked to the reduced risk of breast cancer.[21] However, I do not recommend consuming large quantities of soy products in the hopes of reducing cancer risk. The soybean is not the only bean that contains isoflavones. Most beans are rich in these beneficial anti-cancer compounds, and many different flavonoids with anti-cancer effects are found in beans of all kinds. A healthy diet includes a variety of beans and does not rely on any one food for a disproportionate share of calories. I always recommend the consumption of a broad variety of phytochemical-rich foods to maximize one's health, and beans are no exception

Tofu and frozen soybeans are good sources of omega-3 fat and calcium, but soy nuts, soy milk, and other processed soy products do not retain much of the beneficial compounds found in the natural bean. The more the food is processed, the more the beneficial compounds are destroyed. Most processed soy products can be tasty additions to a plant-based diet, but they are generally high in salt and are not nutrient-dense foods, so you should use them sparingly.

In conclusion, the soybean is a superior food, containing the difficult-to-find omega-3 fats. Beans in general are superior foods that fight against cancer and heart disease, which is why you will benefit from including a variety of beans in your diet.

How much salt is permissible on this nutritional program?

This book is designed for those who want to lose weight and for those who want to maintain excellent health and prevent disease. Any excess salt added to food, outside of what is contained in natural foods, is likely to increase your risk of developing disease. Salt consumption is linked to both stomach cancer and hypertension.[22] For optimal health, I recommend that no salt at all be added to any food. The famous DASH study clearly indicates that Americans consume five to ten times as much sodium as they need and that high sodium levels over the years raise blood pressure.[23] Just because you don't have high blood pressure now doesn't mean that you won't. In fact, you probably will have high blood pressure if you keep eating lots of salt.

Salt also pulls out calcium and other trace minerals in the urine when the excess is excreted, which is a contributory cause of osteoporosis.[24] If that is not enough, high sodium intake is predictive of increased death from heart attacks. In a large prospective trial published in the respected medical journal *Lancet,* there was a frighteningly high correlation between sodium intake and all-cause mortality in overweight men.[25] The researchers concluded, "High sodium intake predicted mortality and risk of coronary heart disease, independent of other cardiovascular risk factors, including high blood pressure. These results provide direct evidence of the harmful effects of high salt intake in the adult population."

This means that salt has significant harmful effects independent of its effects on blood pressure. For instance, it very likely increases the tendency of platelets to clot. I recommend that people resist adding salt to foods and look for no-salt-added products. Since most salt comes from processed foods, bread, and canned goods, it shouldn't be that hard to avoid added sodium.

That said, if you desire to salt your food, do so only after it is on the table and you are ready to eat it. It will taste saltier if the salt is right on the surface of the food. You can add lots of salt to vegetables or soups while they are cooking yet hardly taste it. Use herbs, spices, lemon juice, vinegar, or other no-salt seasonings to flavor food. Condiments such as ketchup, mustard, soy sauce, teriyaki sauce, and relish are very high in sodium, so if you can't resist them, use low-sodium varieties sparingly.

Ideally, all your foods should have less than 1 mg of sodium per calorie. Natural foods contain about 0.5 mg of sodium per calorie. If a food has a serving size of 100 calories and contains 400 mg of sodium, it is a very high-salt food. If the serving has 100 calories and less than 100 mg of sodium, it is a food with hardly any added salt and is an appropriate food for your diet. Try to avoid products with more than 200 mg per 100 calories. Within these guidelines, you should be able to keep your average daily sodium intake around or below 1,000 mg.

If you don't use salt, your taste buds adjust with time and your ability to taste salt improves. When you are using a lot of salt in your diet, it weakens your taste for salt and makes you feel that food tastes bland unless it is heavily seasoned or spiced. The DASH study observed the same phenomenon that I have noted for years—it takes some time for one's salt-saturated taste buds to get used to a low sodium level. If you follow my nutritional recommendations strictly, without compromise, avoiding all processed foods or highly salted foods, your ability to detect and enjoy the subtle flavors in fruits and vegetables will improve as well.

What about coffee?

Clearly, excessive consumption of caffeinated beverages is dangerous. Caffeine addicts are at higher risk of cardiac arrhythmias that could precipitate sudden death.[26] Coffee raises blood pressure, as well as cholesterol and homocysteine, two risk factors for heart disease.[27] One cup of coffee per day is not likely to cause a significant risk, but drinking more than one cup can interfere with your health and even your weight-loss goals.

Besides the increased risk of heart disease, there are two other problems with caffeine. First, it is a stimulant that allows you to get by with less sleep and reduces the depth of sleep. Such sleep deprivation results in higher levels of the stress hormone cortisol and interferes with glucose metabolism, leading to insulin resistance.[28] This insulin resistance, and the subsequent higher baseline glucose level, further promotes heart disease and other problems. Put bluntly, caffeine consumption promotes inadequate sleep, and less sleep promotes disease and premature aging. Adequate sleep is also necessary to prevent overeating. There is no substitute for adequate sleep.

The second issue with caffeine is that eating more frequently and eating more food suppresses caffeine-withdrawal headaches and other withdrawal symptoms. When you are finally finished digesting a meal, the body more effectively cleans house. At this time caffeine addicts experience a drive to eat more to suppress caffeine-withdrawal symptoms. Thus they are prodded to eat more food than they would if they were not addicted to caffeine.

You will never be in touch with your body's true hunger signals while you are addicted to stimulants. For some people giving up coffee is more difficult than following the dietary restrictions I recommend. I suggest that you carefully adhere to my recommendations without caffeinated beverages for the first six weeks. After that time, when the addiction to caffeine is no longer present, you can decide if you really can't give up that one cup of coffee. Keep in mind that it takes four to five days for the caffeine-withdrawal headaches to resolve once you stop drinking coffee. If the symptoms are too severe, try reducing your coffee intake slowly, by about half a cup every three days.

If a little coffee would make it possible for you to remain true to my dietary recommendations, I would not have a strong objection. Losing weight is a more important goal for your overall health. It is just that higher amounts of caffeine do not make it easier to control your appetite and food cravings; they make it harder. It would be much better if you gave this plan a true test. See how well you feel and how much weight you can lose in six weeks. Maybe by then you will have lost your craving for mind-altering substances.

How much alcohol is permissible?

Moderate drinking has been associated with a lower incidence of coronary heart disease in more than forty prospective studies. This applies only to moderate drinking—defined as one drink or less per day for women and two drinks or less for men. More than this is associated with increased fat around the waist and other potential problems.[29] Alcohol consumption also leads to mild withdrawal sensations the next day that are commonly mistaken for hunger. One glass of wine per day is likely insignificant, but I advise against higher levels of alcohol consumption.

Alcohol's anti-clotting properties grant some protective effect against heart attacks, but this protective effect is valuable only in a person or population consuming a heart disease–promoting diet. It is much wiser to avoid the detrimental effects of alcohol completely and protect yourself from heart disease with nutritional excellence. For example, even moderate alcohol consumption is linked to higher rates of breast cancer and to the occurrence of atrial fibrillation.[30] Avoid alcohol and eat healthfully if possible, but if that one drink a day will make you stay with this plan much more successfully, then have it.

I feel best when I eat a high-protein diet, with plenty of animal products. Does that mean these recommendations to eat a plant-based diet are not for me?

I have thousands of patients eating vegetarian or near-vegetarian diets and over the past fifteen years have noted a very small percentage of the total who initially report that they feel better with significant animal products in their diet and worse on a vegetarian diet. Almost all these complaints resolve with time on the new diet. I believe the main reasons for this are as follows.

A diet heavily burdened with animal products places a toxic stress on the detoxification systems of the body. As with stopping caffeine, cigarettes, and heroin, many observe withdrawal symptoms for a short period, usually including fatigue, weakness, headaches, or loose stools. In 95 percent of these cases, these symptoms resolve within two weeks.

It is more common that the temporary adjustment period lasts less than a week, during which you might feel fatigue, have headaches or gas, or experience other mild symptoms as your body withdraws from your prior toxic habits. Don't buy the fallacy that you "need more protein." The menus in this book offer sufficient protein—and protein deficiency does not cause fatigue. Even my vegan menus supply about 50 grams of protein per 1,000 calories, a whopping amount. Stopping dangerous but stimulating foods causes temporary fatigue.

Increased gas and loose stools are also occasionally observed when switching to a diet containing so much fiber and different fibers that the digestive tract has never encountered before. Over many years, the body has adjusted its secretions and peristaltic waves (digestive-related bowel contractions) to a low-fiber diet. These symptoms also improve with time. Chewing extra well, sometimes even blending salads, helps in this period of transition. Some people must avoid beans initially, and then use them only in small amounts, adding more to the diet gradually over a period of weeks to train the digestive tract to handle and digest these new fibers.

Certain people have increased fat requirements, and the type of vegetarian diet they may have been on in the past was not rich enough in certain essential fats for them. This can occur in those eating a plant-based diet that includes lots of low-fat wheat and grain products. Frequently, adding ground flaxseeds or flaxseed oil to the diet to supply additional omega-3 fats is helpful. Some, especially thin individuals, require more calories and more fat to sustain their weight. This is usually "fixed" by including raw nuts, raw nut butters, avocados, and other healthy foods that are nutrient-rich and also high in fat and calories. Even these naturally thin individuals will significantly improve their health and lower their risk of degenerative diseases if they reduce their dependency on animal foods and consume more plant-derived fats, such as nuts, instead.

There is also the rare individual who needs more concentrated sources of protein and fat in his diet because of digestive impairment, Crohn's disease, short gut syndrome, or other uncommon medical conditions. I have also encountered patients on rare occasions who become too thin and malnourished on what I would consider an ideal, nutrient-dense diet. On such occasions, more animal products have been needed to reduce the fiber content, slow transit time in the gut, and aid absorption and concentration of amino acids at each meal. This problem usually is the result of some digestive impairment or difficulty with absorption. I have seen only a handful of such cases in the past twenty years of practice. In other words, not even one in a hundred, in my estimation, requires animal products regularly in his diet. These individuals should still follow my general recommendations for excellent health and can accommodate their individual needs by keeping animal-product consumption down to comparatively low levels.

Do you recommend low-calorie or no-calorie sweeteners?

Sweetening agents such as NutraSweet (aspartame), Sweet'N Low (saccharin), and Splenda (sucralose) are added to thousands of foods and drugs. Many health gurus now recommend substituting stevia in place of artificial sweeteners. Recently approved by the FDA, stevia is made from the leaves of a South American shrub and can be labeled natural.

Many people use these sweeteners in an effort to control their weight. It doesn't work; it just perpetuates your desire for unhealthy food. When researchers compared the caloric intake of women fed aspartame-sweetened drinks with women given higher-calorie beverages, the women given the aspartame merely consumed more calories later.[31] The use of noncaloric sweeteners as a calorie-restriction strategy continues to be criticized by scientists.[32] It has been suggested that consuming something with a sweet taste primes the body for a calorie delivery that doesn't happen. As a result, users of no-calorie sweeteners just seek more sweets to satisfy the body's cravings. Noncaloric sweeteners signal the body that sugar is on the way and stimulate the pancreas to secrete insulin, which is not favorable.

If you are a headache sufferer, beware of products made with aspartame. Studies have shown that migraine sufferers experience more frequent and more severe symptoms after ingesting aspartame.

I recommend playing it safe and sticking to natural foods. The safety of all the artificial sweeteners, as well as of natural sugars, has been questioned in one way or another. Bottom line: try to enjoy your food choices without sweeteners. Fresh fruit and occasionally a little date sugar or ground dates are the safest way to go. I recommend dropping colas, sodas, sweetened teas, and juices. If they don't contain artificial sweeteners, they are loaded with sugar. Eat unrefined foods and drink water. Melons blended with ice cubes make delicious, cooling summer drinks. I certainly believe that if you are significantly overweight, the risk of being overweight probably exceeds any risk associated with these sweeteners. However, I am not convinced that many people have found low-calorie or no-calorie sweeteners to be the solution to their weight problem.

Do you recommend agave nectar as a sweetener?

Agave has become the sweetener of choice for many health enthusiasts, but I do not recommend it. It is just another concentrated, low-nutrient sweetener. In addition, it may pose some significant health problems.

One of its claims to fame is its low glycemic index. That is because agave is approximately 85 percent fructose. Fructose is metabolized differently from other sugars. Instead of going into the bloodstream (where it could raise blood sugar), most of it goes directly to the liver. This is why it has a low glycemic index, but it still promotes fat storage and weight gain. While many see a low glycemic index as a positive, fructose or any concentrated sweetener high in fructose can cause elevated triglycerides and increased risk of heart disease. It may also increase the risk of metabolic syndrome/insulin resistance, particularly in those who are insulin-resistant and/or overweight or obese.[33] These are the same reasons we are given for avoiding products made with high-fructose corn syrup, which has more fructose than regular table sugar.

I eat out frequently, which makes sticking with this plan very difficult. How can I make the transition easier?

Choose restaurants that have healthful options, and know the places that will cater to your needs. When possible, speak to the management or chef in advance. When traveling, look for restaurants that have salad bars. This is not an all-or-nothing plan. Every person exposed to these ideas can improve over his or her current diet. People have a tendency to like best the foods to which they have become accustomed. Keep in mind that eventually you will lose the desire for some of the unhealthful foods you are eating now and you will enjoy the pleasures of healthy, natural foods more. I actually enjoy eating healthy foods more than injurious foods because they taste good and I also feel good. Most of my patients report the same sensation. Food preferences are learned; you can learn to enjoy healthy foods, just as you learned to like unhealthy ones.

You can follow this diet on the road if you are committed to your own success—it just takes more diligence to plan where to eat and to make sure there will be something for you on the menu. Get in the habit of ordering a double-size green salad with the dressing on the side, and use only a tiny amount of dressing or a squeeze of lemon on the salad.

Remember that this is not a temporary diet, it is your life plan. We must consider how our health is affected by what we choose to eat. We all have to make wise choices to get the most out of life. That doesn't mean you must be perfect. It does mean that however you eat, whether you adopt all of my recommendations or just some of them, your health will be better off as a result of those improvements. After a while, it will become a habit. If you give it a good try, you may find, as others have, that it is not as difficult as you thought, and you will likely grow to enjoy it.

Do you think everyone will eventually embrace this way of eating?

No. The social and economic forces that are pulling our population toward obesity and disease will not be defeated by one book preaching about achieving superior health with nutritional excellence. The "good life" will continue to send most Americans to a premature grave. This plan is not for everyone. I do not expect the majority of individuals to live this healthfully. However, they should at least be aware of the facts rather than having their food choices shaped by inaccurate information or food manufacturers. Some people choose to smoke cigarettes, eat unhealthfully, or pursue other reckless habits. They have that inalienable right to live their lives the way they choose. Don't add stress to your life by trying to persuade every person you meet to eat the same way you do. Looking good and feeling healthy will be your best tools of persuasion.

A common criticism of my eating plan, which all knowledgeable authorities agree is healthy, is that most people won't stick to such a restrictive regimen. This is an irrelevant point. Since when is what the "masses" find socially acceptable the criterion for value? Value or correctness is independent of how many will choose to follow my recommendations; that is a separate issue. The critical question is how effective these recommendations are in guaranteeing a slim body, a long life, and enduring health. All those naysayers have missed the point; my plan was not designed to win a popularity contest.

Thousands of enthusiastic individuals who have benefited from this body of knowledge consider this information a special blessing. It is an opportunity to have your life be so much healthier, happier, and more enjoyable. We don't feel deprived; rather, we enjoy fantastic-tasting food that is also healthy. We have developed a distaste for "junk food." At this point in our lives, healthy food simply tastes better. Another question is, how enjoyable is life for those plagued with a multitude of serious medical problems?

Choosing to live a healthful or unhealthful lifestyle is a personal decision, but this is not an all-or-nothing plan. As a health professional, it is my job to encourage people to protect their future health. We can't buy good health; we must earn it. We are given only one body in this lifetime, so I encourage you to take proper care of it. Over time, your health and happiness are inescapably linked. You don't get a new body when you destroy your health with disease-causing foods. I am 100 percent committed to your success and well-being, so please contact me if you encounter roadblocks to recovering your health. I wish you a long life and enduring health. They can be yours.

Glossary

Angiography or catheterization passage of a small catheter into the cardiac circulation to release a radiographic dye permitting visualization of the lumen and detection of cardiac abnormalities

Angioplasty expansion of a blood vessel by means of a balloon catheter inserted into the chosen vessel

Arteriosclerosis or atherosclerosis commonly occurring deposits of yellowish plaques containing lipoid material that thicken and stiffen the vessel walls; these deposits may narrow the lumen, causing chest pain (angina), or rupture, causing clots that lead to heart attacks

Chelation intravenous infusion of a chemical compound that sequesters metallic ions, traditionally used for heavy metal poisoning but controversially promoted as an intervention to reverse atherosclerosis

Detoxification the body's efforts to reduce its toxic load by changing irritants to a less harmful form or one that can be more readily eliminated, or the body's efforts to force the expulsion of such substances through channels of elimination, such as mucus, urine, or skin

Embolus a clot or plug brought by the blood from its original site to a place where it occludes the lumen of a smaller vessel

Epidemiologist one whose field of medicine is the study of factors affecting the frequency and distribution of diseases

Gastric bypass permanent division and separation of the main section (lower segment) of the stomach to create a small stomach pouch with the remaining (upper) segment, which is then reattached to the small intestine

Gastroplasty surgery to reduce the size of the stomach

Homocysteine an intermediate protein in the synthesis of cysteine, which elevates as a result of certain nutritional deficiencies (especially vitamin B_{12} or folate) or because of biochemical variance; the elevation of homocysteine has been implicated in coronary artery disease and heart attacks

Hypertension high blood pressure

Ischemia deficiency of blood flow and subsequent oxygenation secondary to constriction or obstruction of a blood vessel

Ketosis an abnormally high concentration of ketone bodies in the blood, caused by poorly controlled diabetes (high serum glucose) or prolonged carbohydrate insufficiency, such as in fasting or carbohydrate-restricted diets

Lipids a group of water-insoluble fatty substances that serve biological functions in the body: an expression to represent the group of lipoproteins affecting heart disease risk, such as cholesterol, triglycerides, and their component subtypes

Macronutrients fats, carbohydrates, and protein, which supply calories (energy) and are necessary for growth and normal function

Micronutrients essential dietary elements required in small quantities for various bodily needs, but not a source of calories

Nutritarian a person who has a preference for foods and/or an eating style high in micronutrients

Phytochemicals numerous newly discovered micronutrients present in plant foods with substantial ability to maximize the body's defenses against developing disease, including protection from toxins and carcinogens

Receptor a specifically shaped molecule on or within a cell that recognizes or binds with a particular similarly shaped molecule, inducing a specific response within the cell

Revascularization the restoration of normal blood supply by means of a blood vessel graft, as in coronary bypass surgery

Satiated full satisfaction of appetite or thirst without further desire to ingest more food or drink

Sequelae later illnesses or afflictions caused by an initial illness or affliction

Thrombus an aggregation of blood factors forming a clot, frequently causing vascular obstruction at its point of formation

Vascular pertaining to a blood vessel

Acknowledgments

My gratitude and thanks to:

So many wonderful people who have permitted me to use their real names and case histories in this book. They make the book come alive, giving others hope, enthusiasm, and motivation to achieve their own success.

Lisa Fuhrman, my loving wife, who always believed in and encouraged my career dreams, my message, and my vision. Her continual assistance and input in all my work resulted in many contributions to this manuscript.

My four children—Talia, Jenna, Cara, and Sean—all wonderful and uniquely talented. They have all been understanding of my need to frequently work on this manuscript while at home.

Steve Acocella, D.C., my close friend, who spent many tedious hours collecting and compiling disease and food-consumption data from around the world and made phone calls to foreign health officials to clarify or corroborate statistics for me.

The National Health Association, which has

supported my work over the years and contributed a research grant to aid in data collection for this book.

William Harris, M.D., whose insight and scientific advice have greatly aided my work.

Notes

Chapter 1: Digging Our Graves with Forks and Knives

1. Wang Y, Beydoun MA, Liang L, et al. Will all Americans become overweight or obese? Estimating the progression and cost of the US obesity epidemic. *Obesity (Silver Spring)*. 2008 Oct;16(10):2323–30.

2. Centers for Disease Control. National Center for Chronic Disease Prevention and Health Promotion. *Obesity at a Glance*: 2009. http://www.cdc.gov/nccdphp/publications/AAG/pdf/obesity.pdf; United Health Foundation. America's Health Rankings. Direct Health Care Costs Associated with Obesity: 2018. http://www.americashealthrankings.org/2009/obesity/ECO.aspx#2018.

3. Foryet J. Limitations of behavioral treatment of obesity: review and analysis. *J Behav Med*. 1981;4:159–73.

4. Perri MG, Sears SF Jr., Clark JE. Strategies for improving maintenance of weight loss: toward a continuous care model of obesity management. *Diabetes Care*. 1993; 16:200–9.

5. Bouchard C. The causes of obesity: advances in molecular biology but stagnation on the genetic front. *Diabetologia*. 1996; 39(12): 1532–33.

6. Pischon T, Boeing H, Hoffmann K, et al. General and abdominal adiposity and risk of death in Europe. *N Eng J Med*. 2008 Nov 13;359(20):2105–20.

7. Guh DP, Zhang W, Bansback N, et al. The incidence of co-morbidities related to obesity and overweight: a systematic review and meta-analysis. *BMC Public Health*. 2009 Mar 25;9:88; *Clinical guidelines on the identification, evaluation, and treatment of overweight and obesity in adults*. National

Heart, Lung, and Blood Institute reprint. Bethesda, Md.: National Institutes of Health; 1998.

8. Must A, Spadano J, Coakley EH, et al. The disease burden associated with overweight and obesity. *JAMA*. 1999;282(16): 1523–29; Allison DB, Fontaine KR, Manson JE, et al. Annual deaths attributable to obesity in the United States. *JAMA*. 1999;282(16): 1530–38.

9. Melissa J, Christodoulakis M, Spyridakis M, et al. Disorders associated with clinically severe obesity: significant improvement after surgical weight reduction. *South Med J*. 1998; 91(12):1143–48.

10. Lindsey ML, Patterson WL, Gesten FC, et al. Bariatric surgery for obesity: surgical approach and variation in in-hospital complications in New York State. *Obes Surg*. 2009 Jun;19(6):688–700; Choi Y, Frizzi J, Foley A, Harkabus M. Patient satisfaction and results of vertical banded gastroplasty and gastric bypass. *Obes Surg*. 1999;9(1):33–35; *Guidance for treatment of adult obesity*. 2nd ed. Bethesda, Md.: Shape Up America! and the American Obesity Association; 1998.

11. Clinical guidelines on the identification, evaluation, and treatment of overweight and obesity in adults. National Heart, Lung, and Blood Institute reprint. Bethesda, Md.: National Institutes of Health; 1998.

12. Samaras K, Kelly PJ, Chiano MN, et al. Genetic and environmental influences on total-body and central abdominal fat: the effect of physical activity in female twins. *Ann Intern Med*. 1999;130(11):873–82.

13. Maynard M, Gunnell D, Emmett P, et al. Fruit, vegetables, and antioxidants in childhood and risk of adult cancer: the Boyd Orr cohort. *J Epidemiol Community Health*. 2003 Mar; 57(3):218–25. Erratum in: *J Epidemiol Community Health*. 2007 Mar;61(3): 271; Fuemmeler BF, Pendzich MK, Tercyak KP. Weight, dietary behavior, and physical activity in childhood and adolescence: implications for adult cancer risk. *Obes Facts*. 2009; 2(3):179–186; Dieckmann KP, Hartmann JT, Classen J, et al. Tallness is associated with risk of testicular cancer: evidence for the nutrition hypothesis. *Br J Cancer*. 2008 Nov;4;99(9): 1517–21; van der Pols JC, Bain C, Gunnell D, et al. Childhood dairy intake and adult cancer risk: 65-y follow-up of the Boyd Orr cohort. *Am J Clin Nutr*. 2007 Dec;86(6):1722–29; Michels KB, Rosner BA, Chumlea WC, et al. Preschool diet and adult risk of breast cancer. *Int J Cancer*. 2006 Feb 1;118(3):749–54; Stoll BA. Western diet, early

puberty and breast cancer risk. *Breast Cancer Res Treat.* 1998; 49(3): 187–93.

14. Horinger P, Imoberdorf R. Junk food revolution or the cola colonization. *Ther Umsch.* 2000; 57(3): 134–37.

15. Hughes P, Murdock DK, Olson K, et al. School children have leading risk factors for cardiovascular disease and diabetes: the Wausau SCHOOL project. *WMJ.* 2006 Jul;105(5): 32–39.

16. Berenson GS, Wattigney WA, Tracey RE, et al. Atherosclerosis of the aorta and coronary arteries and cardiovascular risk factors in persons aged 6 to 30 years and studied at necropsy (the Bogalusa heart study). *Am J Cardiol.* 1992; 70: 851–58.

17. Berenson GS, Srinivasan SR, Bao W, et al. Association between multiple cardiovascular risk factors and atherosclerosis in children and young adults. *N Eng J Med.* 1998;338:1650–56.

18. Viikari JS, Niinikoski H, Juonala M, et al. Risk factors for coronary heart disease in children and young adults. *Acta Paediatr Suppl.* 2004 Dec;93(446): 34–42; Berenson GS. Childhood risk factors predict adult risk associated with subclinical cardiovascular disease. The Bogalusa Heart Study. *Am J Cardiol.* 2002 Nov 21;90(10C): 3L–7L.

19. Maynard M, Gunnell D, Emmett P, et al. Fruit, vegetables, and antioxidants in childhood and risk of adult cancer: the Boyd Orr cohort. *J Epidemiol Community Health.* 2003 Mar;57 (3):218–25. Erratum in: *J Epidemiol Community Health.* 2007 Mar;61(3):271; Fuemmeler BF, Pendzich MK, Tercyak KP. Weight, dietary behavior, and physical activity in childhood and adolescence: implications for adult cancer risk. *Obes Facts.* 2009;2(3):179–86; Dieckmann KP, Hartmann JT, Classen J, et al. Tallness is associated with risk of testicular cancer: evidence for the nutrition hypothesis. *Br J Cancer.* 2008 Nov 4;99(9):1517–21; van der Pols JC, Bain C, Gunnell D, et al. Childhood dairy intake and adult cancer risk: 65-y follow-up of the Boyd Orr cohort. *Am J Clin Nutr.* 2007 Dec;86(6):1722–29; Michels KB, Rosner BA, Chumlea WC, et al. Preschool diet and adult risk of breast cancer. *Int J Cancer.* 2006 Feb 1;118(3):749–54; Stoll BA. Western diet, early puberty and breast cancer risk. *Breast Cancer Res Treat.* 1998; 49(3):187–93.

20. Ogden CL, Carroll MD, Curtin LR, et al. Prevalence of high body mass index in US children and adolescents, 2007–2008. *JAMA.* 2010;303(3): 235–41.

21. Van Itallie TB. Health implications of overweight and obesity in the United States. *Ann Int Med.* 1985; 103:983–88.

22. Manson JE, Willett WC, Stampfer MJ, et al. Body weight and mortality among women. *N Eng J Med.* 1995;333:677–85.

23. Lee I, Manson JE, Hennekens CH, Paffenbarger RS. Body weight and mortality: a 27-year follow-up of middle-aged men. *JAMA*. 1993; 270(23):2823–28.

24. Manson JE, Stampfer MJ, Hennekens CH, et al. Body weight and longevity: a reassessment. *JAMA*. 1987; 257:353–58.

25. Flegol KM, Carroll MD, Ogden CL, Curtin LR. Prevalence and trends in obesity among U.S. adults, 1999–2008. *JAMA*. 2010; 303(3): 235–41.

26. Folsom AR, Kaye SA, Sellers TA, et al. Body fat distribution and 5-year risk of death in older women. *JAMA*. 1993;269(4): 483–87.

27. Lane MA, Baer DJ, Rumpler WV, et al. Calorie restriction lowers body temperature in rhesus monkeys, consistent with a postulated anti-aging mechanism in rodents. *Proc Natl Acad Sci USA*. 1996; Apr30; 93(9)4159–64.

28. Hansen BC, Bodkin NL, Ortmeyer HK. Calorie restriction in nonhuman primates: mechanism of reduced morbidity and mortality. *Toxicol Sci*. 1999; 52(suppl 2):S56–60; Weindruch R. The retardation of aging by caloric restriction: studies in rodents and primates. *Toxicol Pathol*. 1996; 24(6):742–45; Roth GS, Ingram DK, Lane MA. Caloric restriction in primates: will it work and how will we know? *J Am Geriatric Soc*. 1999;47(7):896–903; McCarter RJ. Role of caloric restriction in the prolongation of life. *Clin Geriatr Med*. 1995; 11(4): 553–65. Weindruch R, Lane MA, Ingram DK, et al. Dietary restriction in rhesus monkeys: lymphopenia and reduced nitrogen-induced proliferation in peripheral blood mononuclear cells. *Aging*. 1997;9(44):304–8; Frame LT, Hart RW, Leakey JE. Caloric restriction as a mechanism mediating resistance to environmental disease. *Environ Health Perspect*. 1998; 106(suppl 1):S313–24; Masoro, EJ. Influence of caloric intake on aging and on the response to stressors. *J Toxicol Environ Health B Crit Rev*. 1998;1(3):243–57; Lane MA, Ingram DK, Roth GS. Calorie restriction in nonhuman primates: effects on diabetes and cardiovascular disease risk. *Toxicol Sci*. 1999; 52(suppl 2):S41–48.

29. Carroll KK. Experimental evidence of dietary factors and hormone-dependent cancers. *Cancer Res*. 1975; 35:3374–83.

30. Fontana L, Weiss EP, Villareal DT, et al. Long-term effects of calorie or protein restriction on serum IGF-1 and IGFBP-3 concentration in humans. *Aging Cell*. 2008 Oct;7(5):681–87.

31. Castro AM, Guerra-Júnior G. [GH/IGF-1 and cancer: what's new in this association]. *Arq Bras Endocrinol Metabol*. 2005 Oct; 49(5):833–42; Papatsoris AG, Karamouzis MV, Papavas-

siliou AG. Novel insights into the implication of the IGF-1 network in prostate cancer. *Trends Mol Med.* 2005 Feb;11(2): 52–55; Kaaks R. Nutrition, insulin, IGF-1 metabolism and cancer risk: a summary of epidemiological evidence. *Novartis Found Symp.* 2004;262: 247–60; discussion 260–68; Lønning PE, Helle SI. IGF-1 and breast cancer. *Novartis Found Symp.* 2004;262:205–12; discussion 212–14, 265–68; Roberts CT Jr. IGF-1 and prostate cancer. *Novartis Found Symp.* 2004;262: 193–99; discussion 199–204, 265–68.

32. Fontana L. The scientific basis of caloric restriction leading to longer life. *Curr Opin Gastroenterol.* 2009 Mar;25(2):144– 50; Fontana L, Klein S. Aging, adiposity, and calorie restriction. *JAMA.* 2007 Mar 7;297(9): 986–94.

33. Butler RN, Fossel M, Pan CX, et al. Anti-aging medicine: efficacy and safety of hormones and antioxidants. *Geriatrics.* 2000; 55:48–58.

34. Lawton CL, Burley VJ, Wales JK, Blundell JE. Dietary fat and appetite control in obese subjects: weak effects on satiation and satiety. *Int J Obes Metab Disord.* 1993;17(7):409–16; Blundell JE, Halford JC. Regulation of nutrient supply: the brain and appetite control. *Proc Nutr Soc.* 1994;53(2):407–18; Stamler J, Dolecek TA. Relation of food and nutrient intakes to body mass in the special intervention and usual care groups on the Multiple Risk Factor Intervention Trial. *Am J Clin Nutr.* 1997; 65(suppl 1):S366–73.

35. Mattes R. Dietary compensation by humans for supplemental energy provided as ethanol or carbohydrates in fluids. *Physiology Behav.* 1996;59:179–87.

36. Dennison BA, Rockwell HL, Baker SL. Excess fruit juice consumption by preschool-aged children is associated with short stature and obesity. *Pediatrics.* 1997;99(1):15–22; Dennison BA. Fruit juice consumption by infants and children: a review. *J Am Coll Nutr.* 1996;15(suppl 5):S4–11.

37. Plymouth Colony. 2000. World Book Millennium.

38. Weinsier RL, Nagy TR, Hunter GR, et al. Do adaptive changes in metabolic rate favor weight regain in weight-reduced individuals? An examination of the set-point theory. *Am J Clin Nutr.* 2000;72: 1088–94.

Chapter 2: Overfed, Yet Malnourished

1. Jedrychowski W, Maugeri U, Popiela T, et al. Case-control study on beneficial effect of regular consumption of apples on colorectal cancer risk in a population with relatively low intake of fruits and vegetables. *Eur J Cancer Prev.* 2010 Jan;

19(1):42–47; Foschi R, Pelucchi C, Dal Maso L, et al. Citrus fruit and cancer risk in a network of case-control studies. *Cancer Causes Control*. 2009 Oct 24. [Epub ahead of print]; van Duijnhoven FJ, Bueno-de-Mesquita HB, Ferrari P, et al. Fruit, vegetables, and colorectal cancer risk: the European Prospective Investigation into Cancer and Nutrition. *Am J Clin Nutr*. 2009 May; 89(5): 1441–52; Maynard M, Gunnell D, Emmett P, et al. Fruit, vegetables and antioxidants in childhood and risk of cancer: the Boyd Orr cohort. *J Epidimiol Community Health*. 2003 Mar; 57(3):219–25; Hebert JR, Landon J, Miller DR. Consumption of meat and fruit in relation to oral and esophageal cancer: a cross-national study. *Nutr Cancer*. 1993; 19(2):169–79; Fraser GE. Association between diet and cancer, ischemic heart disease, and all-cause mortality in non-Hispanic white California Seventh-Day Adventists. *Am J Clin Nutr*. 1999; 70(3)(suppl):532–38; Block G, Patterson B, Subar A. Fruit, vegetable, and cancer prevention: a review of the epidemiological evidence. *Nutr Cancer*. 1992;18(1):1–29.

2. Joseph JA, Shukitt-Hale B, Willis LM. Grape juice, berries, and walnuts affect brain aging and behavior. *J Nutr*. 2009 Sep;139(9)(suppl):S1813–17.

3. Cao G, Shukitt-Hale B, Bickford PC, et al. Hyperoxia-induced changes in antioxidant capacity and the effect of dietary antioxidants. *J Appl Physiol*. 1999;86(6):1817–22.

4. Hertog MG, Bueno-de-Mesquita HB, Fehily AM. Fruit and vegetable consumption and cancer mortality in Caerphilly Study. *Cancer Epidemiol Biomarkers Prevent*. 1996;5(9):673–77.

5. Dietary Assessment of Major Trends in U.S. Food Consumption, 1970–2005. http://www.ers.usda.gov/Publications/EIB33/EIB33_Reportsummary.pdf.

6. Salmeron J, Manson JE, Stampfer MJ, et al. Dietary fiber, glycemic load, and risk of non-insulin-dependent diabetes mellitus in women. *JAMA*. 1997;277(6): 472–77.

7. Salmeron J, Ascherio A, Rimm EB, et al. Dietary fiber, glycemic load, and risk of NIDDM in men. *Diabetes Care*. 1997;20(4): 545–50.

8. Centers for Disease Control. National Diabetes Fact Sheet, 2007. http://www .cdc.gov/diabetes/pubs/pdf/ndfs_2007.pdf.

9. Sahyoun NR, Jacques PF, Zhang XL, et al. Whole-grain intake is inversely associated with the metabolic syndrome and mortality in older adults. *Am J Clin Nutr*. 2006 Jan;83(1): 124–31.

10. Harland JI, Garton LE. Whole-grain intake as a marker of healthy body weight and adiposity. *Public Health Nutr*. 2008 Jun;11(6):554–63; van de Vijver LP, van den Bosch LM, van

den Brandt PA, Goldbohm RA. Whole-grain consumption, dietary fibre intake and body mass index in the Netherlands cohort study. *Eur J Clin Nutr.* 2009 Jan;63(1):31–38; Jacobs DR, Marquart L, Slavin J, Kushi LH. Whole-grain intake and cancer: an expanded review and meta-analysis. *Nutr. Cancer.* 1998; 30(2):85–96; Chatenoud L, Tavani A, La Vecchia C, et al. Whole-grain food intake and cancer risk. *Int J Cancer.* 1998;77(1):24–28.

11. Jacobs DR Jr., Meyer KA, Kushi LH, et al. Whole-grain intake may reduce the risk of ischemic heart disease death in post-menopausal women: the Iowa Women's Health Study. *Am J Clin Nutr.* 1998;68: 248–57.

12. Prentice RL. Future possibilities in the prevention of breast cancer: fat and fiber and breast cancer research. *Breast Cancer Res.* 2000; 2(4):268–76; Park Y, Brinton LA, Subar AF, et al. Dietary fiber intake and risk of breast cancer in postmeno-pausal women: the National Institutes of Health–AARP Diet and Health Study. *Am J Clin Nutr.* 2009 Sep;90(3):664–71; Suzuki R, Rylander-Rudqvist T, Ye W, et al. Dietary fiber intake and risk of postmenopausal breast cancer defined by estrogen and progesterone receptor status—a prospective cohort study among Swedish women. *Int J Cancer.* 2008 Jan 15;122(2): 403–12; McEligot AJ, Largent J, Ziogas A, et al. Dietary fat, fiber, vegetable, and micronutrients are associated with overall survival in postmenopausal women diagnosed with breast cancer. *Nutr Cancer* 2006;55(2):132–40.

13. La Vecchia C. Mediterranean diet and cancer. *Public Health Nutr.* 2004 Oct; 7(7):965–68; Scharlau D, Borowicki A, Habermann N, et al. Mechanisms of primary cancer preven-tion by butyrate and other products formed during gut flora-mediated fermentation of dietary fibre. *Mutat Res.* 2009 Jul–Aug; 682(1):39–53; Bordonaro M, Lazarova DL, Sartorelli AC. Butyrate and Wnt signaling: a possible solution to the puz-zle of dietary fiber and colon cancer risk? *Cell Cycle* 2008 May 1;7(9): 1178–83; Pisani P. Hyper-insulinaemia and cancer, meta-analyses of epidemiological studies. *Arch Physiol Bio-chem.* 2008 Feb;114(1): 63–70; Larsson SC, Bergkvist L, Wolk A. Glycemic load, glycemic index and breast cancer risk in a prospective cohort of Swedish women. *Int J Cancer.* 2009 Jul 1; 125(1):153–57; Wen W, Shu XO, Li H, et al. Dietary carbo-hydrates, fiber, and breast cancer risk in Chinese women. *Am J Clin Nutr.* 2009 Jan;89(1):283–89; Nettleton JA, Steffen LM, Loehr LR, et al. Incident heart failure is associated with lower whole-grain intake and greater high-fat dairy and egg intake in

the Atherosclerosis Risk in Communities (ARIC) study. *J Am Diet Assoc.* 2008 Nov;108(11):1881–87; de Munter JS, Hu FB, Spiegelman D, et al. Whole grain, bran, and germ intake and risk of type 2 diabetes: a prospective cohort study and systematic review. *PLoS Med.* 2007 Aug;4(8): e261; Mellen PB, Liese AD, Tooze JA, et al. Whole-grain intake and carotid artery atherosclerosis in a multiethnic cohort: the Insulin Resistance Atherosclerosis Study. *Am J Clin Nutr.* 2007 Jun;85(6): 1495–502; Mellen PB, Walsh TF, Herrington DM. Whole grain intake and cardiovascular disease: a meta-analysis. *Nutr Metab Cardiovasc Dis.* 2008 May; 18(4):283–90; Zhuo XG, Watanabe S. Factor analysis of digestive cancer mortality and food consumption in 65 Chinese counties. *J Epidemiol.* 1999; 4:275–84; Slattery ML, Benson J, Berry TD, et al. Dietary sugar and colon cancer. *Cancer Epidemiol Biomarkers Prevent.* 1997 Sep; 6(9):677–85; Negri E, Bosetti C, La Vecchia C, et al. Risk factors for adenocarcinoma of the small intestine. *Int J Cancer.* 1999;82(2):171–74; Chatenoud L, La Vecchia C, Franceschi S, et al. Refined-cereal intake and risk of selected cancers in Italy. *Am J Clin Nutr.* 1999; 70(6):1107–10.

14. Pennington JA Intakes of minerals from diets and foods: is there a need for concern? *J Nutr.* 1996; 126(suppl 9):S2304–8.

15. Dargatz DA, Ross PF. Blood selenium concentration in cows and heifers on 253 cow-calf operations in 18 states. *J Anim Sci.* 1996; 74(12):2891–95.

16. Linardakis M, Sarri K, Pateraki MS, et al. Sugar-added beverages consumption among kindergarten children of Crete: effects on nutritional status and risk of obesity. *BMC Public Health.* 2008 Aug 6;8:279; Faith MS, Dennison BA, Edmunds LS, Stratton HH. Fruit juice intake predicts increased adiposity gain in children from low-income families: weight status–by–environment interaction. *Pediatrics.* 2006 Nov; 118(5): 2066–75.

17. Dennison BA. Fruit juice consumption by infants and children: a review. *J Am Coll Nutr.* 1995;15(5)(suppl):S4–11.

18. Ames BN. DNA damage from micronutrient deficiencies is likely to be a major cause of cancer. *Mutat Res.* 2001 Apr 18;475(1–2):7–20; Lonsdale D, Shamberger RJ. Red cell transketolase as an indicator of nutritional deficiency. *Am J Clin Nutr.* 1980;33:205–11; Lane BC. Myopia prevention and reversal: new data confirms the interaction of accommodative stress and deficit inducing nutrition. *J Int Acad Prev Med.* 1982; 7(3):28.

19. Dietary Assessment of Major Trends in U.S. Food Consumption, 1970–2005. http://www.ers.usda.gov/Publications/EIB33/EIB33_Reportsummary.pdf.

20. Romanski SA, Nelson RM, Jensen MD. Meal fatty acid uptake in adipose tissue: gender effects in nonobese humans. *Am J Physiol Endocrinol Metab.* 2000; 279(2): E445–62.

21. Popp-Snijders C, Blonk MC. Omega-3 fatty acids in adipose tissue of obese patients with non-insulin dependent diabetes mellitus reflect long-term dietary intake of eicosapentaenoic and docosahexaenoic acid. *Am J Clin Nutr.* 1995;61(2):360–65.

22. Karalis IK, Alegakis AK, Kafatos AG, et al. Risk factors for ischaemic heart disease in a Cretan rural population: a twelve year follow-up study. *BMC Public Health.* 2007 Dec 18;7:351; Kafatos A, Diacatou A, Voukik G, et al. Heart disease risk factor status and dietary changes in the Cretan population over the past 30 years: the Seven Countries Study. *Am J Clin Nutr.* 1997; 65(6):1882–86.

23. Katan MB, Grundy SM, Willett WC. Should a low-fat, high-carbohydrate diet be recommended for everyone? Beyond low-fat diets. *N Eng J Med.* 1997; 337(8):563–67.

24. Han JH, Yang YX, Feng MY. Contents of phytosterols in vegetables and fruits commonly consumed in China. *Biomed Environ Sci.* 2008 Dec;21(6):449–53; Chen CY, Blumberg JB. Phytochemical composition of nuts. *Asia Pac J Clin Nutr.* 2008;17 (suppl 1): S329–32; Ryan E, Galvin K, O'Connor TP, et al. Phytosterol, squalene, tocopherol content and fatty acid profile of selected seeds, grains, and legumes. *Plant Foods Hum Nutr.* 2007 Sep;62(3):85–91; Segura R, Javierre C, Lizarraga MA, Ros E. Other relevant components of nuts: phytosterols, folate and minerals. *Br J Nutr.* 2006 Nov;96 (suppl 2):S36–44.

25. Micheli A, Gatta G, Sant M, et al. Breast cancer prevalence measured by the Lombardy Cancer Registry. *Tumori.* 1997; 83(6): 875–79.

26. Link LB, Potter JD. Raw versus cooked vegetables and cancer risk. *Cancer Epidemiol Biomarkers Prevent.* 2004 Sep;13(9): 1422–35; Rungapamestry V, Duncan AJ, Fuller Z, Ratcliffe B. Effect of cooking brassica vegetables on the subsequent hydrolysis and metabolic fate of glucosinolates. *Proc Nutr Soc.* 2007 Feb;66(1):69–81; Tang L, Zirpoli GR, Guru K, et al. Consumption of raw cruciferous vegetables is inversely associated with bladder cancer risk. *Cancer Epidemiol Biomarkers Prevent.* 2008 Apr;17(4):938–44; Steinmetz KA, Potter JD.

Vegetables, fruit and prevention: a review. *J Am Diet Assoc.* 1996; 96(10): 1027–39; Hertog MG, Bueno-de-Mesquita HB, Fehily AM, et al. Fruit and vegetable in the Caerphilly Study. *Cancer Epidemiol Biomarkers Prevent.* 1996; 5(9):673–77; Block G, Patterson B, Subar A. Fruit, vegetables, and cancer: a review of the epidemiological evidence. *Nutr Cancer.* 1992;18(10):1–29; Steinmetz KA, Potter JD. Food-group consumption and colon cancer in the Adelaide Case-Control Study. I. Vegetables and fruit. *Int J Cancer.* 1993; 53(5):711–19; Steinmetz KA, Potter JD. Vegetables, fruit and cancer. I. Epidemiology. *Cancer Causes Control.* 1991;2(5): 325–57; Franceschi S, Parpinel M, La Vecchia C, et al. Role of different types of vegetables and fruit in the prevention of cancer of the colon, rectum, and breast. *Epidemiology.* 1998; 9(3):338–41.

27. Linking plants to people: a visit to the laboratory of Dr. Paul Talalay. *American Institute for Cancer Research Newsletter.* 1995; 46:10–11.

28. Douglass JM, Rasgon IM, Fleiss PM, et al. Effects of raw food diet on hypertension and obesity. *South Med J.* 1995; 78(7):841–44.

29. Prochaska LJ, Piekutowski WV. On the synergistic effects of enzymes in food with enzymes in the human body. A literature survey and analytical report. *Med Hypotheses.* 1994;42(6): 355–62.

30. Rumm-Kreuter D, Demmel I. Comparison of vitamin losses in vegetables due to various cooking methods. *J Nutr Sci Vitaminol.* 1990; 36(suppl):S7–15.

31. Kimura M, Itokawa Y. Cooking losses of minerals in foods and its nutritional significance. *J Nutr Sci Vitaminol.* 1990;36(suppl 1): 25–32.

32. Franceschi S. Nutrients and food groups and large bowel cancer in Europe. *Eur J Cancer Prev.* 1999;9 (suppl 1):S49–52.

33. Bazzano LA. Effects of soluble dietary fiber on low-density lipoprotein cholesterol and coronary heart disease risk. *Curr Atheroscler Rep.* 2008 Dec;10(6):473–77.

34. Schatzkin A, Lanza E, Corle D. Lack of effect of a low-fat, high-fiber diet on the recurrence of colorectal adenomas. *New Eng J Med.* 2000;342:1149–55; Alberts DS, Martinez ME, Roe DJ, et al. Lack of effect of a high-fiber cereal supplement on the recurrence of colorectal adenomas. *New Eng J Med.* 2000;342:1156–62.

35. Byers T. Diet, colorectal adenomas, and colorectal cancer (editorial). *New Eng J Med.* 2000; 342(16): 1206–7.

36. Ludwig DS, Pereira MA, Kroenke CH, et al. Dietary fiber, weight gain and cardiovascular disease risk factors in young adults. *JAMA*. 1999;282(16): 1539–46.

Chapter 3: Phytochemicals

1. USDA Economic Research Service. Loss-Adjusted Food Availability. http://www.ers.usda.gov/Data/FoodConsumption/FoodGuideIndex.htm.

2. Williams CD, Satia JA, Adair LS, et al. Dietary patterns, food groups, and rectal cancer risk in whites and African-Americans. *Cancer Epidemiol Biomarkers Prevent*. 2009 May;18(5):1552–61; Flood A, Rastogi T, Wirfält E, et al. Dietary patterns as identified by factor analysis and colorectal cancer among middle-aged Americans. *Am J Clin Nutr*. 2008 Jul;88(1):176–84.

3. USDA Economic Research Service. Dietary Assessment of Major Trends in U.S. Food Consumption, 1970–2005. http://www.ers.usda.gov/publications/EIB33; USDA Economic Research Service. Loss-Adjusted Food Availability. http://www.ers.usda.gov/Data/FoodConsumption/FoodGuideIndex.htm#calories.

4. USDA Food Availability (per capita) Data System. http://www.ers.usda.gov/amberwaves/February 05/findings/cheese consumption.htm.

5. Agudo A, Cabrera L, Amiano P, et al. Fruit and vegetable intakes, dietary antioxidant nutrients, and total mortality in Spanish adults: findings from the Spanish cohort of the European Prospective Investigation into Cancer and Nutrition (EPIC-Spain). *Am J Clin Nutr*. 2007 Jun; 85(6):1634–42; Nagura J, Iso H, Watanabe Y, et al. Fruit, vegetable and bean intake and mortality from cardiovascular disease among Japanese men and women: the JACC Study. *Br J Nutr*. 2009 Jul;102(2): 285-92; Tobias M, Turley M, Stefanogiannis N, et al. Vegetable and fruit intake and mortality from chronic disease in New Zealand. *Aust N Z J Public Health*. 2006 Feb;30(1): 26–31.

6. Heron M, Tejada-Vera B. Deaths: Leading Causes for 2005. *National Vital Statistics Reports*. 2009;58(8). Available online at http://www.cdc.gov/nchs/data/nvsr/nvsr58/nvsr58_08.pdf.

7. USDA Economic Research Service. Loss-Adjusted Food Availability. http://www.ers.usda.gov/Data/FoodConsumption/Food GuideIndex.htm.

8. Original chart: data compiled from 1960s mortality data from the World Health Organization and National Institutes of

Health (no longer available online), food balance sheets from the Food and Agriculture Organization of the United Nations (http://faostat.fao.org/site/368/default.aspx#ancor), and communication with health authorities in several of the countries listed.

9. Radhika G, Sudha V, Mohan Sathya R, et al. Association of fruit and vegetable intake with cardiovascular risk factors in urban south Indians. *Br J Nutr.* 2008 Feb;99(2):398–405; Nöthlings U, Schulze MB, Weikert C, et al. Intake of vegetables, legumes, and fruit, and risk for all-cause, cardiovascular, and cancer mortality in a European diabetic population. *J Nutr.* 2008 Apr;138(4):775–81.

10. Zhang CX, Ho SC, Chen YM, et al. Greater vegetable and fruit intake is associated with a lower risk of breast cancer among Chinese women. *Int J Cancer.* 2009 Jul 1;125(1):181–188; Sandoval M, Font R, Mañós M, et al. The role of vegetable and fruit consumption and other habits on survival following the diagnosis of oral cancer: a prospective study in Spain. *Int J Oral Maxillofac Surg.* 2009 Jan;38(1):31–139; Nomura AM, Wilkens LR, Murphy SP, et al. Association of vegetable, fruit, and grain intakes with colorectal cancer: the Multiethnic Cohort Study. *Am J Clin Nutr.* 2008 Sep; 88(3):730–137; Kirsh VA, Peters U, Mayne ST, et al. Prostate, Lung, Colorectal and Ovarian Cancer Screening Trial. Prospective study of fruit and vegetable intake and risk of prostate cancer. *J Natl Cancer Inst.* 2007 Aug 1;99(15):1200–9; Satia-Abouta J, Galanko JA, Martin CF, et al. Food groups and colon cancer risk in African-Americans and Caucasians. *Int J Cancer.* 2004 May 1;109(5): 728–136; Franceschi S, Parpinel M, La Vecchia C, et al. Role of different types of vegetables and fruit in the prevention of cancer of the colon, rectum and breast. *Epidemiology.* 1998;9(3):338–41; Van Den Brandt PA. Nutrition and cancer: causative, protective, and therapeutc aspects. *Ned Tijdschr Geneeskd.* 1999; 143(27):1414–20; Fraser GE. Association between diet and cancer, ischemic heart disease, and all-cause mortality in non-Hispanic white California Seventh-Day Adventists. *Am J Clin Nutr.* 1999;70(Suppl 3):S532-38.

11. Bjelakovic G, Nikolova D, Gluud LL, et al. Mortality in randomized trials of antioxidant supplements for primary and secondary prevention: systematic review and meta-analysis. *JAMA.* 2007 Feb 28;297(8): 842–57.

12. Goodman GE. Prevention of lung cancer. *Curr Opini Oncol.* 1998; 10(2): 122–26.

13. Omenn GS, Goodman GE, Thornquist MD, et al. Effects of a combination of beta carotene and vitamin A on lung cancer and cardiovascular disease. *N Eng J Med.* 1996;334(18):1150–55; Hennekens CH, Buring JE, Manson JE, et al. Lack of effect of long-term supplementation with beta-carotene on the incidence of malignant neoplasms and cardiovascular disease. *N Eng J Med.* 1996;334(18): 1145–49.

14. Albanes D, Heinonen OP, Taylor PR, et al. Alpha-tocopherol and beta-carotene supplements lung cancer incidence in the alpha-tocopherol, beta-carotene prevention study: effects of baseline characteristics and study compliance. *J Natl Cancer Inst.* 1996; 8(21):1560–70; Rapola JM, Virtamo J, Ripatti S, et al. Randomized trial of alpha-tocopherol and beta-carotene supplements on incidence of major coronary events in men with previous myocardial infarction. *Lancet.* 1997; 349(9067): 1715–20.

15. Bjelakovic G, Nikolova D, Gluud LL, et al. Mortality in randomized trials of antioxidant supplements for primary and secondary prevention: systematic review and meta-analysis. *JAMA.* 2007 Feb 28;297(8): 842–57.

16. Nelson NJ. Is chemoprevention research overrated or underfunded? *Primary Care and Cancer.* 1996; 16(8):29.

17. Cohen JH, Kristal AR, Stanford JL. Fruit and vegetable intakes and prostate cancer risk. *J Natl Cancer Inst.* 2000;92(1):61–68.

18. Forte A, De Sanctis R, Leonetti G, et al. Dietary chemoprevention of colorectal cancer. *Ann Ital Chir.* 2008 Jul–Aug;79(4): 261–67; Harikumar KB, Aggarwal BB. Resveratrol: a multitargeted agent for age-associated chronic diseases. *Cell Cycle.* 2008 Apr 15;7(8):1020–35; Juge N, Mithen RF, Traka M. Molecular basis for chemoprevention by sulforaphane: a comprehensive review. *Cell Mol Life Sci.* 2007 May;64(9):1105–27; Lee ER, Kang GH, Cho SG. Effect of flavonoids on human health: old subjects but new challenges. *Recent Pat Biotechnol.* 2007;1(2): 139–50; Messina M, Kucuk O, Lampe JW. An overview of the health effects of isoflavones with an emphasis on prostate cancer risk and prostate-specific antigen levels. *J AOAC Int.* 2006 Jul–Aug;89(4):1121–34.

19. Roa I, Araya JC, Villaseca M, et al. Preneoplastic lesions and gallbladder cancer: an estimate of the period required for progression *Gastroenterology.* 1996;111(1):232–36; Kashayap V, Das BC. DNA aneuploidy and infection of human papillomavirus type 16 in preneoplastic lesions of the uterine cervix: correlation with progression to malignancy. *Cancer Lett.* 1998; 123(1):47–52.

20. Higdon JV, Delage B, Williams DE, Dashwood RH. Cruciferous vegetables and human cancer risk: epidemiologic evidence and mechanistic basis. *Pharmacol Res.* 2007 Mar; 55(3): 224–36; Srivastava SK, Xiao D, Lew KL, et al. Allyl isothiocyanate, a constituent of cruciferous vegetables, inhibits growth of PC-3 human prostate cancer xenografts in vivo. *Carcinogenesis.* 2003 Oct; 24(10):1665–70; Rose P, Huang Q, Ong CN, Whiteman M. Broccoli and watercress suppress matrix metalloproteinase-9 activity and invasiveness of human MDA-MB-231 breast cancer cells. *Toxicol Appl Pharmacol.* 2005 Dec 1;209(2):105–13; Ray A. Cancer preventive role of selected dietary factors. *Indian J Cancer.* 2005 Jan–Mar;42(1):15–24; Keck AS, Finley JW. Cruciferous vegetables: cancer protective mechanisms of glucosinolate hydrolysis products and selenium. *Integr Cancer Ther.* 2004 Mar;3(1):5–12; Seow A, Yuan JM, Sun CL, et al. Dietary isothiocyanates, glutathione S-transferase polymorphisms and colorectal cancer risk in the Singapore Chinese Health Study. *Carcinogenesis.* 2002 Dec;23 (12):2055–61; Johnston N. Sulforaphane halts breast cancer cell growth. *Drug Discov Today.* 2004 Nov 1;9(21):908.
21. Based on USDA standard reference data for broiled porterhouse steak and chopped frozen broccoli.
22. Nutritionist Pro Nutrition Analysis Software, Versions 2.5, 3.1, Axxya Systems, Stafford TX, 2006. Based on USDA standard reference data for cooked frozen broccoli, broiled porterhouse steak, chopped romaine lettuce, and boiled kale.
23. Kahn HA, Phillips RL, Snowdon DA, Choi W. Association between reported diet and all-cause mortality: twenty-one-year follow-up on 27,530 adult Seventh Day Adventists. *Am J Epid.* 1984; 119(5): 775–87.
24. Steinmetz KA, Potter JD. Vegetables, fruit and cancer prevention: a review. *J Am Diet Assoc.* 1996;96: 1027–39.
25. A pyramid topples at the USDA. *Consumer Reports.* 1991 Oct: 663–66.
26. Harris W. *The scientific basis of vegetarianism.* Honolulu: Hawaii Health Publishers, 1995. pp. 101–6.
27. Hausman, P. *Jack Sprat's legacy: the science and politics of fat and cholesterol.* New York: Center for Science in the Public Interest; 1981.
28. USDA Fiscal Year 2007 Budget of the U.S. Government: Mid-Session Review. http://www.fsa.usda.gov/Internet/FSA_File/07midsessionrev.pdf.
29. Hebert JR, Hurley TG, Olendzki BC, et al. Nutritional and socioeconomic factors in relation to prostate cancer mortality:

a cross national study. *J Nati Cancer Inst.* 1998;90(21): 1637–47.

Chapter 4: The Dark Side of Animal Protein

1. Brody J. Huge study of diet indicts fat and meat. *New York Times.* 1990 May 8: Science Times:1.

2. Chen J, Campbell TC, Li J, Peto R. *Diet, life-style and mortality in China: a study of the characteristics of 65 Chinese counties.* Oxford: Oxford University Press; 1990. p. 894.

3. Campbell TC, Parpia B, Chen J. Diet, lifestyle, and the etiology of coronary artery disease: the Cornell China Study. *Am J Cardiol.* 1998;82(10B):18–21T.

4. Thiébaut AC, Jiao L, Silverman DT, et al. Dietary fatty acids and pancreatic cancer in the NIH-AARP diet and health study. *J Natl Cancer Inst.* 2009 Jul 15;101(14): 1001–11; Brock KE, Gridley G, Chiu BC, et al. Dietary fat and risk of renal cell carcinoma in the USA: a case-control study. *Br J Nutr.* 2009 Apr;101(8): 1228–38; Sieri S, Krogh V, Ferrari P, et al. Dietary fat and breast cancer risk in the European Prospective Investigation into Cancer and Nutrition. *Am J Clin Nutr.* 2008 Nov;88(5): 1304–12; Jakobsen MU, O'Reilly EJ, Heitmann BL, et al. Major types of dietary fat and risk of coronary heart disease: a pooled analysis of 11 cohort studies. *Am J Clin Nutr.* 2009 May;89(5):1425–32; Wiviott SD, Cannon CP. Update on lipid-lowering therapy and LDL-cholesterol targets. *Nat Clin Pract Cardiovasc Med.* 2006 Aug; 3(8):424–36; Simopoulos AP. The omega-6/omega-3 fatty acid ratio, genetic variation, and cardiovascular disease. *Asia Pac J Clin Nutr.* 2008;17 (suppl 1): 131–134; Simopoulos AP. Evolutionary aspects of diet, the omega-6/omega-3 ratio and genetic variation: nutritional implications for chronic diseases. *Biomed Pharmacother.* 2006 Nov;60(9):502–7.

5. Castro AM, Guerra-Júnior G. [GH/IGF-1 and cancer: what's new in this association]. *Arq Bras Endocrinol Metabol.* 2005 Oct;49(5): 833–42; Papatsoris AG, Karamouzis MV, Papavassiliou AG. Novel insights into the implication of the IGF-1 network in prostate cancer. *Trends Mol Med.* 2005 Feb;11(2): 52–55; Kaaks R. Nutrition, insulin, IGF-1 metabolism and cancer risk: a summary of epidemiological evidence. *Novartis Found Symp.* 2004;262:247–60; discussion 260–68; Lønning PE, Helle SI. IGF-1 and breast cancer. *Novartis Found Symp.* 2004;262:205–12; discussion 212–14, 265–68; Roberts CT Jr. IGF-1 and prostate cancer. *Novartis Found Symp.* 2004;262: 193–99; discussion 199–204, 265–68.

6. Campbell, TC, Parpia B, Chen J. A plant-enriched diet and long-term health, particularly in reference to China. *Hort Science.* 1990; 25(12):1512–14.

7. Andrikoula M, McDowell IF. The contribution of ApoB and ApoA1 measurements to cardiovascular risk assessment. *Diabetes Obes Metab.* 2008 Apr;10(4): 271–78; Kampoli AM, Tousoulis D, Antoniades C, Siasos G, Stefanadis C. Biomarkers of premature atherosclerosis. *Trends Mol Med.* 2009 Jul;15(7): 323–32.

8. Van Ee JH. Soy constituents: modes of action in low-density lipoprotein management. *Nutr Rev.* 2009 Apr;67(4):222–34; Kris-Etherton PM, Hu FB, Ros E, Sabaté J. The role of tree nuts and peanuts in the prevention of coronary heart disease: multiple potential mechanisms. *J Nutr.* 2008 Sep;138(9)(suppl):S1746–51; Harland JI, Haffner TA. Systematic review, meta-analysis and regression of randomised controlled trials reporting an association between an intake of circa 25 g soya protein per day and blood cholesterol. *Atherosclerosis.* 2008 Sep;200(1):13–27; Plant-based proteins lower LDL and overall cholesterol. Plant-based proteins are higher in fiber, with far less fat and cholesterol than animal protein. *Duke Medicine Health News.* 2009 Sep;15(9):3.

9. Singh PN, Fraser GE. Dietary risk factors for colon cancer in a low-risk population. *Am J Epidemiol.* 1998;148:761–74.

10. U.S. Department of Agriculture. Agricultural Research Service. USDA National Nutrient Database for Standard Reference, release 13. 1999. Nutrient Data Laboratory home page, http://www.nal.usda.gov/fnic/foodcomp.

11. Sinha R, Rothman N, Brown ED, et al. High concentrations of the carcinogen 2-amino-1-methyl-6-phenylimidazo-[4,5-b] pyridine (PhIP) occur in chicken but are dependent on the cooking method. *Cancer Res.* 1995;55(20): 4516–19.

12. Thomson B. Heterocyclic amine levels in cooked meat and the implication for New Zealanders. *Eur J Cancer Prev.* 1999; 8(3): 201–6.

13. Davidson MH, Hunninghake D, Maki KC, et al. Comparison of the effects of lean red meat vs. lean white meat on serum lipid levels among free-living persons with hypercholesterolemia: a long-term, randomized clinical trial. *Arch Intern Med.* 1999;159(12): 1331–38.

14. Campbell TC. Why China holds the key to your health. *Nutrition Advocate.* 1995;1(1):7–8.

15. World Health Statistics Annual, 1999. Available online at http://www.who .int/whosis.

16. Singh PN, Sabaté J, Fraser GE. Does low meat consumption increase life expectancy in humans? *Am J Clin Nutr.* 2003 Sep; 78(suppl 3):S526–32; Fraser, GE, Lindsted KD, Beeson WL. Effect of risk factor values on lifetime risk of and age at first coronary event: the Adventist Health Study. *Am J Epidemiol.* 1995;142(7):746–58; Fraser, GE. Associations between diet and cancer, ischemic heart disease, and all-cause mortality in non-Hispanic white California Seventh-Day Adventists. *Am J Clin Nutr.* 1999;70 (suppl 3): S532–38.

17. Willett, WC, Hunter DJ, Stampfer MJ, et al. Dietary fat and fiber in relation to risk of breast cancer: an eight-year follow-up. *JAMA.* 1992;268:2037–44.

18. Campbell TC, Junshi C. Diet and chronic degenerative diseases: perspective from China. *Am J Clin Nutr.* 1994;59(suppl 5): S1153–61.

19. Key TJ, Thorogood AM, Appleby PN, Burr ML. Dietary habits and mortality in 11,000 vegetarians and health conscious people: results of a 17-year follow up. *BMJ.* 1996;313: 775–79.

20. Nelson NJ. Is chemo prevention research overrated or underfunded? *Primary Care and Cancer* 168: 29–30.

21. Shu XO, Zheng Y, Cai H, et al. Soy food intake and breast cancer survival. *JAMA.* 2009 Dec 9;302(22): 2437–43; Hwang YW, Kim SY, Jee SH, et al. Soy food consumption and risk of prostate cancer: a meta-analysis of observational studies. *Nutr Cancer.* 2009;61(5):598–606; Aune D, De Stefani E, Ronco A, et al. Legume intake and the risk of cancer: a multisite case-control study in Uruguay. *Cancer Causes Control.* 2009 Nov;20(9): 1605–15; Korde LA, Wu AH, Fears T, et al. Childhood soy intake and breast cancer risk in Asian American women. *Cancer Epidemiol Biomarkers Prevent.* 2009 Apr;18 (4):1050–59; Park SY, Murphy SP, Wilkens LR, et al. Multiethnic Cohort Study. Legume and isoflavone intake and prostate cancer risk: the Multiethnic Cohort Study. *Int J Cancer.* 2008 Aug 15;123(4):927–32; Nöthlings U, Schulze MB, Weikert C, et al. Intake of vegetables, legumes, and fruit, and risk for all-cause, cardiovascular, and cancer mortality in a European diabetic population. *J Nutr.* 2008 Apr;138(4):775–81.

22. Chang-Claude J, Frentzel-Beyme R. Dietary and lifestyle determinants of mortality among German vegetarians. *Int J Epidemiol.* 1993;22(2):228–36; Kahn HA, Phillips RI, Snowdon DA, Choi W. Association between reported diet and all-cause mortality: twenty-one-year follow-up on 27,530 adult Seventh-Day Adventists. *Am J Epidemiol.* 1984;119(5):775–87; Nestle M. Animal v. plant foods in human diets and health:

is the historical record unequivocal? *Proc Nutr Soc.* 1999; 58(2):211–28.

23. Barnard ND, Nicholson A, Howard JL. The medical costs attributed to meat consumption. *Prev Med.* 1995;24:646–55; Segasothy M, Phillips PA. Vegetarian diet: panacea for modern lifestyle disease? *QJM.* 1999;92(9):531–44.

24. Rucker C, Hoffman J. *The Seventh-Day Diet.* New York: Random House; 1991.

25. Kahn HA, Phillips RI, Snowdon DA, Choi W. Association between reported diet and all-cause mortality: twenty-one-year follow-up on 27,530 adult Seventh-Day Adventists. *Am J Epidemiol.* 1984;119(5):775–87.

26. Rodriguez C, Calle EE, Tatheam LM, Wingo PA, et al. Family history of breast cancer as a predictor for fatal prostate cancer. *Epidemiology.* 1998;9(5): 525–29.

27. Russo J, Russo IH. Differentiation and breast cancer. *Medicina.* 1997;57(suppl 2):81–91.

28. Lautenbach A, Budde A, Wrann CD, et al. Obesity and the associated mediators leptin, estrogen and IGF-I enhance the cell proliferation and early tumorigenesis of breast cancer cells. *Nutr Cancer.* 2009; 61(4):484–91; Pike MC, Spicer DV, Dahmoush L, Press MF. Estrogens, progestogens, normal breast cell proliferation, and breast cancer risk. *Epidemiol Rev.* 1993;15(1):17–35.

29. Vandeloo MJ, Bruckers LM, Janssens JP. Effects of lifestyle on the onset of puberty as determinant for breast cancer. *Eur J Cancer Prev.* 2007 Feb;16(1):17–25; Hamilton AS, Mack TM. Puberty and genetic susceptibility to breast cancer in a case-control study in twins. *N Engl J Med.* 2003 Jun 5;348 (23):2313–22; Leung AW, Mak J, Cheung PS, Epstein, RJ. Evidence for a programming effect of early menarche on the rise of breast cancer incidence in Hong Kong. *Cancer Detect Prev.* 2008;32(2):156–61.

30. Anderson AS, Caswell S. Obesity management—an opportunity for cancer prevention. *Surgeon.* 2009 Oct;7(5):282–85; Brown KA, Simpson ER. Obesity and breast cancer: progress to understanding the relationship. *Cancer Res.* 2010 Jan 1;70(1):4–7.

31. Diamandis EP, Yu H. Does prostate cancer start at puberty? *J Clin Lab Anal.* 1996;10(6):468–69; Weir HK, Kreiger N, Marrett LD. Age at puberty and risk of testicular germ cell cancer. *Cancer Causes Control.* 1998;9(3):253–58; United Kingdom Testicular Cancer Study Group. Aetiology of testicular cancer: association with congenital abnormalities, age at

puberty, infertility, and exercise. *BMJ*. 1994;308(6941):
1393–99.

32. Ross MH, Lustbader ED, Bras G. Dietary practices of early life
    and spontaneous tumors of the rat. *Nutr Cancer*. 1982;3(3):
    150–67.

33. Tanner JM. Trend toward earlier menarche in London, Oslo,
    Copenhagen, the Netherlands and Hungary. *Nature*. 1973;243:
    75–76.

34. Beaton G. *Practical population indicators of health and nutri-
    tion*. World Health Organization monograph 1976;62:500.

35. Register, UD, Sonneberg, JA. The vegetarian diet. *J Am Diet
    Assoc*. 1973;45: 537; Hardinge MG, Sanchez A, Waters D,
    et al. Possible factors associated with the prevalence of acne
    vulgaris. *Fed Proc*. 1971;30: 300.

36. Cheek DB. Body composition, hormones, nutrition, and ado-
    lescent growth. In: Grumbach, MM, Brace, GD, Mayers, FE,
    editors. *Control of the onset of puberty*. New York: John
    Wiley and Sons; 1973. p. 424.

37. Apter D, Reinila M, Vihko R. Some endocrine characteristics
    of early menarche, a risk factor for breast cancer, are preserved
    into adulthood. *Int J Cancer*. 1989; 44(5):783–87.

38. Chiaffarino F, Parazzini F, LaVecchia C, et al. Diet and uterine
    myomas. *Obstet Gynecol*. 1999; 94(3): 395–98.

39. Kralj-Cercek L. The influence of food, body build, and social
    origin on the age of menarche. *Hum Bio*. 1956;28:393; San-
    chez A, Kissinger DG, Phillips RI. A hypothesis on the etiologi-
    cal role of diet on age of menarche. *Med Hypothese*. 1981;
    7:1339–45.

40. Burell RJW, Healy MJR, Tanner JM. Age at menarche in South
    African Bantu schoolgirls living in the Transkei reserve. *Hum
    Bio*. 1961;33: 250.

41. Guo WD, Chow WH, Zheng W, et al. Diet, serum markers and
    breast cancer mortality in China. *Japan J Cancer Res*. 1994;85:
    572–77.

42. Hill P, Garbeczewski L, Kasumi F. Plasma testosterone and
    breast cancer. *Eur J Cancer Clin Oncol*. 1985; 21:1265–66.

43. USDA Food Availability (Per Capita) Data System. http://
    www.ers.usda.gov/amberwaves/february05/findings/Cheese
    Consumption.htm.

44. De Waard F, Trichopoulos D. A unifying concept of the aetiol-
    ogy of breast cancer. *Int J Cancer*. 1998;41: 666–69.

45. Decarli A, Favero A, La Vecchia C, et al. Macronutrients,
    energy intake, and breast cancer risk: implications from differ-
    ent models. *Epidemiology*. 1997;8:425–28.

46. Nicholson A. Diet and the prevention and treatment of breast cancer, *Altern Ther Health Med.* 1996;2(6):32–38.

47. Wynder EL, Cohen LA, Muscat JE, et al. Breast cancer: weighing the evidence for a promoting role of dietary fat. *J Natl Cancer Inst.* 1997;89:766–75.

48. Ross MH, Lustbader E, Bras G. Dietary practices and growth responses as predictors of longevity. *Nature.* 1976;262(5569): 548–53.

49. Comments in: Gunnell DJ, Smith GD, Holly JM, Frankel S. Leg length and risk of cancer in the Boyd Orr cohort. *BMJ.* 1998; 317 (7169):1950–51.

50. Cheng Z, Hu J, King J, Campbell TC. Inhibition of hepatocellular carcinoma development in hepatitis B virus transfected mice by low dietary casein. *Hepatology.* 1997;26(5):1351–54; Torosian MH Effect of protein intake on tumor growth and cell cycle kinetics. *J Surg Res.* 1995; 59(2):225–28; Youngman LD, Park JY, Ames BN. Protein oxidation associated with aging is reduced by dietary restriction of protein calories. *Proc Nat Acad Sci.* 1992;89(19): 9112–16.

51. Hebert JR, Hurley TG, Olendzki BC, et al. Nutritional and socioeconomic factors in relation to prostate cancer mortality: a cross-national study. *J Natl Cancer Inst.* 1998; 90(21): 1637–47.

52. Frentzel-Beyme R, Chang-Claude J. Vegetarian diets and colon cancer: the German experience. *Am J Clin Nutr.* 1994; 59(suppl.): S1143–52.

53. Berkel J, deWaard F. Mortality pattern and life expectancy of Seventh-Day Adventists in the Netherlands. *Int J Epidemiol.* 1983;12:455–59; Phillips RL, Snowdon DA. Dietary relationships with fatal colorectal cancer among Seventh-Day Adventists. *J Natl Cancer Inst.* 1985;74: 307–17.

54. Corliss J. Pesticide metabolites linked to breast cancer. *J Natl Cancer Inst.* 1993;85:602.

55. Dietary carcinogens linked to breast cancer. *Medical World News.* 1993 May:13.

56. Fraser GE. Association between diet and cancer, ischemic heart disease, and all-cause mortality in non-Hispanic white California Seventh-Day Adventists. *Am J Clin Nutr.* 1999; 70(suppl 3):S532–38; Sarasua S, Savitz DA. Cured and broiled meat consumption in relation to childhood cancer. *Cancer Causes Control.* 1994;5(2): 141–48; Favero A, Parpinel M, Franceschi S. Diet and risk of breast cancer: major findings from an Italian case-control study. *Biomed Pharmacother.* 1998;52(3):109–15; Levi F, Pasche C, La Vecchia C, Lucchini

F, Franceschi S. Food groups and colorectal cancer risk. *Br J Cancer.* 1999;79(7–8):1283–87; Steinmetz KA, Potter JD. Food-group consumption and colon cancer in the Adelaide Case-Control Study: meat, poultry, seafood, dairy foods and eggs. *Int J Cancer.* 1993;53(5): 720–27; Levi F, Franceschi S, Negri E, La Vecchia C. Dietary factors and the risk of endometrial cancer. *Cancer.* 1993;71(11):3575–81; Negri E, Bosetti C, La Vecchia C, et al. Risk factors for adenocarcinoma of the small intestine. *Int J Cancer.* 1999;82(2):171–74; Chow WH, Gridley G, McLoughlin JK, et al. Protein intake and risk of renal cell cancer. *J Natl Cancer Inst.* 1994;86:1131–39; Kwiatkowski A. Dietary and other environmental risk factors in acute leukemias: a case-control study of 119 patients. *Eur J Cancer Prev.* 1993;2(2):139–46; National Institutes of Health. National Cancer Institute. *Cancer rates and risks: cancer death rates among 50 countries (age adjusted to the world standard).* 4th ed. U.S. Department of Health and Human Services; 1996. Lung cancer, p. 39. Source: World Health Organization data as adapted by the American Cancer Society; Deneo-Pelligrini H, De Stefani E, Ronco A, et al. Meat consumption and risk of lung cancer; a case-control study from Uruguay. *Lung Cancer.* 1996;14(2–3):195–205; Zhang S, Hunter DJ, Rosner BA, et al. Greater intake of meats and fats associated with higher risk of non-Hodgkins lymphoma. *J Natl Cancer Inst.* 1999;91(20):1751–58; Cunningham AS. Lymphomas and animal-protein consumption. *Lancet.* 1976;27:1184–86; Franceschi S, Favero A, Conti E, et al. Food groups, oils and butter, and cancer of the oral cavity and pharynx. *Br J Cancer.* 1999;80(3–4): 614–20; Tominaga S, Aoki K, Fujimoto I, et al. *Cancer mortality and morbidity statistics. Japan and the world—1994.* Boca Raton, Fla.: CRC Press; 1994. p. 196; Soler M, Chatenoud L, La Vecchia C, et al. Diet, alcohol, coffee and pancreatic cancer: final results from an Italian study. *Eur J Cancer Prev.* 1998;7(6): 455–60; Sung JF, Lin RS, Pu YS, et al. Risk factors for prostate carcinoma in Taiwan: a case-control study in a Chinese population. *Cancer.* 1999;86(3): 484–91; Black HS, Herd JA, Goldberg LH, et al. Effect of a low-fat diet on the incidence of actinic keratosis. *New Eng J Med.* 1994;330:1272–75.

57. Peer PG, van Dijck JA, Hendriks JH, et al. Age dependent growth rate of primary breast cancer. *Cancer.* 1993;71(11): 3547–51.

58. Esserman L, Shieh Y, Thompson I. Rethinking screening for breast cancer and prostate cancer: *JAMA.* 2009 Oct 21;

302(15):1685–92; Wright CJ, Mueller CB. Screening mammography and public health policy: the need for perspective. *Lancet.* 1995; 346(8966):29–32; Neugut AI, Jacobson JS. The limitations of breast cancer screening for first-degree relatives of breast cancer patients. *Am J Public Health* 1995;85(6):832–34; Olsen O, Gotzzsche PC. Cochrane review on screening for breast cancer with mammography. *Lancet.* 2001;358:1340–42.

59. Le Marchand L, Hankin JH, Bach F, et al. An ecological study of diet and lung cancer in the South Pacific. *Int J Cancer.* 1995; 63(1):18–23.

60. Gao CM, Tajima K, Kuroishi T, et al. Protective effects of raw vegetables and fruit against lung cancer among smokers and ex-smokers: a case-control study in the Tokai area of Japan. *Japan J Cancer Res.* 1993;84(6):594–600.

61. Verreault R, Brisson J, Deschenes L, et al. Dietary fat in relation to prognostic indicators in breast cancer. *J Natl Cancer Inst.* 1988; 89:819–25.

62. Gregorio DI, Emrich LJ, Graham S, et al. Dietary fat consumption and survival among women with breast cancer. *J Natl Cancer Inst.* 1985;75:37–41.

63. Kwan ML, Weltzien E, Kushi LH, et al. Dietary patterns and breast cancer recurrence and survival among women with early-stage breast cancer. *J Clin Oncol.* 2009 Feb 20;27(6): 919–26; Dal Maso L, Zucchetto A, Talamini R, et al. Effect of obesity and other lifestyle factors on mortality in women with breast cancer. *Int J Cancer.* 2008 Nov 1;123(9):2188–94; Kellen E, Vansant G, Christiaens MR, et al. Lifestyle changes and breast cancer prognosis: a review. *Breast Cancer Res Treat.* 2009 Mar;114(1):13–22.

64. Berkow SE, Barnard ND, Saxe GA, Ankerberg-Nobis T. Diet and survival after prostate cancer diagnosis. *Nutr Rev.* 2007 Sep; 65(9):391–403.

65. Giem P, Beeson WL, Fraser GE. The incidence of dementia and intake of animal products: preliminary findings from the Adventist Health Study. *Neuroepidemiology.* 1993;12:28–36.

66. Wynn E, Krieg MA, Lanham-New SA, et al. Postgraduate symposium: positive influence of nutritional alkalinity on bone health. *Proc Nutr Soc.* 2010 Feb;69(1):166–73; Siener R. Impact of dietary habits on stone incidence. *Urol Res.* 2006 Apr; 34(2):131–33; Motokawa M, Fukuda M, Muramatsu W, et al. Regional differences in end-stage renal disease and amount of protein intake in Japan. *J Ren Nutr.* 2007 Mar;17(2):118–25; Frank H, Graf J, Amann-Gassner U, et al. Effect of short-term high-protein compared with normal-

protein diets on renal hemodynamics and associated variables
in healthy young men. *Am J Clin Nutr.* 2009 Dec;90(6): 1509–16;
Blumenthal JA, Babyak MA, Hinderliter A, et al. Effects of the
DASH diet alone and in combination with exercise and weight
loss on blood pressure and cardiovascular biomarkers in men
and women with high blood pressure: the ENCORE study.
Arch Intern Med. 2010 Jan 25;170(2):126–35; Todd AS, Mac-
ginley RJ, Schollum JB, et al. Dietary salt loading impairs arterial vascular reactivity. *Am J Clin Nutr.* 2010 Mar;91(3):
557–64; Sluijs I, Beulens JW, van der A DL, et al. Dietary
intake of total, animal, and vegetable protein and risk of type 2
diabetes in the European Prospective Investigation into Cancer
and Nutrition (EPIC)-NL Study. *Diabetes Care.* Jan 2010;
33(1):43–48; Bogardus ST Jr. What do we know about diver-
ticular disease? A brief overview. *J Clin Gastroenterol.* 2006
Aug;40 (suppl 3): S108–11; Chiaffarino F, Parazzini F, La Vecchia C, et al. Diet and uterine myomas. *Obstet Gynecol.* 1999
Sep;94(3):395–98; Nordoy A, Goodnight SH. Dietary lipids
and thrombosis: relationship to atherosclerosis. *Arteriosclerosis.* 1990;10(2):149–63.

67. Maggi S, Kelsey JL, Litvak J, Hayes SP. Incidence of hip fractures in the elderly: a cross-national analysis. *Osteoporosis* Int.
1991; 1:232–41.

68. Feskanich D, Willett WC, Stampfer MJ, Colditz GA. Milk,
dietary calcium, and bone fractures in women: a 12-year prospective study. *Am J Public Health.* 1997; 87:992–97.

69. Chen YM, Ho SC, Woo JL. Greater fruit and vegetable intake
is associated with increased bone mass among postmenopausal
Chinese women. *Br J Nutr.* 2006 Oct; 96(4):745–51; Prynne
CJ, Mishra GD, O'Connell MA, et al. Fruit and vegetable
intakes and bone mineral status: a cross sectional study in 5
age and sex cohorts. *Am J Clin Nutr.* 2006 Jun;83(6):1420–28;
McGartland CP, Robson PJ, Murray LJ, et al. Fruit and vegetable consumption and bone mineral density: the Northern Ire-
land Young Hearts Project. *Am J Clin Nutr.* 2004 Oct;
80(4):1019–23; Tylavsky FA, Holliday K, Danish R, et al. Fruit
and vegetable intakes are an independent predictor of bone size
in early pubertal children. *Am J Clin Nutr.* 2004 Feb;
79(2):311–17; Tucker KL, Hannan MT, Chen H, et al. Potassium, magnesium, and fruit and vegetable intakes are associated with greater bone mineral density in elderly men and
women. *Am J Clin Nutr.* 1999;68(4):727–36.

70. Kerstetter JE, Wall DE, O'Brien KO, et al. Meat and soy protein affect calcium homeostasis in healthy women. *J Nutr.*

2006 Jul;136(7):1890–5; Massey LK. Dietary animal and plant protein and human bone health: a whole foods approach. *J Nutr.* 2003 Mar;133(3)(suppl):S862–65; Nowson CA, Patchett A, Wattanapenpaiboon N. The effects of a low-sodium base-producing diet including red meat compared with a high-carbohydrate, low-fat diet on bone turnover markers in women aged 45–75 years. *Br J Nutr.* 2009 Oct;102(8): 1161–70; Teucher B, Dainty JR, Spinks CA. Sodium and bone health: impact of moderately high and low salt intakes on calcium metabolism in postmenopausal women. *J Bone Miner Res.* 2008 Sep;23(9): 1477–85; Siener R, Schade N, Nicolay C, et al. The efficacy of dietary intervention on urinary risk factors for stone formation in recurrent calcium oxalate stone patients. *J Urol.* 2005 May;173(5):1601–5; Yildirim ZK, Büyükavci M, Eren S, et al. Late side effects of high-dose steroid therapy on skeletal system in children with idiopathic thrombocytopenic purpura. *J Pediatr Hematol Oncol.* 2008 Oct;30(10): 749–53; Karner I, Hrgović Z, Sijanović S, et al. Bone mineral density changes and bone turnover in thyroid carcinoma patients treated with supraphysiologic doses of thyroxine. *Eur J Med Res.* 2005 Nov 16;10(11):480–88; Lim LS, Harnack LJ, Lazovich D, Folsom AR. Vitamin A intake and the risk of hip fracture in postmenopausal women: the Iowa Women's Health Study. *Osteoporos Int.* 2004 Jul;15(7): 552–59; Caire-Juvera G, Ritenbaugh C, Wactawski-Wende J, et al. Vitamin A and retinol intakes and the risk of fractures among participants of the Women's Health Initiative Observational Study. *Am J Clin Nutr.* 2009 Jan;89(1): 323–30; Massey LK, Whiting SJ. Caffeine, urinary calcium, calcium metabolism and bone. *J Nutr.* 1993 Sep;123(9):1611–14; Harris SS, Dawson-Hughes B. Caffeine and bone loss in healthy postmenopausal women. *Am J Clin Nutr.* 1994;60(4):573–78; Nguyen NU, Dumoulin G, Wolf JP, Berthelay S. Urinary calcium and oxalate excretion during oral fructose or glucose load in man. *Horm Metab Res.* 1989; 21(2):96–99; Sampson HW. Alcohol, osteoporosis, and bone regulating hormones. *Alcohol Clin Exp Res.* 1997;21(3):400–3; Wolinsky-Friedland M. Drug-induced metabolic bone disease. *Endocrinol Metab Clin North Am.* 1995;24(2):395–420; Melhus H, Michaelson K, Kindmark A, et al. Excessive dietary intake of vitamin A is associated with reduced bone mineral density and increased risk of hip fracture. *Ann Intern Med.* 1998;129(10):770–78.

71. Sellmeyer DE, Stone KL, Sebastian A, Cummings SR. A high ratio of dietary animal to vegetable protein increases the rate of

bone loss and the risk of fracture in postmenopausal women: study of Osteoporotic Fractures Research Group. *Am J Clin Nutr.* 2001 Jan;73(1): 118–22.

72. Jajoo R, Song L, Rasmussen H, et al. Dietary acid-base balance, bone resorption, and calcium excretion. *J Am Coll Nutr.* 2006 Jun; 25(3):224–30; Nowson CA, Patchett A, Wattanapenpaiboon N. The effects of a low-sodium base-producing diet including red meat compared with a high-carbohydrate, low-fat diet on bone turnover markers in women aged 45–75 years. *Br J Nutr.* 2009 Oct;102(8): 1161–70; Barzel US, Massey LK. Excess dietary protein can adversely affect bone. *J Nutr.* 1998;128(6): 1051–53; Remer T, Mantz F. Estimation of the renal net acid excretion by adults consuming diets containing variable amounts of protein. *Am J Clin Nutr.* 1994;59: 1356–61.

73. Feskanich D, Willett WC, Stampfer MJ, Colditz GA. Milk, dietary calcium, and bone fractures in women: a 12-year prospective study. *Am J Public Health.* 1997; 87:992–97.

74. Abelow BJ, Holford TR, Insogna KL. Cross-cultural association between dietary animal protein and hip fracture: a hypothesis. *Calcif Tissue Int.* 1992; 50(1):14–18.

75. Wynn E, Krieg MA, Lanham-New SA, et al. Postgraduate symposium: positive influence of nutritional alkalinity on bone health. *Proc Nutr Soc.* 2010 Feb;69(1):166–73.

76. Dawson-Hughes B. Interaction of dietary calcium and protein in bone health in humans. *J Nutr.* 2003 Mar;133(3) (suppl): S852–54; Dawson-Hughes B. Calcium and protein in bone health. *Proc Nutr Soc.* 2003 May;62(2):505–9.

77. Whiting SJ, Lemke B. Excess retinol intake may explain the high incidence of osteoporosis in northern Europe. *Nutr Rev.* 1999;57(6):192–95.

78. Mazess RB, Mather W. Bone mineral content of North Alaskan Eskimos. *Am J Clin Nutr.* 1997; 27(9):916–25; Pawson IG. Radiographic determination of excessive bone loss in Alaskan Eskimos. *Hum Biol.* 1974;46(3):369–80.

79. Weaver CM. Choices for achieving adequate dietary calcium with a vegetarian diet. *Am J Clin Nutr.* 1999;70(suppl): S543–48.

80. Tucker KL. Osteoporosis prevention and nutrition. *Curr Osteoporos Rep.* 2009 Dec;7(4):111–17; Lanou AJ. Should dairy be recommended as part of a healthy vegetarian diet? Counterpoint. *Am J Clin Nutr.* 2009 May;89(5)(suppl): S1638–42; Yang Z, Zhang Z, Penniston KL, et al. Serum carotenoid concentrations in postmenopausal women from the United

States with and without osteoporosis. *Int J Vitam Nutr Res.* 2008 May; 78(3): 105–11; Tucker KL, Hannan MT, Chen H, et al. Potassium, magnesium, and fruit and vegetable intakes are associated with greater mineral density in elderly men and women. *Am J Clin Nutr.* 1999; 69(4):727–36; New SA, Robins SP, Campbell MK, et al. Dietary influences on bone mass and bone metabolism: further evidence of a positive link between fruit and vegetable consumption and bone health? *Am J Clin Nutr.* 2000;71(1):142–51.

81. Bügel S. Vitamin K and bone health in adult humans. *Vitam Horm.* 2008;78:393–416; Feskanich D, Weber P, Willett WC, et al. Vitamin K intake and hip fractures in women: a prospective study. *Am J Clin Nutr.* 1999; 69(1):74–79.

82. Bischoff-Ferrari H. Vitamin D: what is an adequate vitamin D level and how much supplementation is necessary? *Best Pract Res Clin Rheumatol.* 2009 Dec;23(6):789–95.

83. Reginster J. The high prevalence of inadequate serum vitamin D levels and implications for bone health. *Curr Med Res Opin.* 2005;21(4):579–85.

84. Bischoff-Ferrari HA, Willet WC, Wong JB, et al. Fracture prevention with vitamin D supplementation: a meta-analysis of randomized controlled trials. *JAMA.* 2005;292(18): 2257–64.

85. Jain P, Jain P, Bhandari S, Siddhu A. A case-control study of risk factors for coronary heart disease in urban Indian middle-aged males. *Indian Heart J.* 2008 May–Jun;60(3):233–40; Grant WB. Milk and other dietary influences on coronary heart disease. *Altern Med Rev.* 1998;3: 281–94; Segall JJ. Epidemiological evidence for the link between dietary lactose and atherosclerosis. In: Colaco, C., editor. *The glycation hypothesis of atherosclerosis.* Austin, Tex.: Landes Bioscience; 1997. pp. 185–209; Artad-Wild SM, Connor SL, Sexton G, et al. Differences in coronary mortality can be explained by differences in cholesterol and saturated fat intakes in 40 countries but not in France and Finland: a paradox. *Circulation.* 1993;88:2771–79.

86. Keszei AP, Schouten LJ, Goldbohm RA, et al. Dairy intake and the risk of bladder cancer in the Netherlands Cohort Study on Diet and Cancer. *Am J Epidemiol.* 2009 Dec 30; Kurahashi N, Inoue M, Iwasaki M, et al. Dairy product, saturated fatty acid, and calcium intake and prostate cancer in a prospective cohort of Japanese men. *Cancer Epidemiol Biomarkers Prevent.* 2008 Apr;17(4):930–37; van der Pols JC, Bain C, Gunnell D, et al. Childhood dairy intake and adult cancer risk: 65-y follow-up of the Boyd Orr cohort. *Am J Clin Nutr.* 2007 Dec;86(6): 1722–29; Park Y, Mitrou PN, Kipnis V, et al. Calcium, dairy

foods, and risk of incident and fatal prostate cancer: the NIH-AARP Diet and Health Study. *Am J Epidemiol.* 2007 Dec 1;166(11):1270–79; Rohrmann S, Platz EA, Kavanaugh CJ, et al. Meat and dairy consumption and subsequent risk of prostate cancer in a US cohort study. *Cancer Causes Control.* 2007 Feb;18(1):41–50; Davies TW, Palmer CR, Ruja E, Lipscombe JM. Adolescent milk, dairy products and fruit consumption and testicular cancer. *Br J Cancer.* 1996; 74(4):657–60.

87. Charnley G, Doull J. Human exposure to dioxins from food, 1999–2002. *Food Chem Toxicol.* 2005 May;43(5):671–79.

88. U.S. Environmental Protection Agency. National Center for Environmental Assessment. Dioxin. http://cfpub.epa.gov/ncea/CFM/nceaQFind.cfm?keyword= Dioxin; Skrzycki C, Warrick J. EPA report ratchets up dioxin peril. *Washington Post* 2000 May 17.

89. Welch AA, Mulligan A, Bingham SA, et al. Urine pH is an indicator of dietary acid-base load, fruit and vegetables and meat intakes: results from the European Prospective Investigation into Cancer and Nutrition (EPIC)–Norfolk population study. *Br J Nutr.* 2008 Jun;99(6):1335–43; Alexy U, Kersting M, Remer T. Potential renal acid load in the diet of children and adolescents: impact of food groups, age and time trends. *Public Health Nutr.* 2008 Mar; 11(3):300–6.

90. Ma RW, Chapman K. A systematic review of the effect of diet in prostate cancer prevention and treatment. *J Hum Nutr Diet.* 2009 Jun;22(3):187–99; quiz 200–2; Kurahashi N, Inoue M, Iwasaki M. Dairy product, saturated fatty acid, and calcium intake and prostate cancer in a prospective cohort of Japanese men. *Cancer Epidemiol Biomarkers Prevent.* 2008 Apr;17(4): 930–37; Allen NE, Key TJ, Appleby PN, et al. Animal foods, protein, calcium and prostate cancer risk: the European Prospective Investigation into Cancer and Nutrition. *Br J Cancer.* 2008 May 6;98(9): 1574–81; Ahn J, Albanes D, Peters U, et al. Dairy products, calcium intake, and risk of prostate cancer in the prostate, lung, colorectal, and ovarian cancer screening trial. *Cancer Epidemiol Biomarkers Prevent.* 2007 Dec;16(12): 2623–30; Qin LQ, Xu JY, Wang PY, et al. Milk consumption is a risk factor for prostate cancer in Western countries: evidence from cohort studies. *Asia Pac J Clin Nutr.* 2007; 16(3):467–76; Ganmaa D, Sato A. The possible role of female sex hormones in milk from pregnant cows in the development of breast, ovarian and corpus uteri cancers. *Med Hypotheses.* 2005;65(6):1028–37; Genkinger JM, Hunter DJ, Spiegelman D, et al. Dairy products and ovarian cancer: a pooled analysis

of 12 cohort studies. *Cancer Epidemiol Biomarkers Prevent.* 2006 Feb;15(2):364–72; Larsson SC, Orsini N, Wolk A. Milk, milk products and lactose intake and ovarian cancer risk: a meta-analysis of epidemiological studies. *Int J Cancer.* 2006 Jan 15; 118(2):431–41; Qin LQ, Xu JY, Wang PY, et al. Milk/ dairy products consumption, galactose metabolism and ovarian cancer: meta-analysis of epidemiological studies. *Eur J Cancer Prev.* 2005 Feb;14(1):13–19; Larsson SC, Bergkvist L, Wolk A. Milk and lactose intakes and ovarian cancer risk in the Swedish Mammography Cohort. *Am J Clin Nutr.* 2004 Nov;80(5):1353–57; Fairfield KM, Hunter DJ, Colditz GA, et al. A prospective study of dietary lactose and ovarian cancer. *Int J Cancer.* 2004 Jun 10; 110(2):271–77.

91. Chan JM, Stampfer MJ, Ma J, et al. Dairy products, calcium, and prostate cancer risk in the Physicians' Health Study. Presentation. American Association for Cancer Research, San Francisco, April 2000.

92. Bosetti C, Tzonou A, Lagiou P, et al. Fraction of prostate cancer attributed to diet in Athens, Greece. *Eur J Cancer Prev.* 2000; 9(2):119–23.

93. Tseng M, Breslow RA, Graubard BI, Ziegler RG. Dairy, calcium and vitamin D intakes and prostate cancer risk in the National Health and Nutrition Examination Epidemiologic Follow-up Study cohort. *Am J Clin Nutr.* 2005;(81)1147–54. Park S, Murphy S, Wilkens L, Stram D, et al. Calcium, vitamin D, and dairy product intake and prostate cancer risk: the Multiethnic Cohort Study. *Am J Epidemiol.* 2007; 166(11) 1259–69.

94. Voskuil DW, Vrieling A, van't Veer LJ, Kampman E, Rookus MA. The insulin-like growth factor system in cancer prevention: potential of dietary intervention strategies. *Cancer Epidemiol Biomarkers Prevent.* 2005 Jan;14(1):195–203.

95. Cohen P. Serum insulin-like growth factor 1 levels and prostate cancer risk—interpreting the evidence. *J Natl Cancer Inst.* 1998(90): 876–79.

96. Chan JM, Stampfer MJ, Giovannucci E, et al. Plasma insulin-like growth factor-I and prostate risk: a prospective study. *Science* 1998(279):563–65.

97. Fairfield K. Annual meeting of the Society for General Internal Medicine: Dairy products linked to ovarian cancer risk. *Family Practice News.* 2000 Jun 11: 8.

Chapter 5: Nutritional Wisdom Makes You Thin

1. Rolls BJ. The relationship between dietary energy density and energy intake. *Physiol Behav.* 2009 Jul 14;97(5):609–15; Dun-

can K. The effects of high- and low-energy-density diets of satiety, energy intake, and eating time of obese and non-obese subjects. *Am J Clin Nutr.* 1983;37:763

2. Bernstein PS, Delori FC, Richer S, et al. The value of measurement of macular carotenoid pigment optical densities and distributions in age-related macular degeneration and other retinal disorders. *Vision Res.* 2010 Mar 31;50(7): 716–28; Carpentier S, Knaus M, Suh M. Associations between lutein, zeaxanthin, and age-related macular degeneration: an overview. *Crit Rev Food Sci Nutr.* 2009 Apr; 49(4):313–26.

3. Mangels AR, Holden JM, Beecher GR, et al. Carotenoid content of fruits and vegetables: an evaluation of analytic data. *J Am Diet Assoc.* 1993;93(3):284–96.

4. Dwyer JH, Paul-Labrador MJ, Fan J, et al. Progression of carotid intima-media thickness and plasma antioxidants: the Los Angeles Atherosclerosis Study. *Arterioscler Thromb Vasc Biol.* 2004 Feb;24(2):313–19; Dwyer JH, Navab M, Dwyer KM, et al. Oxygenated carotenoid lutein and progression of early atherosclerosis: the Los Angeles Atherosclerosis Study. *Circulation.* 2001; 103(24): 2922–27.

5. Harris W. Less grains, more greens. VigSource.com. Posted 2000 Jun 11. No longer available online.

6. Harris W. *The scientific basis of vegetarianism.* Honolulu: Hawaii Health Publishers; 2000. pp. 98–100.

7. Lee JH, O'Keefe JH, Lavie CJ, Harris WS. Omega-3 fatty acids: cardiovascular benefits, sources and sustainability. *Nat Rev Cardiol.* 2009 Dec;6(12): 753–58; Lavie CJ, Milani RV, Mehra MR, Ventura HO. Omega-3 polyunsaturated fatty acids and cardiovascular diseases. *J Am Coll Cardiol.* 2009 Aug 11;54(7):585–94; Cole GM, Ma QL, Frautschy SA. Omega-3 fatty acids and dementia. *Prostaglandins Leukot Essent Fatty Acids.* 2009 Aug–Sep; 81(2–3):213–21; Wendel M, Heller AR. Anticancer actions of omega-3 fatty acids— current state and future perspectives. *Anti Canc Agents Med Chem.* 2009 May;9(4):457–70; Calder PC, Yaqoob P. Omega-3 polyunsaturated fatty acids and human health outcomes. *Biofactors.* 2009 May–Jun;35(3): 266–72; Yashodhara BM, Umakanth S, Pappachan JM, et al. Omega-3 fatty acids: a comprehensive review of their role in health and disease. *Postgrad Med J.* 2009 Feb; 85(1000):84–90; Cakiner-Egilmez T. Omega 3 fatty acids and the eye. *Insight.* 2008 Oct–Dec; 33(4):20–5; quiz 26–27; Das UN. Essential fatty acids—a review. *Curr Pharm Biotechnol.* 2006 Dec;7(6): 467–82; Smith WL. Nutritionally essential fatty acids and biologically

indispensable cyclooxygenases. *Trends Biochem Sci.* 2008 Jan;33(1):27–37.

8. Simopoulos AP. The importance of the omega-6/omega-3 fatty acid ratio in cardiovascular disease and other chronic diseases. *Exp Biol Med (Maywood).* 2008 Jun;233(6):674–88; Miyake Y, Sasaki S, Tanaka K, et al. Relationship between dietary fat and fish intake and the prevalence of atopic eczema in pregnant Japanese females: baseline data from the Osaka Maternal and Child Health Study. *Asia Pac J Clin Nutr.* 2008;17(4):612–19; Koch C, Dölle S, Metzger M, et al. Docosahexaenoic acid (DHA) supplementation in atopic eczema: a randomized, double-blind, controlled trial. *Br J Dermatol.* 2008 Apr;158(4): 786–92; Freeman MP. Omega-3 fatty acids in major depressive disorder. *J Clin Psychiatry.* 2009;70(suppl 5):S7–11; Thiébaut AC, Chajès V, Gerber M, et al. Dietary intakes of omega-6 and omega-3 polyunsaturated fatty acids and the risk of breast cancer. *Int J Cancer.* 2009 Feb 15;124(4):924–31; Berquin IM, Edwards IJ, Chen YQ. Multi-targeted therapy of cancer by omega-3 fatty acids. *Cancer Lett.* 2008 Oct 8;269(2): 363–77.

9. Simopoulos AP. The importance of the omega-6/omega-3 fatty acid ratio in cardiovascular disease and other chronic diseases. *Exp Biol Med (Maywood).* 2008 Jun;233(6):674–88; Sartorelli DS, Damião R, Chaim R, et al. Dietary omega-3 fatty acid and omega-3: omega-6 fatty acid ratio predict improvement in glucose disturbances in Japanese Brazilians. *Nutrition.* 2010 Feb;26(2): 184–91; Simopoulos AP. Essential fatty acids in health and chronic disease. *Am J Clin Nutr.* 1999;70(3): 560–69.

10. CBS News: Health-Lawsuit: Disclose PCB Levels in Fish Oil. March 2, 2010; http://www.cbsnews.com/stories/2010/03/02/health/main6259938.shtml.

11. Waitzberg DL, Torrinhas RS. Fish oil lipid emulsions and immune response: what clinicians need to know. *Nutr Clin Pract.* 2009 Aug–Sep;24(4):487–99; Mori TA, Beilin LJ. Omega-3 fatty acids and inflammation. *Curr Atheroscler Rep.* 2004 Nov;6(6):461–67; Fernandes G. Progress in nutritional immunology. *Immunol Res.* 2008;40(3): 244–61. Huges DA, Pinder AC. N-3 polyunsaturated fatty acids inhibit the antigen-presenting function of human monocytes. *Am J Clin Nutr.* 2000;71(suppl 1):S357–60; Purasiri P, McKechnie A, Heys SD, Eremin O. Modulation in vitro of human natural cytotoxicity, lymphocyte proliferation response to mitogens and cytokine production by essential fatty acids. *Immunology.* 1997; 92(2): 166–72.

12. Sijben JW, Calder PC. Differential immunomodulation with long-chain n-3 PUFA in health and chronic disease. *Proc Nutr Soc.* 2007 May;66(2):237–59; Simopoulos AP. Omega-3 fatty acids in inflammation and autoimmune diseases. *J Am Coll Nutr.* 2002 Dec; 21(6):495–505.

13. Joseph A. Manifestations of coronary atherosclerosis in young trauma victims—an autopsy study. *J Am Coll Cardiol.* 1993; 22:459.

14. Virtanen JK, Mozaffarian D, Chiuve SE, Rimm EB. Fish consumption and risk of major chronic disease in men. *Am J Clin Nutr.* 2008 Dec;88(6):1618–25; Harris WS, Kris-Etherton PM, Harris KA. Intakes of long-chain omega-3 fatty acid associated with reduced risk for death from coronary heart disease in healthy adults. *Curr Atheroscler Rep. 2008* Dec; 10(6): 503–9.

15. Vrablík M, Prusíková M, Snejdrlová M, Zlatohlávek L. Omega-3 fatty acids and cardiovascular disease risk: do we understand the relationship? *Physiol Res.* 2009;58 (suppl 1):S19–26; Lee JH, O'Keefe JH, Lavie CJ, Harris WS. Omega-3 fatty acids: cardiovascular benefits, sources and sustainability. *Nat Rev Cardiol.* 2009 Dec;6(12): 753–58; Lavie CJ, Milani RV, Mehra MR, Ventura HO. Omega-3 polyunsaturated fatty acids and cardiovascular diseases. *J Am Coll Cardiol.* 2009 Aug 11;54(7):585–94; Holub BJ. Docosahexaenoic acid (DHA) and cardiovascular disease risk factors. *Prostaglandins Leukot Essent Fatty Acids.* 2009 Aug–Sep;81(2–3): 199–204.

16. Siguel EN. Dietary sources of long-chain n-3 polyunsaturated fatty acids. *JAMA.* 1996;275:836.

17. Marangoni F, Colombo C, Martiello A, et al. Levels of the n-3 fatty acid eicosapentaenoic acid in addition to those of alpha linolenic acid are significantly raised in blood lipids by the intake of four walnuts a day in humans. *Nutr Metab Cardiovasc Dis.* 2007 Jul; 17(6):457–61; Harnack K, Andersen G, Somoza V. Quantitation of alpha-linolenic acid elongation to eicosapentaenoic and docosahexaenoic acid as affected by the ratio of n6/n3 fatty acids. *Nutr Metab (Lond).* 2009 Feb 19;6:8; Siguel EN, Macture M. Relative enzyme activity of unsaturated fatty acid metabolic pathways in humans. *Metabolism.* 1987;36: 664–69.

18. Mozaffarian D, Rimm EB. Fish intake, contaminants, and human health: evaluating the risks and the benefits. *JAMA.* 2006 Oct 18; 296(15):1885–99; Salonen JT, Seppanen K, Nyyssonen K, et al. Intake of mercury from fish, lipid

peroxidation, and the risk of myocardial infarction and coronary, cardiovascular, and any death in eastern Finnish men. *Circulation*. 1995;91:645–55.

19. Virtanen JK, Voutilainen S, Rissanen TH, et al. Mercury, fish oils, and risk of acute coronary events and cardiovascular disease, coronary heart disease, and all-cause mortality in men in eastern Finland. *Arterioscler Thromb Vasc Biol*. 2005 Jan;25(1):228–33; Ihanainen M, Salonen R, Seppanen R, Salonen JT. Nutrition data collection in the Kuopio Ischaemic Heart Disease Risk Factor Study: nutrient intake of middle-aged eastern Finnish men. *Nutr Res*. 1989;9:597–604; WHO Monica Project: assessing CHD mortality and morbidity. *Int J Epidemiol*. 1989;18(suppl):S38–45; Salonen JT, Seppanen K, Nyyssonen K, et al. Intake of mercury from fish, lipid peroxidation, and the risk of myocardial infarction and coronary, cardiovascular, and any death in eastern Finnish men. *Circulation*. 1995;91:645–55.

20. Wiggers GA, Peçanha FM, Briones AM, et al. Low mercury concentrations cause oxidative stress and endothelial dysfunction in conductance and resistance arteries. *Am J Physiol Heart Circ Physiol*. 2008 Sep;295(3):H1033–43.

21. Black JJ, Bauman PC. Carcinogens and cancers in freshwater fishes. *Environ Health Perspec*. 1991; 90:27–33.

22. Oken E, Bellinger DC. Fish consumption, methylmercury and child neurodevelopment. *Curr Opin Pediatr*. 2008 Apr;20(2):178–83; Murata K, Dakeishi M, Shimada M, et al. Assessment of intrauterine methylmercury exposure affecting child development: messages from the newborn. *Tohoku J Exp Med*. 2007 Nov; 213(3):187–202; Jedrychowski W, Perera F, Jankowski J, et al. Fish consumption in pregnancy, cord blood mercury level and cognitive and psychomotor development of infants followed over the first three years of life: Krakow epidemiologic study. *Environ Int*. 2007 Nov;33(8):1057–62; Gilbertson M. Male cerebral palsy hospitalization as a potential indicator of neurological effects of methylmercury exposure in Great Lakes communities. *Environ Res*. 2004 Jul;95(3): 375–84; Rylander L, Stromberg U, Hagmar L. Dietary intake of fish contaminated with persistent organochlorine compounds in relation to low birthweight. *Scand J Work Environ Health*. 1996; 2(4):260–66; Does methylmercury have a role in causing developmental disabilities in children? *Environ Health Perspect*. 2000;108(suppl. 3):S413–20.

23. Clarkson TW. The toxicology of mercury. *Crit Rev Clin Lab Sci*. 1997;34(4): 369–403.

24. Calder PC. Immunomodulation by omega-3 fatty acids. *Prostaglandins Leukot Essent Fatty Acids*. 2007 Nov–Dec;77(5–6): 327–35; Wang H, Hao Q, Li QR, et al. Omega-3 polyunsaturated fatty acids affect lipopolysaccharide-induced maturation of dendritic cells through mitogen- activated protein kinases p38. *Nutrition*. 2007 Jun; 23(6):474–82; Meydani SN, Lichtenstein AH, Cornwall S, et al. Immunologic effects of national cholesterol education panel step-2 diets with and without fish-derived n-3 fatty acid enrichment. *J Clin Invest*. 1993;92(1):105–13.

25. Roy J, Pallepati P, Bettaieb A, et al. Acrolein induces a cellular stress response and triggers mitochondrial apoptosis in A549 cells. *Chem Biol Interact*. 2009 Oct 7;181(2):154–67; Dung CH, Wu SC, Yen GC. Genotoxicity and oxidative stress of the mutagenic compounds formed in fumes of heated soybean oil, sunflower oil and lard. *Toxicol In Vitro*. 2006 Jun;20(4):439–47; Chiang TA, Wu PF, Wang LF, et al. Mutagenicity and polycyclic aromatic hydrocarbon content of fumes from heated cooking oils produced in Taiwan. *Mutat Res*. 1997;381(2):157–61; Sheerin AN, Silwood C, Lynch E, Grootveld M. Production of lipid peroxidation products in culinary oils and fats during episodes of thermal stressing: a high field 1H NMR investigation. *Biochem Soc Trans*. 1997;25(3) Supplement: 5495. Warner K. Impact of high-temperature food processing on fats and oils. *Adv Exp Med Biol*. 1999;459:67–77.

26. Kurth T, Moore SC, Gaziano JM, et al. Healthy lifestyle and the risk of stroke in women. *Arch Intern Med*. 2006 Jul 10; 166(13):1403–9; Posner B, Cobb JL, Belanger A, et al. Dietary lipid predictors of coronary heart disease in men. *Arch Intern Med*. 1991;151:1181–87; Gillman MW, Cupples LA, Millen BE, et al. Inverse association of dietary fat with development of ischemic stroke in men. *JAMA*. 1997;278:2145–50; Iso H, Stampfer MJ. A study of fat and protein intake and risk of intraparenchymal hemorrhage in women. *Circulation*. 2001; 103:856.

27. Dauchet L, Amollye P, Dallongeville J. Fruit and vegetable consumption and risk of stroke: a meta-analysis of cohort studies. *Neurology*. 2005 Oct 25;65(8):1193–97; Mizrahi A, Knekt P, Montonen J, et al. Plant foods and the risk of cerebrovascular diseases: a potential protection of fruit consumption. *Br J Nutr*. 2009 Oct;102(7):1075–83; Nagura J, Iso H, Watanabe Y, et al. Fruit, vegetable and bean intake and mortality from cardiovascular disease among Japanese men and women: the JACC Study. *Br J Nutr*. 2009 Jul;102(2): 285–92.

28. Woo D, Haverbusch M, Sekar P, et al. Effect of untreated hypertension on hemorrhagic stroke. *Stroke.* 2004 Jul;35(7): 1703–8; Perry HM Jr., Davis BR, Price TR, et al. Effects of treating isolated systolic hypertension on the risk of developing various types and subtypes of stroke: the Systolic Hypertension in the Elderly Program (SHEP). *JAMA.* 2000;284(4): 465–71.

29. Park Y, Park S, Yi H, et al. Low level of n-3 polyunsaturated fatty acids in erythrocytes is a risk factor for both acute ischemic and hemorrhagic stroke in Koreans. *Nutr Res.* 2009 Dec;29(12):825–30; Simon JA, Fong J, Bernert JT Jr., Browner WS. Serum fatty acids and the risk of stroke. *Stroke.* 1995;26:778–82; Shimokawa T, Moriuchi A, Hori T, et al. Effect of dietary alpha-linolenate/linoleate balance on mean survival time, incidence of stroke and blood pressure of spontaneously hypertensive rats. *Life Sci.* 1988; 43:2067–75.

30. Kurth T, Moore SC, Gaziano JM, et al. Healthy lifestyle and the risk of stroke in women. *Arch Intern Med.* 2006 Jul 10; 166(13):1403–9; Sasaki S, Zhang XH, Kesteloot H. Dietary sodium, potassium, saturated fat, alcohol, and stroke mortality. *Stroke.* 1995;26(5): 783–89.

31. Bos MB, de Vries JH, Feskens EJ, et al. Effect of a high monounsaturated fatty acids diet and a Mediterranean diet on serum lipids and insulin sensitivity in adults with mild abdominal obesity. *Nutr Metab Cardiovasc Dis.* 2009 Aug 17. [Epub ahead of print]; Rallidis LS, Lekakis J, Kolomvotsou A, et al. Close adherence to a Mediterranean diet improves endothelial function in subjects with abdominal obesity. *Am J Clin Nutr.* 2009 Aug; 90(2):263–68; Perez-Jimenez F, Castro P, Lopez-Miranda J, et al. Circulating levels of endothelial function are modulated by dietary monounsaturated fat. *Atherosclerosis* 1999; 145(2):351–58.

32. Nettleton JA, Polak JF, Tracy R, et al. Dietary patterns and incident cardiovascular disease in the Multi-Ethnic Study of Atherosclerosis. *Am J Clin Nutr.* 2009 Sep;90(3):647–54; Sinha R, Cross AJ, Graubard BI, et al. Meat intake and mortality: a prospective study of over half a million people. *Arch Intern Med.* 2009 Mar 23; 169(6):562–71; Sabaté J, Ang Y. Nuts and health outcomes: new epidemiologic evidence. *Am J Clin Nutr.* 2009 May;89(5)(suppl): S1643–48; Ros E. Nuts and novel biomarkers of cardiovascular disease. *Am J Clin Nutr.* 2009 May; 89(5)(suppl):S1649–56; Nash SD, Nash DT. Nuts as part of a healthy cardiovascular diet. *Curr Atheroscler Rep.* 2008 Dec;10(6):529–35; Fraser GE. Association between diet and cancer, ischemic heart disease, and all-cause mortality in

non-Hispanic white California Seventh-Day Adventists. *Am J Clin Nutr.* 1999; 70(supp. 3): S532–38.

33. Hu FB, Stampfer MJ. Nut consumption and risk of coronary heart disease: a review of epidemiologic evidence. *Curr Atheroscler Rep.* 1999 Nov;1(3):204–9.

34. Mukuddem-Petersen J, Oosthuizen W, Jerling JC. A systematic review of the effects of nuts on blood lipid profiles in humans. *J Nutr.* 2005;135(9):2082–89.

35. Lamarche B, Desroche S, Jenkins DJ, et al. Combined effects of a dietary portfolio of plant sterols, vegetable protein, viscous fiber and almonds on LDL particle size. *Br J Nutr.* 2004; 92(4):654–63.

36. Ellsworth JL, Kushi LH, Folsom AR. Frequent nut intake and risk of death from coronary heart disease and all causes in postmenopausal women: the Iowa Women's Health Study. *Nutr Metab Cardiovasc Dis.* 2001;11(6):372–77.

37. Yuen AW, Sander JW. Is omega-3 fatty acid deficiency a factor contributing to refractory seizures and SUDEP? A hypothesis. *Seizure.* 2004 Mar;13(2): 104–7.

38. Coates AM, Howe PR. Edible nuts and metabolic health. *Curr Opin Lipidol.* 2007;18(1):25–30; Segura R, Javierre C, Lizarraga MA, Ros E. Other relevant components of nuts: phytosterols, folate and minerals. *Br J Nutr.* 2006:96 (suppl 2):S36–44.

39. Rajaram S, Sabat AJ. Nuts, body weight and insulin resistance. *Br J Nutr.* 2006;96 (suppl 2):S79–86; Sabat ÃJ. Nut consumption and body weight. *Am J Clin Nutr.* 2003;78(suppl 3): S647–50; Bes-Rastrollo M, Sabat ÃJ, Gamez-Gracia E, et al. Nut consumption and weight gain in a Mediterranean cohort: the SUN study. *Obesity.* 2007;15(1):107–16; Garca-Lorda P, Megias Rangil I, Salas-Salvada J. Nut consumption, body weight and insulin resistance. *Eur J Clin Nutr.* 2003;57 (suppl 1):S8–11; Megas-Rangil I, Garca-Lorda P, Torres-Moreno M, et al. Nutrient content and health effects of nuts. *Arch Latinoam Nutr.* 2004; 54(2) (suppl 1):83–6.

40. Ascherio A, Willett WC. Health effects of trans fatty acids. *Am J Clin Nutr.* 1997;66(suppl 4):S1006–10.

41. Mozaffarian D, Aro A, Willett WC. Health effects of trans-fatty acids: experimental and observational evidence. *Eur J Clin Nutr.* 2009 May;63 (suppl 2):S5–21.

42. Willett WC. Trans fatty acids and cardiovascular disease—epidemiological data. *Atheroscler Suppl.* 2006 May;7(2):5–8; de Roos NM, Bots ML, Katan MB. Replacement of dietary saturated fatty acids by trans fatty acids lowers serum HDL cholesterol and impairs endothelial function in healthy men

and women. *Arterioscler Thromb Vasc Biol.* 2001 Jul; 21(7): 1233–37.

43. Mozaffarian D, Aro A, Willett WC. Health effects of trans-fatty acids: experimental and observational evidence. *Eur J Clin Nutr.* 2009 May;63 (suppl 2):S5–21; Willett WC, Stampfer MJ, Manson JE, et al. Intake of trans fatty acids and risk of coronary heart disease among women. *Lancet.* 1993;341:581–85; Ascherio A, Hennekens CH, Buring JE, et al. Trans-fatty acids intake and risk of myocardial infarction. *Circulation.* 1994;89(1):94–101; Lichtenstein AH. Trans fatty acids and cardiovascular disease risk. *Curr Opin Lipidol.* 2000;11(1): 37–42.

44. Chajès V, Thiébaut AC, Rotival M, et al. Association between serum trans-monounsaturated fatty acids and breast cancer risk in the E3N-EPIC Study. *Am J Epidemiol.* 2008 Jun 1; 167(11):1312–20.

45. National Academy of Sciences, Food and Nutrition Board. Dietary Reference Intakes for Energy, Carbohydrates, Fiber, Fat, Protein and Amino Acids (Macronutrients). 2005:500–589.

46. Hegsted D. Minimum protein requirements of adults. *Am J Clin Nutr.* 1968;21: 3520.

47. Suárez López MM, Kizlansky A, López LB. [Assessment of protein quality in foods by calculating the amino acids score corrected by digestibility]. *Nutr Hosp.* 2006 Jan–Feb;21(1):47–51; Schaafsma G. The protein digestibility–corrected amino acid score. *J Nutr.* 2000;130(7)(suppl):S1865–67; Henley EC, Kuster JM. Protein quality evaluation by protein digestibility corrected amino acid scoring. *Food Technol.* 1994; 48(4):74–77.

Chapter 6: Breaking Free of Food Addiction

1. Vives-Bauza C, Anand M, Shirazi AK, et al. The age lipid A2E and mitochondrial dysfunction synergistically impair phagocytosis by retinal pigment epithelial cells. *J Biol Chem.* 2008; 283(36): 24770–80.

2. Chinmay P, Husam G, Shreyas R, et al. Prolonged reactive oxygen species generation and nuclear factor-B activation after a high-fat, high-carbohydrate meal in the obese. *J Clin Endocrinol Metab.* 2007;92(11): 4476–79.

3. Peairs AT, Rankin JW. Inflammatory response to a high-fat, low-carbohydrate weight loss diet: effect of antioxidants. *Obesity* 2008;16(7):1573–78.

4. Scanlan N. Compromised hepatic detoxification in companion animals and its correction via nutritional supplementation and modified fasting. *Altern Med Rev.* 2001;6(suppl):S24–37.

5. Bes-Rastrollo M, Sanchez-Villegas A, Basterra-Gortari FJ. Prospective study of self-reported usual snacking and weight gain in a Mediterranean cohort: the SUN Project. *Clin Nutr.* 2010 Jun; 29(3):323–30.

6. Mattson MP, Wan R. Beneficial effects of intermittent fasting and caloric restriction on the cardiovascular and cerebrovascular systems. *J Nutr Biochem.* 2005; 16(3):129–37.

7. Preboth MA, Wright S. Quantum sufficit. *Am Fam Physician.* 1998: 58(3);639.

8. Mokdad, AH, Serdula MK, Dietz WH, et al. The spread of the obesity epidemic in the United States, 1991–1998. *JAMA.* 1999;282(16): 1519–22.

9. Food and Agriculture Organization and World Health Organization. *Human vitamin and mineral requirements.* Report 2002. Available online at http://www.fao.org/docrep/004/Y2809E/y2809e08.htm#bm08.

10. Golay A, Guy-Grand B. Are diets fattening? *Ann Endocrinol.* 2002; 63(6):2.

11. Hernandez TL, Sutherland JP, Wolfe P, et al. Lack of suppression of circulating free fatty acids and hypercholesterolemia during weight loss on a high-fat, low-carbohydrate diet. *Am J Clin Nutr.* 2010; 91(3):578–85; Brinkworth GD, Noakes M, Buckley JD, et al. Long-term effects of a very-low-carbohydrate weight loss diet compared with an isocaloric low-fat diet after 12 mo. *Am J Clin Nutr.* 2009;90(1):23–32; Wycherley TP, Brinkworth GD, Keogh JB, et al. Long-term effects of weight loss with a very low carbohydrate and low fat diet on vascular function in overweight and obese patients. *J Intern Med.* 2010 May; 267(5): 452–61.

12. Key TJA, Thorogood M, Appleby PN, Burr ML. Dietary habits and mortality in 11,000 vegetarians and health conscious people: results of a 17-year follow up. *BMJ.* 1996;313: 775–79.

13. Stevens A, Robinson DP, Turpin J, et al. Sudden cardiac death of an adolescent during [Atkins] dieting. *South Med J.* 2002: 95:1047.

14. Zhang ZJ, Croft JB, Gilles WH, Mensah GA. Sudden cardiac death in the United States, 1989 to 1998. *Circulation.* 2001 Oct 30; 104(18):2158–63.

15. Surawicz B, Waller BF. The enigma of sudden cardiac death related to diet. *Can J Cardiol.* 1995; 11(3): 228–31.

16. Best TH, Franz DN, Gilbert DL, et al. Cardiac complications in pediatric patients on the ketogenic diet. *Neurology.* 2000; 54(12): 2328–30.

17. De Stefani E, Fierro L, Mendilaharsu M, et al. Meat intake, "mate" drinking and renal cell cancer in Uruguay: a case-control study. *Br J Cancer.* 1998;78(9): 1239–43; Risch HA, Jain M, Marrett LD, Howe GR. Dietary fat intake and risk of epithelial ovarian cancer. *J Natl Cancer Inst.* 1994;86(18): 1409–15; Pillow PC, Hursting SD, Duphorne CM, et al. Case-control assessment of diet and lung cancer risk in African Americans and Mexican Americans. *Nutr Cancer.* 1997;29(2):169–73; Alavanja MC, Brown CC, Swanson C, Brownson RC. Saturated fat intake and lung cancer risk among nonsmoking women in Missouri. *J Natl Cancer Inst.* 1993;85(23): 1906–16.

18. Nöthlings U, Wilkens, LR, Murphy SP, et al. Meat and fat intake as risk factors for pancreatic cancer: the Multiethnic Cohort Study. *J Natl Cancer Inst.* 2005 Oct 5;97(19):1458–65.

19. O'Keefe SJ, Kidd M, Espitalier NG, Owira P. Rarity of colon cancer in Africans is associated with low animal product consumption, not fiber. *Am J Gastroenterol.* 1999;94(5):1373–80.

20. Brown LM, Swanson CA, Gridley G, et al. Dietary factors and the risk of squamous cell esophageal cancer among black and white men in the United States. *Cancer Causes Control.* 1998;9(5):467–74; Cheng KK, Day NE. Nutrition and esophageal cancer. *Cancer Causes Control.* 1996;7(1): 33–40; Hirohata T, Kono S. Diet/nutrition and stomach cancer in Japan. *Int J Cancer.* 1997;(suppl 10): 34–36; Kono S, Hirohata T. Nutrition and stomach cancer. *Cancer Causes Control.* 1996;7(1):41–45; Terry P, Nyren O, Yuen J. Protective effect of fruits and vegetables on stomach cancer in a cohort of Swedish twins. *Int J Cancer.* 1998; 76(1):35–37.

21. Willett WC, Trichopoulos D. Nutrition and cancer: a summary of the evidence. *Cancer Causes Control.* 7: 178–80; La Vecchia C, Tavani A. Fruit and vegetables, and human cancer. *Eur J Cancer Prev.* 1998; 7(1):3–8; Tavani A, La Vecchia C. Fruit and vegetable consumption and cancer risk in a Mediterranean population. *Am J Clin Nutr.* 1995;61(6)(suppl): S1374–77.

22. Torosian MH. Effect of protein intake on tumor growth and cell cycle kinetics. *J Surg Res.* 1995; 59(2):225–28; Youngman LD, Park JY, Ames BN. Protein oxidation associated with aging is reduced by dietary restriction of protein or calories. *Proc Nat Acad Sci.* 1992;89(19): 9112–16; Carroll KK. Hypercholesterolemia and atherosclerosis: effects of dietary protein. *Fed Proc.* 1982;41(11):2792–96; Carroll KK. Dietary proteins and amino acids—their effects on cholesterol metabolism. In: Gibney MJ, Kritchevshy D, editors. *Animal and vegetable pro-*

teins in lipid metabolism and atherosclerosis. New York: Liss; 1993. pp. 9–17; Willett WC. Nutrition and cancer. *Salud Publica Mex.* 1997; 39(4):298–309.

23. Tavani A, La Vecchia C, Gallus S, et al. Red meat and cancer risk: a study in Italy. *Int J Cancer.* 2000; 86(3):425–28; Kuller LH. Dietary fat and chronic diseases: epidemiologic overview. *J Am Diet Assoc.* 1997;97(suppl 7):S9–15; Willett WC. Nutrition and cancer. *Salud Publica Mex.* 1997;39(4):298–309; La Vecchia C. Cancer associated with high-fat diets. *J Natl Cancer Inst Monogr.* 1992; 12:79–85; Steinmetz KA, Potter JD. Vegetables, fruit, and cancer prevention: a review. *J Am Diet Assoc.* 1996;96(10): 1027–39.

24. Fontana L, Weiss EP, Villareal DT, et al. Long-term effects of calorie or protein restriction on serum IGF-1 and IGFBP-3 concentration in humans. *Aging Cell.* 2008:7:681–87.

25. Sherwood NE, Jeffery RW, French SA, et al. Predictors of weight gain in the Pound of Prevention study. *Int J Obes Relat Metab Disord.* 2000;24(4):395–403; Astrup A. Macronutrient balances and obesity: the role of diet and physical activity. *Public Health Nutr.* 1999;2(3A):341–47.

26. Kahn HS, Tatham LM, Rodriguez C, et al. Stable behaviors associated with adults' 10-year change in body mass index and likelihood of gain at the waist. *Am J Public Health.* 1997; 87(5):747–57.

27. Kasiske BL, Lakatua JD, Ma JZ, Louis TA. A meta-analysis of the effects of dietary protein restriction on the rate of decline in renal function. *Am J Kidney Dis.* 1998;31(6):954–61; Holm EA, Solling K. Dietary protein restriction and the progression of chronic renal insufficiency: a review of the literature. *J Intern Med.* 1996;239(2): 99–104; Brenner BM, Meyer TW, Hostetter TH. Dietary protein intake and the progressive nature of kidney disease: the role of the hemodynamically mediated glomerular injury in the pathogenisis of progressive glomerular sclerosis in aging, renal ablation and intrinsic renal disease. *N Eng J Med.* 1982;307(11): 652–59.

28. Licata AA, Bow E, Bartler FC, et al. Effect of dietary protein on urinary calcium in normal subjects and in patients with nephrolithiasis. *Metabolism.* 1979;28: 895; Robertson WG, Heyburn J, Peacock M, et al. The effect of high animal protein intake on the risk of calcium stone formation in the urinary tract. *Clin Sci.* 1979; 57:285; Brokis JG, Levitt AS, Cruthers SM. The effects of vegetable and animal protein diets on calcium, urate and oxalate excretion. *Br J Urol.* 1982; 54:590; Robertson WG, Peacock M, Heyburn PJ, et al. The risk of

calcium stone formation in relation to affluence and dietary animal protein. In: Brokis JG, Finlayson B, editors. *Urinary calculus: International Urinary Stone Conference.* Littleton, Mass.: PSG Publishing; 1981. p. 3; Atkins diet raises concerns. *Cortland Forum* 2004 Apr:22.

29. Knight EL, Stampfer MJ, Hankinson SE, et al. The impact of protein on renal function decline in women with normal renal function or mild renal insufficiency. *Ann Int Med.* 2003:138: 460–67.

30. Gin H, Rigalleau V, Aparicio M. Lipids, protein intake, and diabetic nephropathy. *Diabetes Metab.* 2000;26(suppl 4): S45–53.

31. Pedrini MT, Levey AS, Lau J, et al. The effect of dietary protein on the progression of diabetic and nondiabetic renal disease: a meta-analysis. *Ann Intern Med.* 1996; 124(7):627–32.

32. Jenkins DJ, Kendall CW, Popovich DG, et al. Effect of a very-high-fiber vegetable, fruit, and nut diet on serum lipids and colonic function. *Metabolism.* 2001 Apr; 50(4):494–503.

33. Sarter B, Campbell TC, Fuhrman J. Effect of a high nutrient diet on long term weight loss: a retrospective chart review. *Altern Ther Health Med.* 2008;14(3): 48–53; Foster GD, Wyatt HR, Hill JO, et al. Weight and metabolic outcomes after 2 years on a low-carbohydrate versus low-fat diet: a randomized trial. *Ann Intern Med.* 2010 Aug 3;153(3):147–57. Brinkworth GD, Noakes M, Buckley JD, et al. Long-term effects of a very-low-carbohydrate weight loss diet compared with an isocaloric low-fat diet after 12 mo. *Am J Clin Nutr.* 2009 Jul;90(1):23–32. Sacks FM, Bray GA, Carey VJ, et al. Comparison of weight-loss diets with different compositions of fat, protein, and carbohydrates. *N Eng J Med.* 2009 Feb 26;360(9): 859–73. Jiménez-Cruz A, Jiménez AB, Pichardo-Osuna A, et al. Long term effect of Mediterranean diet on weight loss. *Nutr Hosp.* 2009 Nov-Dec; 24(6): 753–54.

Chapter 7: Eat to Live Takes On Disease

1. Allen S, Britton JR, Leonardi-Bee JA. Association between antioxidant vitamins and asthma outcome measures: systematic review and meta-analysis. *Thorax.* 2009 Jul;64(7): 610–19; Wood LG, Gibson PG. Dietary factors lead to innate immune activation in asthma. *Pharmacol Ther.* 2009 Jul;123(1):37–53; Bacopoulou F, Veltsista A, Vassi I, et al. Can we be optimistic about asthma in childhood? A Greek cohort study. *J Asthma.* 2009 Mar;46(2):171–47; Delgado J, Barranco P, Quirce S. Obesity and asthma. *J Investig Allergol Clin*

Immunol. 2008;18(6):420–52; Carnargro CA, Weiss DY, Zhang D, et al. Prospective study of body mass index, weight change, and risk of adult-onset asthma in women. *Arch Intern Med.* 1999;159:2582–88.

2. American Heart Association. Heart Attack and Angina Statistics. 2006. http://www.americanheart.org/presenter.jhtml ?identifier=4591.

3. Berenson GS, Wattigney WA, Bao W, Srinivasan SR, Radhakrishnamurthy B. Rationale to study the early natural history of heart disease: the Bogalusa Heart Study. *Am J Med Sci.* 1995; 310(suppl):S22–28.

4. Marrugat J, Sala J, Masia R, et al. Mortality differences between men and women following first myocardial infarction. *JAMA.* 1998;280:1405–9.

5. Hanekamp C, Koolen J, Bonnier H, et al. Randomized comparison of balloon angioplasty versus silicon carbon-coated stent implantation for de novo lesions in small coronary arteries. *Am J Cardiol.* 2004 May 15;93(10): 1233–37.

6. Ramsey LE, Yeo WW, Jackson PR. Dietary reduction of serum cholesterol concentration: time to think again. *BMJ.* 1991;303: 953–57.

7. Ferdowsian HR, Barnard ND. Effects of plant-based diets on plasma lipids. *Am J Cardiol.* 2009 Oct 1;104(7): 947–56; Dod HS, Bhardwaj R, Sajja V, et al. Effect of intensive lifestyle changes on endothelial function and on inflammatory markers of atherosclerosis. *Am J Cardiol.* 2010 Feb 1;105(3): 362–76; Frattaroli J, Weidner G, Merritt-Worden TA, et al. Angina pectoris and atherosclerotic risk factors in the multisite cardiac lifestyle intervention program. *Am J Cardiol.* 2008 Apr 1;101(7):911–18; Ornish D, Brown SE, Scherwitz LW, et al. Can lifestyle changes reverse coronary heart disease? *Lancet.* 1990; 336(8708):129–33; Ellis F. Angina and vegan diet. *Am Heart J.* 1997;93(6):803–5.

8. Davidson MH, Hunninghake D, Maki KC, et al. Comparison of the effects of lean red meat vs. lean white meat on serum lipid levels among free-living persons with hypercholesterolemia: a long-term, randomized clinical trial. *Arch Intern Med.* 1999; 159(12):1331–38.

9. Fraser GE. Association between diet and cancer, ischemic heart disease, and all-cause mortality in non-Hispanic white California Seventh-Day Adventists. *Am J Clin Nutr.* 1999; 70(suppl 3):S532–38.

10. Ros E. Nuts and novel biomarkers of cardiovascular disease. *Am J Clin Nutr.* 2009 May;89(5)(suppl): S1649–56; Nash SD,

Nash DT. Nuts as part of a healthy cardiovascular diet. *Curr Atheroscler Rep.* 2008 Dec;10(6):529–35; Gebauer SK, West SG, Kay CD, et al. Effects of pistachios on cardiovascular disease risk factors and potential mechanisms of action: a dose-response study. *Am J Clin Nutr.* 2008 Sep;88(3):651–59; Ma Y, Njike VY, Millet J, et al. Effects of walnut consumption on endothelial function in type 2 diabetic subjects: a randomized controlled crossover trial. *Diabetes Care.* 2010 Feb;33(2): 227–32; Banel DK, Hu FB. Effects of walnut consumption on blood lipids and other cardiovascular risk factors: a meta-analysis and systematic review. *Am J Clin Nutr.* 2009 Jul;90(1): 56–63; Spaccarotella KJ, Kris-Etherton PM, Stone WL, et al. The effect of walnut intake on factors related to prostate and vascular health in older men. *Nutr J.* 2008 May 2;7:13; Ros E, Mataix J. Fatty acid composition of nuts—implications for cardiovascular health. *Br J Nutr.* 2006 Nov;96(suppl 2):S29–35.

11. Mozaffarian D. Does alpha-linolenic acid intake reduce the risk of coronary heart disease? A review of the evidence. *Altern Ther Health Med.* 2005 May–Jun;11(3): 24–30; quiz 31, 79.

12. Stefanick ML, Mackey S, Sheehan M, et al. Effects of diet and exercise in men and postmenopausal women with low levels of HDL cholesterol and high levels of LDL cholesterol. *N Eng J Med.* 339:12–20.

13. Kodama S, Saito K, Tanaka S, et al. Influence of fat and carbohydrate proportions on the metabolic profile in patients with type 2 diabetes: a meta-analysis. *Diabetes Care.* 2009 May;32(5): 959–65; Lichtenstein AH, Van Horn L. Very low fat diets. *Circulation.* 1998 Sep 1;98(9):935–39.

14. McKeown NM, Meigs JB, Liu S, et al. Dietary carbohydrates and cardiovascular disease risk factors in the Framingham offspring cohort. *J Am Coll Nutr.* 2009 Apr; 28(2):150–58; Siri-Tarino PW, Sun Q, Hu FB, Krauss RM. Saturated fat, carbohydrate, and cardiovascular disease. *Am J Clin Nutr.* 2010 Mar; 91(3):502–9.

15. De Natale C, Annuzzi G, Bozzetto L, et al. Effects of a plant-based high-carbohydrate/high-fiber diet versus high-monounsaturated fat/low-carbohydrate diet on postprandial lipids in type 2 diabetic patients. *Diabetes Care.* 2009 Dec; 32(12):2168–73; Anderson JW. Dietary fiber prevents carbohydrate-induced hypertriglyceridemia. *Curr Atheroscler Rep.* 2000 Nov;2(6):536–41; Turley ML, Skeaff CM, Mann JI, Cox B. The effect of low-fat, high-carbohydrate diet on serum high density lipoprotein cholesterol and triglycerides. *Eur J Clin Nutr.* 1998;52(10):728–32.

16. Jenkins DJ, Kendall CW, Popovich DG. Effects of a very-high-fiber vegetable, fruit, and nut diet on serum lipids and colonic function. *Metabolism*. 2001;50 (4):494–503.

17. Lichtenstein AH, Van Horn L. Very low fat diets. *Circulation*. 1998 Sep 1;98(9): 935–39.

18. Ivanov AN, Medkova IL, Mosiakina LI. The effect of anti-atherogenic vegetarian diet on the clinico-hemodynamic and biochemical indices in elderly patients with ischemic heart disease. *Ter Arkh*. 1999; 71(2):75–78.

19. Ishikawa T. Postprandial lipemia as an atherosclerotic risk factor and fat tolerance test. *Nippon Rinsho* 1999;57(12): 2668–72.

20. Koeford BC, Gullov AL, Peterson P. Cerebral complications of surgery using cardiopulmonary bypass. *Ugeskr Laeger*. 1995; 157(6)728–34.

21. Joshi B, Brady K, Lee J, et al. Impaired autoregulation of cerebral blood flow during rewarming from hypothermic cardiopulmonary bypass and its potential association with stroke. *Anesth Analg*. 2010 Feb; 110(2):321–28; Chauhan S. Brain, cardiopulmonary bypass and temperature: what should we be doing? *Ann Card Anaesth*. 2009 Jul–Dec;12(2):104–6; Brain damage and open-heart surgery. *Lancet*. 1989 Aug 12;2 (8659):364–66.

22. Hanekamp C, Koolen J, Bonnier H, et al. Randomized comparison of balloon angioplasty versus silicon carbon-coated stent implantation for de novo lesions in small coronary arteries. *Am J Cardiol*. 2004 May 15;93(10):1233–37.

23. Agostoni P, Valgimigli M, Biondi-Zoccai GG, et al. Clinical effectiveness of bare-metal stenting compared with balloon angioplasty in total coronary occlusions: insights from a systematic overview of randomized trials in light of the drug-eluting stent era. *Am Heart J*. 2006 Mar; 151(3):682–89.

24. Stähli BE, Camici GG, Tanner FC. Drug-eluting stent thrombosis. *Ther Adv Cardiovasc Dis*. 2009 Feb;3(1):45–52; Lüscher TF, Steffel J, Eberli FR, et al. Drug-eluting stent and coronary thrombosis: biological mechanisms and clinical implications. *Circulation*. 2007 Feb 27; 115(8):1051–58.

25. Bates B. Angiograms miss most atheromas. *Family Practice News*. 2001 Jul 15;31(14):1, 4.

26. Nissen SE. Pathobiology, not angiography, should guide management in acute coronary syndrome/non-ST-segment elevation myocardial infarction: the non-interventionist's perspective. *J Am Coll Cardiol*. 2003 Feb 19;41(4) (suppl S): S103–12; Schoenhagen P, Ziada KM, Vince DG, Nissen SE,

Tuzcu EM. Arterial remodeling and coronary artery disease: the concept of "dilated" versus "obstructive" coronary atherosclerosis. *J Am Coll Cardiol.* 2001 Aug;38(2)297–306.

27. Shrihari JS, Roy A, Prabhakaran D, Reddy KS. Role of EDTA chelation therapy in cardiovascular diseases. *Natl Med J India.* 2006 Jan–Feb;19(1):24–26; Seely DM, Wu P, Mills EJ. EDTA chelation therapy for cardiovascular disease: a systematic review. *BMC Cardiovasc Disord.* 2005 Nov 1;5:32.

28. Gould KL. New concepts and paradigms in cardiovascular medicine: the noninvasive management of coronary artery disease. *Am J Med.* 1998;104(6A)(suppl):S2–17; Franklin BA, Kahn JK. Delayed progression or regression of coronary atherosclerosis with intensive risk factor modification: effects of diet, drugs, and exercise. *Sports Med.* 1996;22(5):306–20.

29. Kannel WB. Range of serum cholesterol values in the population developing coronary artery disease. *Am J Cardiol.* 1995; 76(9):69c–77c; Castelli WP, Anderson K, Wilson PW, Levy D. Lipids and the risk of coronary heart disease: the Framingham Study. *Ann Epidemiol.* 1992;2(1–2):23–28.

30. Cooper R, Rotimi C, Ataman S, et al. The prevalence of hypertension in seven populations of west African origin. *Am J Public Health.* 1997 Feb;87(2):160–8. He J, Klag MJ, Whelton PK, et al. Body mass and blood pressure in a lean population in southwestern China. *Am J Epidemiol.* 1994 Feb 15;139(4):380–9.

31. Fogari R, Zoppi A, Corradi L, et al. Effect of body weight loss and normalization on blood pressure in overweight non-obese patients with stage 1 hypertension. *Hypertens Res.* 2010 Mar;33(3):236–42; Sacks FM, Svetkey LP, Vollmer WM, et al. Effects on blood pressure of reduced dietary sodium and the Dietary Approaches to Stop Hypertension (DASH) diet. *N Eng J Med.* 2001 Jan 4;344(1):3–10; Haddy FJ, Vanhoutte PM, Feletou M. Role of potassium in regulating blood flow and blood pressure. *Am J Physiol Regul Integr Comp Physiol.* 2006 Mar; 290(3):R546–52; Wu G, Tian H, Han K, et al. Potassium magnesium supplementation for four weeks improves small distal artery compliance and reduces blood pressure in patients with essential hypertension. *Clin Exp Hypertens.* 2006 Jul;28(5):489–97; Houston MC, Harper KJ. Potassium, magnesium, and calcium: their role in both the cause and treatment of hypertension. *J Clin Hypertens (Greenwich).* 2008 Jul; 10(7)(suppl 2):S3–11; Sesso HD, Cook NR, Buring JE, et al. Alcohol consumption and the risk of hypertension in women and men. *Hypertension.* 2008 Apr;51(4): 1080–7; Beilin LJ, Puddey IB. Alcohol and hypertension: an

update. *Hypertension*. 2006 Jun; 47(6):1035–38; Uiterwaal CS, Verschuren WM, Bueno-de-Mesquita HB, et al. Coffee intake and incidence of hypertension. *Am J Clin Nutr.* 2007 Mar; 85(3):718–23; Winkelmayer WC, Stampfer MJ, Willett WC, et al. Habitual caffeine intake and the risk of hypertension in women. *JAMA*. 2005 Nov 9;294(18):2330–35; Flint AJ, Hu FB, Glynn RJ, et al. Whole grains and incident hypertension in men. *Am J Clin Nutr.* 2009 Sep;90(3): 493–98; Utsugi MT, Ohkubo T, Kikuya M, et al. Fruit and vegetable consumption and the risk of hypertension determined by self measurement of blood pressure at home: the Ohasama study. *Hypertens Res*. 2008 Jul;31(7):1435–43; Owen A, Wiles J, Swaine I. Effect of isometric exercise on resting blood pressure: a meta analysis. *J Hum Hypertens*. 2010 Feb 25. [Epub ahead of print]; Chen YL, Liu YF, Huang CY, et al. Normalization effect of sports training on blood pressure in hypertensives. *J Sports Sci*. 2010 Feb;19:1–7.

32. Jablonski KL, Gates PE, Pierce GL, Seals DR. Low dietary sodium intake is associated with enhanced vascular endothelial function in middle-aged and older adults with elevated systolic blood pressure. *Ther Adv Cardiovasc Dis*. 2009 Oct;3(5):347–56; Padiyar A. Nonpharmacologic management of hypertension in the elderly. *Clin Geriatr Med*. 2009 May;25(2):213–19; Whelton PK, Appel LI, Espeland MA, et al. Sodium reduction and weight loss in the treatment of hypertension in older persons: a randomized controlled trial of nonpharmacologic interventions in the elderly. *JAMA*. 1998;279:839–46.

33. Stafford RS, Blumenthal D. Specialty differences in cardiovascular disease prevention practices. *J Am Coll Cardiol*. 1998; 32(5): 1238–43.

34. American Diabetes Association: Diabetes Statistics. http://www.diabetes.org/diabetes-basics/diabetes-statistics.

35. American Diabetes Association. Diabetes Statistics. http://www.diabetes.org/diabetes-basics/diabetes-statistics/.

36. Eppens MC, Craig ME, Cusumano J, et al. Prevalence of diabetes complications in adolescents with type 2 compared with type 1 diabetes. *Diabetes Care*. 2006. Jun 29:1300–6; Gaster B, Hirsh IB. The effects of improved glucose control on complications in type 2 diabetes. *Arch Intern Med*. 1998; 158:34–40.

37. Ioacara S, Lichiardopol R, Ionescu-Tirgoviste C, et al. Improvements in life expectancy in type 1 diabetes patients in the last six decades. *Diabetes Res Clin Pract*. 2009 Nov;86(2): 146–51; Barr EL, Zimmet PZ, Welborn TA, et al. Risk of cardiovascular and all-cause mortality in individuals with

diabetes mellitus, impaired fasting glucose, and impaired glucose tolerance: the Australian Diabetes, Obesity, and Lifestyle Study (AusDiab). *Circulation*. 2007 Jul 10;116(2):151–57; Siscovick DS, Sotoodehnia N, Rea TD, et al. Type 2 diabetes mellitus and the risk of sudden cardiac arrest in the community. *Rev Endocr Metab Disord*. 2010 Mar;11(1):53–59; Stamler J, Stamler O, Vaccaro JD. Diabetes, other risk factors, and 12-year cardiovascular mortality for men screened in the multiple risk factor intervention trial. *Diabetes Care*. 1993;16: 434–44; Haffner SM, Lehto S, Ronnemaa T, et al. Mortality from coronary heart disease in subjects with type 2 diabetes and in nondiabetic subjects with and without prior myocardial infarction. *N Eng J Med*. 1998;339(4):229–34; Janka HU. Increased cardiovascular morbidity and mortality in diabetes mellitus: identification of the high risk patient. *Diabetes Res Clin Pract*. 1996;30(suppl):585–88.

38. Crane M. Regression of diabetic neuropathy with total vegetarian (vegan) diet. *J Nutr Med*. 1994; 4:431.

39. Rector RS, Warner SO, Liu Y, et al. Exercise and diet induced weight loss improves measures of oxidative stress and insulin sensitivity in adults with characteristics of the metabolic syndrome. *Am J Physiol Endocrinol Metab*. 2007 Aug;293(2): E500–6; Dengel DR, Kelly AS, Olson TP, et al. Effects of weight loss on insulin sensitivity and arterial stiffness in overweight adults. *Metabolism*. 2006 Jul;55(7):907–11; Rosenfalck AM, Almdal T, Viggers L, et al. A low-fat diet improves peripheral insulin sensitivity in patients with type 1 diabetes. *Diabetic Med*. 2006 Apr;23(4):384–92.

40. Williamson DF, Thompson TJ, Thun M, et al. Intentional weight loss and mortality among overweight individuals with diabetes. *Diabetes Care*. 2000;23(10):1499–1504; Fujioka K. Benefits of moderate weight loss in patients with type 2 diabetes. *Diabetes Obes Metab*. 2010 Mar;12(3):186–94.

41. Hinton EC, Parkinson JA, Holland AJ, Arana FS, Roberts AC, Owen AM. Neural contributions to the motivational control of appetite in humans. *Eur J Neurosci*. 2004 Sep;20(5): 1411–18; Tataranni, PA, Gautier JF, Chen K, et al. Neuroanatomical correlates of hunger and satiation in humans using positron emission tomography. *Proc Natl Acad Sci. U S A*. 1999;96(8):4569–74; Friedman MI, Ulrich P, Mattes RD. A figurative measure of subjective hunger sensations. *Appetite* 1999;32(3):395–404.

42. Fukui PT, Gonçalves TR, Strabelli CG, et al. Trigger factors in migraine patients. *Arq Neuropsiquiatr*. 2008 Sep;66(3A): 494–99; Millichap JG, Yee MM. The diet factor in pediatric and

adolescent migraine. *Pediatr Neurol.* 2003 Jan;28(1):9–15; Diamond S. Migraine headache: recognizing its peculiarities, precipitants, and prodromes. *Consultant.* 1995 Aug; 1190–95.

43. Fuhrman, J. *Fasting and eating for health: a medical doctor's program for conquering disease.* New York: St. Martin's Press; 1995.

44. Katsarava Z, Holle D, Diener HC. Medication overuse headache. *Curr Neurol Neurosci Rep.* 2009 Mar;9(2):115–19; Stephenson, J. Detox is crucial in chronic daily headache. *Family Practice News.* 1993 Jul:1, 2.

45. Hagen KB, Byfuglien MG, Falzon L, et al. Dietary interventions for rheumatoid arthritis. *Cochrane Database Syst Rev.* 2009 Jan 21; (1):CD006400; Proudman SM, Cleland LG, James MJ. Dietary omega-3 fats for treatment of inflammatory joint disease: efficacy and utility. *Rheum Dis Clin North Am.* 2008 May;34(2):469–79; Calder PC, Albers R, Antoine JM, et al. Inflammatory disease processes and interactions with nutrition. *Br J Nutr.* 2009 May; 101(suppl 1):S1–45; O'Sullivan M. Symposium on "The challenge of translating nutrition research into public health nutrition." Session 3: Joint Nutrition Society and Irish Nutrition and Dietetic Institute Symposium on "Nutrition and autoimmune disease." Nutrition in Crohn's disease. *Proc Nutr Soc.* 2009 May;68(2):127–34; Calder PC. Session 3: Joint Nutrition Society and Irish Nutrition and Dietetic Institute Symposium on "Nutrition and autoimmune disease." PUFA, inflammatory processes and rheumatoid arthritis. *Proc Nutr Soc.* 2008 Nov;67(4):409–18; Fujita A, Hashimoto Y, Nakahara K, et al. Effects of a low-calorie vegan diet on disease activity and general condition in patients with rheumatoid arthritis. *Rinsho Byori* 1999;47(6): 554–60; Haugen MA, Kjeldsen-Kragh J, Bjerve KS, et al. Changes in plasma phospholipid fatty acids and their relationship to disease activity in rheumatoid arthritis patients treated with a vegetarian diet. *Br J Nutr.* 1994; 72(4):555–66; Peltonen R, Nenonen M, Helve T, et al. Faecal microbial flora and disease activity in rheumatoid arthritis during a vegan diet. *Br J Rheumatol.* 1997; 36(1): 64–68; Kjeldsen-Kragh J. Rheumatoid arthritis treated with vegetarian diets. *Am J Clin Nutr.* 1999; 70(suppl 3):S594–600; Haddad EH, Berk LS, Kettering JD, et al. Dietary intake and biochemical, hematologic, and immune status of vegans compared with nonvegetarians. *Am J Clin Nutr.* 1999;70(suppl 3):S586–93.

46. Stapel SO, Asero R, Ballmer-Weber BK, et al. EAACI Task Force. Testing for IgG4 against foods is not recommended as a diagnostic tool: EAACI Task Force report. *Allergy* 2008

Jul;63(7):793–96; Kurowski K, Boxer RW. Food allergies: detection and management. *Am Fam Physician.* 2008 Jun 15;77(12):1678–86; Kjeldsen-Kragh J, Hvatum M, Haugen, et al. Antibodies against dietary antigens in rheumatoid arthritis patients treated with fasting and a one-year vegetarian diet. *Clin Exp Rheumatol.* 1995; 13(2):167–72.

47. Scott D, Symmons DP, Coulton BL, Popert AJ. Long-term outcome of treating rheumatoid arthritis: results after 20 years. *Lancet.* 1987;1(8542):1108–11.

48. Jones M, Symmons D, Finn J, Wolfe F. Does exposure to immunosuppressive therapy increase the 10-year malignancy and mortality risk? *Br J Rheum.* 1996; 35(8):738–45.

49. Barnard, ND, Scialli AR, Hurlock D, Berton P. Diet and sex-hormone binding globulin, dysmenorrhea, and premenstrual symptoms. *Obstet Gynecol.* 2000; 92(2):245–50.

50. Does what you eat cause IBS? Common foods, including chicken, eggs, milk and wheat, may be the culprits. *Health News.* 2005 Dec; 11(12):7–8; King TS, Elia M, Hunter JO. Abnormal colonic fermentation in irritable bowel syndrome. *Lancet.* 1998; 352(9135): 1187–89.

Chapter 8: Your Plan for Substantial Weight Reduction

1. Gustafsson K, Asp NG, Hagander B, et al. Influence of processing and cooking of carrots in mixed meals on satiety, glucose and hormonal reponse. *Int J Food Sci Nutr.* 1995;46(1):3–12.

2. Blackberry I, Kouris-Blazos A, Wahlqvist ML, et al. Legumes: the most important dietary predictor of survival in older people of different ethnicities. *Asia Pac J Clin Nutr.* 2004; 13(suppl): S126.

3. Abdelrahaman SM, Elmaki HB, Idris WH, et al. Antinutritional factor content and hydrochloric acid extractability of minerals in pearl millet cultivars as affected by germination. *Int J Food Sci Nutr.* 2007 Feb;58(1):6–17; Kariluoto S, Liukkonen KH, Myllymäki O, et al. Effect of germination and thermal treatments on folates in rye. *J Agricult Food Chem.* 2006 Dec 13;54(25):9522–28; Xu JG, Tian CR, Hu QP, et al. Dynamic changes in phenolic compounds and antioxidant activity in oats (Avena nuda L.) during steeping and germination. *J Agricult Food Chem.* 2009 Nov 11;57(21):10392–98; Lintschinger J, Fuchs N, Moser H, et al. Uptake of various trace elements during germination of wheat, buckwheat and quinoa. *Plant Foods Hum Nutr.* 1997;50(3):223–37.

4. Wang L, Huang H, Wei Y, et al. Characterization and antitumor activities of sulfated polysaccharide SRBPS2a obtained

from defatted rice bran. *Int J Biol Macromol.* 2009 Nov 1;45(4):427–31; Phutthaphadoong S, Yamada Y, Hirata A, et al. Chemopreventive effects of fermented brown rice and rice bran against 4-(methylnitrosamino)-1-3-pyridyl)-1-butanone-induced lung tumorigenesis in female A/J mice. *Oncol Rep.* 2009 Feb;21(2):321–27; Kannan A, Hettiarachchy N, Johnson MG, Nannapaneni R. Human colon and liver cancer cell proliferation inhibition by peptide hydrolysates derived from heat-stabilized defatted rice bran. *J Agricult Food Chem.* 2008 Dec 24;56(24):11643–37; Hudson EA, Dinh PA, Kokubun T, et al. Characterization of potentially chemopreventive phenols in extracts of brown rice that inhibit the growth of human breast and colon cancer cells. *Cancer Epidemiol. Biomarkers Prevent.* 2000;9(11):1163–70.

5. Flood JE, Rolls BJ. Soup preloads in a variety of forms reduce meal energy intake. *Appetite.* 2007 Nov;49(3):626–34; Jordan HA, Levitz LS, Utgoff KL, et al. Role of food characteristics in behavioral change and weight loss. *J Am Diet Assoc.* 1981;79:24; Foreyt JP, Reeves RS, Darnell LS, et al. Soup consumption as a behavioral weight-loss strategy. *J Am Diet Assoc.* 1986;86:524–26.

6. Yashodhara BM, Umakanth S, Pappanchan JM, et al. Omega-3 fatty acids: a comprehensive review of their role in health and disease. *Postgrad Med J.* 2009 Feb;85(1000):84–90.

7. Sabaté J, Ang Y. Nuts and health outcomes: new epidemiologic evidence. *Am J Clin Nutr.* 2009 May;89(5)(suppl):S1643–48; Ros E. Nuts and novel biomarkers of cardiovascular disease. *Am J Clin Nutr.* 2009 May;89(5)(suppl): S1649–56.

8. Jedrychowski W, Maugeri U, Popieta T, et al. Case-control study on beneficial effect of regular consumption of apples on colorectal cancer risk in a population with relatively low intake of fruits and vegetables. *Eur J Cancer Prev.* 2010 Jan;19(1):42–47; Foschi R, Pelucchi C, Dal Maso L, et al. Citrus fruit and cancer risk in a network of case-control studies. *Cancer Causes Control.* 2010 Feb;21(2):237–42; van Duijnhoven FJ Buenn-de-Plesquita HB, Ferrori P, et al. Fruit, vegetables, and colorectal cancer risk: the European Prospective Investigation into Cancer and Nutrition. *Am J Clin Nutr.* 2009 May;89(5):1441–52; Maynard M, Gunnell D, Emmett P, et al. Fruit, vegetables and antioxidants in childhood and risk of cancer: the Boyd Orr cohort. *J Epidimiol Community Health.* 2003; 57:219–25.

9. National Heart, Lung, and Blood Institute. National Institute of Diabetes and Digestive and Kidney Diseases. *Clinical guidelines on the identification, evaluation, and treatment of*

overweight and obesity in adults. National Heart, Lung, and Blood Institute reprint. Bethesda, Md.: National Institutes of Health. http://www.nhlbi.nih.gov/guidelines/obesity/ob_gdlns .htm.

Chapter 10: Frequently Asked Questions

1. Ginde AA, Lill MC, Camargo CA Jr. Demographic differences and trends of vitamin D insufficiency in the US population, 1988–2004. *Arch Intern Med.* 2009; 169(6):626–32.

2. Oregon State University. Linus Pauling Institute. Micronutrient Information Center. Vitamin D. http:1pi .oregonstate.edu/ infocenter/vitamins/vitaminD.

3. Chen P, Hup, Xie D, Qin Y, Wang F, Wang H. Meta-analysis of vitamin D, calcium and the prevention of breast cancer. *Breast Cancer Res Treat.* 2009 Oct 23. [Epub ahead of print]

4. Zhou G, Stoitzfus J, Swan BA. Optimizing vitamin D status to reduce colorectal cancer risk: an evidentiary review. *Clin J Oncol Nurs.* 2009 Aug;13(4):E3–17.

5. National Institutes of Health. Office of Dietary Supplements. Dietary Supplement Fact Sheet: Vitamin B12. 2010.

6. Mayne ST. Beta-carotene, carotenoids, and disease prevention in humans. *FASEB J.* 1996;10(7):690–701; Goodman GE. Prevention of lung cancer. *Curr Opin Oncol.* 1998;10(2): 122–26; Kolata G. Studies find beta carotene, taken by millions, can't forestall cancer or heart disease. *New York Times.* 1996 Jan 19. Omenn GS, Goodman GE, Thornquist MD, et al. Effects of a combination of beta carotene and vitamin A on lung cancer and cardiovascular disease. *N Eng J Med.* 1996; 334(18);1150–55; Hennekens CH, Buring JE, Manson JE, et al. Lack of effect of long-term supplementation with beta carotene on the incidence of malignant neoplasms and cardiovascular disease. *N Eng J Med.* 1996; 334(18):1145–49; Albanes D, Heinonen OP, Taylor PR, et al. Alpha-tocopherol and beta-carotene supplements and lung cancer incidence in the alpha-tocopherol, beta-carotene cancer prevention study: effects of baseline characteristics and study compliance. *J Natl Cancer Inst.* 1996;88(21):1560–70; Rapola JM, Virtamo J, Ripatti S, et al. Randomized trial of alpha-tocopherol and beta-carotene supplements on incidence of major coronary events in men with previous myocardial infarction. *Lancet.* 1997;349(9067): 1715–20; Bjelakovic G, Nikolova D, Gluud LL, et al. Antioxidant supplements for prevention of mortality in healthy participants and patients with various diseases. *Cochrane Database Syst Rev.* 2008 Adr 16;(2): CD007176.

7. Harvard School of Public Health. The Nutrition Source. Keep the Multi, Skip the Heavily Fortified Foods. http://www.hsph.harvard.edu/nutritionsource/what-should-you-eat/folic-acid/.

8. Yi K. Does a high folate intake increase the risk of breast cancer? *Nutr Rev.* 2006; 64(10 Pt 1): 468–75; Cole B, Baron J, Sandler R, et al. Folic acid for the prevention of colorectal adenomas. *JAMA.* 2007; 297(21): 2351–59; Stolzenberg-Solomon R, Chang S, Leitzman M. Folate intake, alcohol use and post-menopausal breast cancer risk in the Prostate, Lung, Colorectal and Ovarian Cancer Screening Trial. *Am J Clin Nutr.* 2006;83:895–904; Smith AD, Kim Y, Refsuh H. Is folic acid good for everyone? *Am J Clin Nutr.* 2008; 87(3):517; Kim Y. Role of folate in colon cancer development and progression. *J Nutr.* 2003;133(11) (suppl 1):S3731–39; Guelpen BV, Hultdin J, Johansson I, et al. Low folate levels may protect against colorectal cancer. *Gut.* 2006;55:1461–66.

9. Heymsfield SB, Allison DB, Vasselli JR, et al. Garcinia cambogia (hydroxycitric acid) as a potential antiobesity agent. *JAMA.* 1998; 280(18):1596–1600.

10. Jull AB, Ni Mhurchu C, Bennett DA, et al. Chitosan for overweight or obesity. *Cochrane Database Syst Rev.* 2008 Jul 16;(3):CD003892.

11. Andraws R, Chawla P, Brown DL. Cardiovascular effects of ephedra alkaloids: a comprehensive review. *Prog Cardiovasc Dis.* 2005 Jan–Feb;47(4):217–25.

12. Robinson JR, Niswender KD. What are the risks and the benefits of current and emerging weight-loss medications? *Curr Diab Rep.* 2009 Oct;9(5):368–75; Bray GA. Medications for obesity: mechanisms and applications. *Clin Chest Med.* 2009 Sep;30(3): 525–38, ix.

13. Chiesa A, Serretti A. Mindfulness-based stress reduction for stress management in healthy people: a review and meta-analysis. *J Altern Complement Med.* 2009 May;15(5):593–600; Walton KG, Schneider RH, Nidich S. Review of controlled research on the transcendental meditation program and cardiovascular disease. Risk factors, morbidity, and mortality. *Cardiol Rev.* 2004 Sep–Oct; 12(5):262–66; Everly GS. *A clinical guide to the treatment of the human stress response.* New York: Plenum Press; 1989.

14. Butryn ML, Phelan S, Hill JO, Wing RR. Consistent self-monitoring of weight: a key component of successful weight loss maintenance. *Obesity (Silver Spring).* 2007 Dec;15(12): 3091–96; Boutelle, KN, Kirschenbaum DS Further support for

consistent self-monitoring as a vital component of successful weight control. *Obes Res.* 1998; 6:219–24.

15. Mangat I. Do vegetarians have to eat fish for optimal cardio-vascular protection? *Am J Clin Nutr.* 2009 May;89(5)(suppl):S1597–1601; Davis BC, Kris-Etherton PM. Achieving optimal essential fatty acid status in vegetarians: current knowledge and practical implications. *Am J Clin Nutr.* 2003 Sep;78(Suppl 3):S640-46; Pauletto P, Puato, M Caroli MG, et al. Blood pressure and atherogenic lipoprotein profiles of fish-diet and vegetarian villagers in Tanzania: the Lugaiawa Study. *Lancet* 1996; 348: 784–88; Key TJ, Fraser GE, Thorogood M, et al. Mortality in vegetarians and nonvegetarians: detailed findings from a collaborative analysis of 5 prospective studies. *Am J Clin Nutr.* 1999; 70(3)(suppl):S516–24.

16. Steenland K, Bertazzi P, Baccarelli A, Kogevinas M. Dioxin revisited: developments since the 1997 IARC classification of dioxin as a human carcinogen. *Environ Health Perspect.* 2004 Sep;112(13):1265–68; EPA report ratchets up dioxin peril. *Washington Post.* 2000 May 17.

17. Environmental Working Group. Shopper's Guide to Pesticides. http://www.foodnews.org/walletguide .php.

18. Bjelakovic G, Nikolova D, Gluud LL, et al. Antioxidant supplements for prevention of mortality in healthy participants and patients with various diseases. *Cochrane Database Syst Rev* 2008 Apr 16;(2):CD007176.

19. Report from Loma Linda University's Carbophobia Conference. *Vegetarian Nutrition and Health Letter,* 2000;3(5):4.

20. Lichtenstein AH, Ausman LM, Jalbert SM, Schaefer EJ. Effects of different forms of dietary hydrogenated fats on serum lipoprotein cholesterol levels. *N Eng J Med.* 1999;340:1933–40.

21. Lee S, Xiao-Ou S, Honglan L, et al. Adolescent and adult soy food intake and breast cancer risk: results from the Shanghai Women's Health Study. *Am J Clin Nutr.* 2009;89:1920–26.

22. Tsugane S, Sasazuki S. Diet and the risk of gastric cancer. Gastric Cancer 2007; 10(2):75–83; Strazzullo P, D'Elia L, Ngianga-Bakwin K, Cappucio FP. Salt intake, stroke, and cardiovascular disease: meta-analysis of prospective studies *BMJ.* 2009;339: b4567

23. Obarzanek E, Sacks FM, Moore TJ, et al. Dietary approaches to stop hypertension (DASH)—sodium trial. Paper. American Society of Hypertension, New York, May 17, 2000.

24. Nowson CA, Patchett A, Wattanapenpaiboon N. The effects of a low-sodium base-producing diet including red meat compared with a high-carbohydrate, low-fat diet on bone turnover

markers in women aged 45–75 years. *Br J Nutr.* 2009 Oct;102(8):1161–70; Itoh R, Suyama Y. Sodium excretion in relation to calcium and hydroxyproline excretion in a healthy Japanese population. *Am J Clin Nutr.* 1996;63(5):735–40.

25. Tuomilehto J, Jousilahti P, Rastenyte D, et al. Urinary sodium excretion and cardiovascular mortality in Finland: a prospective study. *Lancet.* 2001;357(9259): 848–51.

26. Mehta A, Jain AC, Mehta MC, Billie M. Caffeine and cardiac arrhythmias: an experimental study in dogs with review of literature. *Acta Cardiol.* 1997;52(3): 273–83.

27. Riksen NP, Rongen GA, Smits P. Acute and long-term cardiovascular effects of coffee: implications for coronary heart disease. *Pharmacol Ther.* 2009 Feb;121(2):185–91; Nurminen ML, Niittymen L, Korpela R, Vapaatalo H. Coffee, caffeine and blood pressure: a critical review. *Eur J Clin Nutr.* 1999; 53(11):831–39; Christensen B, Mosdol A, Retterstol L, et al. Abstention from filtered coffee reduces the concentration of plasma homocysteine and serum cholesterol—a randomized controlled trial. *Am J Clin Nutr.* 2001;74(3):302–7.

28. Van Cauter E, Spiegel K, Tasali E, Leproult R. Metabolic consequences of sleep and sleep loss. *Sleep Med.* 2008 Sep;9 (Suppl 1): S23–28.

29. Ferreira MG, Valente JG, Gonçalves-Silva RM, Sichieri R. Alcohol consumption and abdominal fat in blood donors. *Rev Saude Publica.* 2008 Dec;42(6): 1067–73; Sesso HD, Cook NR, Buring JE, et al. Alcohol consumption and the risk of hypertension in women and men. *Hypertension.* 2008 Apr;51(4): 1080–7.

30. Singletary KW, Gapstur SM. Alcohol and breast cancer: review of epidemiologic and experimental evidence and potential mechanisms. *JAMA.* 2001 Nov 7;286(17): 2143–51; George A, Figueredo VM. Alcohol and arrhythmias: a comprehensive review. *J Cardiovasc Med (Hagerstown).* 2010 Apr;11(4): 221–28.

31. Lavin JH, French SJ, Read NW. The effect of sucrose- and aspartame-sweetened drinks on energy intake, hunger and food choice of female, moderately restrained eaters. *Int J Obes Relat Metab Disord.* 1997;21(1):37–42.

32. Swithers SE, Martin AA, Davidson TL. High-intensity sweeteners and energy balance. *Physiol Behav.* 2010 Apr 26; 100(1):55–62. Bellisle F, Drewnowski A. Intense sweeteners, energy intake and the control of body weight. *Eur J Clin Nutr.* 2007 Jun;61(6):691–700; Mattes RD, Popkin BM. Nonnutritive sweetener consumption in humans: effects on appetite and

food intake and their putative mechanisms. *Am J Clin Nutr.* 2009 Jan;89(1):1–14.

33. Bray G. How bad is fructose? *Am J Clin Nutr.* 2007;86(4):895–96; Tappy L, Lê KA. Metabolic effects of fructose and the worldwide increase in obesity. *Physiol Rev.* 2010 Jan; 90(1): 23–46.

Index